Drug Delivery Devices

DRUGS AND THE PHARMACEUTICAL SCIENCES

A Series of Textbooks and Monographs

Edited by

James Swarbrick
School of Pharmacy
University of North Carolina
Chapel Hill, North Carolina

Additional Volumes in Preparation

Drug Delivery Devices

FUNDAMENTALS AND APPLICATIONS

edited by

Praveen Tyle

SANDOZ PHARMACEUTICAL CORPORATION
LINCOLN, NEBRASKA

MARCEL DEKKER, INC.   New York and Basel

Library of Congress Cataloging-in-Publication Data

Drug delivery devices : fundamentals and applications / edited by
  Praveen Tyle.
    p.   cm. -- (Drugs and the pharmaceutical sciences ; v. 32)
  Includes index.
  ISBN 0-8247-7836-7
  1. Drug delivery devices. I. Tyle, Praveen. II. Series.
RS210.D78 1988
615.5'8--dc 19   87-33156
                                                                CIP

MARCEL DEKKER, INC.
270 Madison Avenue, New York, New York 10016

Current printing (last digit):
10   9   8   7   6   5   4   3   2   1

PRINTED IN THE UNITED STATES OF AMERICA

To the memory

of

Professor Takeru Higuchi

Foreword

With the great advances made during the past several decades in our understanding of the pharmacological and toxicological effects of drug action and with our ever-increasing awareness and appreciation of the practical advantages associated with using "novel" methods of drug delivery in therapy, it is only natural that the field of drug delivery devices has been receiving more and more attention. The first generation devices for transdermal, peroral, and parenteral drug delivery have already become a significant part of the armamentaria for drug therapy. So have the pumps, including the implantable pumps. Wideranging interest has been shown by academic and industrial researchers in the various physical, biological, and clinical sciences and in the engineering disciplines, and research support from governmental sources and industrial sponsors has been increasing exponentially.

A plateau in the level of activity in this field is not in sight. The second- and third-generation systems will involve more as well as newer biological/pharmacodynamical considerations and additional physical and engineering concepts and methods. The future may well have many examples utilizing concepts such as the feedback principle as drug delivery devices become tailored to specific pharmacodynamics of the drug and are aimed at optimizing therapy while maximizing patient comfort and convenience.

William I. Higuchi
Distinguished Professor
Department Chairman
Department of Pharmaceutics
The University of Utah
Salt Lake City, Utah

Preface

The salient aspect of conventional methods of drug delivery—including tablets, capsules, liquids, and eye drops—is the fluctuation in concentration between dosages. With some drugs, this fluctuation causes no problem, but with drugs that cause toxic reactions when administered above a narrow therapeutic concentration range, such variations can cause undesirable side effects. There are two ways to improve the situation: first, the development of new and better drugs, and second, more effective and safer use of the drugs.

Until recently, the method of choice for the development of new drugs was to either change the structure of the drug or synthesize a new chemical entity. Today, though, due to increased awareness in the medical and pharmaceutical community of the importance of safe, effective use of drugs, development of novel delivery methods and techniques is at the forefront of research and development. In addition, the rapidly expanding field of genetically engineered drugs by recombinant DNA techniques has led to an urgent need for adequate systems for delivering drugs to specific sites of action. These new drugs present a considerable challenge to those developing delivery systems because of their potency, high molecular weight, sensitivity to environmental agents, and poor oral activity.

Despite many obstacles, however, investigators are developing many potential solutions to the delivery problems posed by these new drugs. Among the various avenues being explored, devices used for drug delivery represent an entirely new and rapidly developing area.

Devices represent a means by which a pharmacologically active moiety may be continuously delivered or monitored either systematically or to a target site in an effective, reliable, repeatable, and safe manner. These devices are also capable of delivering the desired concentration of a drug in a fixed, predetermined pattern for a definite time period. Thus, unnecessary side effects are avoided and the delivery of a desired concentration at a precise time is made possible.

Considering the number of recently published papers dealing with drug delivery devices, it is clear that interest in the development of such systems is rapidly increasing. Nevertheless, as far as I know, there is no book covering the subject. The aim of this work is to partially fill this gap and I hope it will act as a stimulus and basis for research in this mostly unexplored area. The book describes the principles of innovative drug delivery devices and examines the various possibilities suggested by these devices. The concept in the development of these devices ranges from very simple infusion pumps to highly complex microprocessor controlled devices. The book is organized to first present selected basic physical pharmacy, pharmacokinetic, biopharmaceutical and regulatory considerations that influence drug delivery device design and its performance. The systems based on implantable infusion technology are gaining increasing popularity for drug delivery. These are presented in Part Two of the book. These types of systems allow a wide range of delivery rates and minimize the chance of infection by maintaining the body's natural barriers. The devices based on access ports into the vascular system are already commercially available and are included in Part Two along with osmotic pumps, infusors, implantable systems, and a programmable implantable medication system being developed at Johns Hopkins University. Implantable pumps and access ports offer several advantages over external drug delivery systems, including their long life, programmability, site-specific delivery, and the need for minimal patient training. They are therefore, expected to double in number in the market over the next four years. They are also generally well accepted by the patients. Part Three of the book covers specialized devices for drug delivery. These include magnetically controlled, ultrasonically modulated, transdermal therapeutic, iontophoretic, ophthalmic, intrauterine, intranasal, and dental devices. This section is focused more on the systems presently being investigated by various research laboratories. New product performance standards to ensure safety and efficacy will have to be developed for these devices. However, some therapeutic systems, such as transdermal, iontophoretic, intrauterine, and intranasal devices, presently are available in the market. The final section,

Part Four, presents various devices being utilized in the animal health industry. These include ectoparasitic, rumen lodging, and other special devices required for drug delivery and used widely in the veterinary field.

This book is designed for individuals of diverse backgrounds who are interested in the design, development, use and/or optimization of drug delivery devices, and in carrying the product from R & D to the marketplace. Scientists and management involved in clinical practice and research and development, and marketing personnel responsible for innovative developments in the drug delivery device systems and their use in the future, should find this book useful.

I am indebted to specialists in several areas of drug delivery who prepared chapters and persevered through several revisions and deadlines. I would also like to extend my thanks to Drs. Vincent H. L. Lee, Robert Langer, Joseph Robinson, and Richard Toothill for reviewing some important chapters in this book. I am also grateful to my brother Navin for his guidance and encouragement and his wife, Alka, for preparing the index for this book. Special appreciation is extended to Sandra Beberman and Carol Mayhew of Marcel Dekker, Inc., for their expert assistance in the preparation of this book.

The late Professor Takeru Higuchi of the University of Kansas was originally scheduled to write the foreword for this book. In his place, Professor William Higuchi has provided the foreword in memory of his esteemed brother. In view of his many contributions to the field during his lifetime, I dedicate this work to Professor Takeru Higuchi, the father of physical pharmacy.

Praveen Tyle

Contents

Contributors

Amir Ansari, M.D. Department of Obstetrics and Gynecology, Shady-side Hospital, Pittsburgh, Pennsylvania and Medical College of Georgia, Augusta, Georgia

Alex Bell, B.Sc. [*] Dispensing System Application Department, Perfect-Valois UK Ltd., Aylesbury, Buckinghamshire, United Kingdom

Perry J. Blackshear, M.D., D. Phil. Department of Medicine, Duke University Medical Center, Durham, North Carolina

Serap Büyükyaylaci, Ph.D. Animal Formulation Development, Merck Sharp & Dohme Research Laboratories, Division of Merck & Co., Inc., Rahway, New Jersey

Henry Buchwald, M.D., Ph.D. Department of Surgery and Biomedical Engineering, University of Minnesota, Minneapolis, Minnesota

---

[*]*Current affiliation*: Research and Development Department, Valois S.A., Le Neubourg, France

John W. Fara, Ph.D. New Product Opportunities, ALZA Corporation, Palo Alto, California

Robert E. Fischell, BSME, M.S. Space Department, The Johns Hopkins University Applied Physics Laboratory, Laurel, Maryland

Michael Friedman, Ph.D. School of Pharmacy, The Hebrew University of Jerusalem, Jerusalem, Israel

Sharad K. Govil, Ph.D. Transdermal Formulation & Development, Schering-Plough Corporation, Miami, Florida

Robert J. Gyurik, B.A. Pharmaceutical Development and Nutrition Departments, SmithKline Beckman Animal Health Products, West Chester, Pennsylvania

Bruce Kari, Ph.D. Biomedical Research Center, Children's Hospital, St. Paul, Minnesota

Louis Kopito, M.S. Clinical Research Department, Shiley Infusaid Inc., Norwood, Massachusetts

Joseph Kost, Ph. D. Department of Chemical Engineering, Ben-Gurion University of the Negev, Beer-Sheva, Israel

Lilian Chong Kwan, Ph.D. Pharmaceutical Development, SmithKline Beckman Animal Health Products, West Chester, Pennsylvania

Mark A. Longer, M.S. School of Pharmacy, University of Wisconsin, Madison, Wisconsin

Peter Lukacsko, Ph.D. Hospital Products Division, Pharmacia Deltec Inc., Piscataway, New Jersey

Graham S. May, M.D. Hospital Products Division, Pharmacia Deltec Inc., Piscataway, New Jersey

David L. Middleton, M.S. School of Pharmacy, University of Wisconsin, Madison, Wisconsin

Ashim K. Mitra, Ph.D. Department of Industrial and Physical Pharmacy, School of Pharmacy and Pharmacal Sciences, Purdue University, West Lafayette, Indiana

David F. Ranney, M.D. Laboratory of Targeted Diagnosis and Therapy, Department of Pathology, The University of Texas Health Science Center, Dallas, Texas

Nigel Ray, B.Sc. New Product Opportunitites, ALZA Corporation, Palo Alto, California

Thomas D. Rohde, M.S. Department of Surgery, University of Minnesota, Minneapolis, Minnesota

Wolfgang A. Ritschel, Ph.D., Dr. Univ., F.A.S.A., F.C.P. College of Pharmacy, University of Cincinnati Medical Center, Cincinnati, Ohio

Joseph R. Robinson, Ph.D. School of Pharmacy, University of Wisconsin, Madison, Wisconsin

Brij B. Saxena, Ph.D., D.Sc. Division of Reproductive Endocrinology, Department of Obstetrics and Gynecology, Cornell University Medical College, New York, New York

Mukul Singh, M.D. Division of Reproductive Endocrinology, Department of Obstetrics and Gynecology, Cornell University Medical College, New York, New York

Doron Steinberg, M.Sc. School of Pharmacy, The Hebrew University of Jerusalem, Jerusalem, Israel

John Stigi, MBA Division of Small Manufacturers Assistance, Food and Drug Administration, Washington, D.C.

Frank M. Sturtevant, Ph.D. Department of Medical and Scientific Information, Searle Research and Development, G. D. Searle & Co., Skokie, Illinois

Joel A. Tune, MBA Parenterals Division, Baxter Healthcare Corporation, Round Lake, Illinois

Praveen Tyle, Ph.D.* Formulations Research Section, American Cyanamid Company, Princeton, New Jersey

Paul K. Wilkinson, Ph.D. Animal Formulation Development, Merck Sharp & Dohme Laboratories, Division of Merck & Co., Inc., Rahway, New Jersey

---

Current affiliation: Pharmaceutical Research, Sandoz Consumer Health Care Group, Sandoz Pharmaceutical Corporation, Lincoln, Nebraska

David A. Winchell, B.S., M.S. Parenterals Division, Baxter Health-Care Corporation, Round Lake, Illinois

Joel R. Zingerman, B.S. Animal Formulation Development, Merck Sharp & Dohme Research Laboratories, Division of Merck & Co., Inc., Rahway, New Jersey

Drug Delivery Devices

Part One
GENERAL CONSIDERATIONS

1

Conventional Routes of Delivery and the Need for Devices

MARK A. LONGER, DAVID L. MIDDLETON, and
JOSEPH R. ROBINSON / University of Wisconsin, Madison, Wisconsin

I. INTRODUCTION

Since the introduction of the SKF Spansule system in the early 1950s, substantial advances in sustained release drug delivery technology have occurred. However, it is still not possible to accurately modulate

the delivery of most drugs, unless an external pump is employed. For
this reason, utilization of external pumps to regulate drug delivery
has become increasingly popular, especially for long-term therapy.
Additionally, these controllable systems are being used as research
tools because of their ability to accurately deliver small amounts of
drugs in small volumes to specific locations in the body.

The reason so very few sustained release systems have enjoyed the
relative success of the external pump is rather obvious if one considers
the nature of the biological constraints, commonly referred to collec-
tively as "the biological barrier," imposed on traditional dosage forms
(Table 1).* These factors impart some rather strict limitations on accurate, predictable drug delivery. Indeed, an area of great activity
in drug delivery research involves identifying and understanding the
mechanisms of those biological factors that limit controlled drug delivery. The use of devices is an attempt to circumvent the biological
barrier. The relative success or failure of a drug delivery system,
irrespective of whether it is a device, rests on its ability to achieve
this, while at the same time minimizing bioincompatibility or interaction
of the delivery system with its site of administration. Common to all
routes of administration is the problem of the effect of pathological
disease states and drug-induced pathologies on subsequent drug-blood
levels, due to alteration in expected rates of absorption, distribution,
metabolism, or excretion.

This introductory chapter is intended to provide nomenclature
and definitions, establish a baseline of information and, to the greatest extent possible, describe the issues that need to be considered in
assessing drug delivery systems. To set the stage for such a discussion, it is worthwhile to briefly pause and examine the purpose of developing a sustained release product. Clearly, a number of such products have been introduced for the sole purpose of obtaining a patented
line extension, and perhaps to help protect an important drug that
is due to go off patent. In every case these extended duration products can claim a reduction in dosing frequency, a corresponding improvement in patient compliance, and thus improved therapy. Inargu-
ably, the greatest potential for sustained release products lies in their
ability to optimize drug utilization, that is, to reduce local or systemic
side effects and to cure or control the condition in the shortest time
possible, employing the smallest quantity of drug. Optimization of
drug use (i.e., drug delivery) is a future objective of all drugs and
delivery systems and presently appears to be applied only to a small
number of important drugs with either serious side effects or substantial requirements for maintaining constant tissue-drug levels. It is

---

*
The terms "dosage form" and "delivery system" are used interchange-
ably in this chapter without bias to either term.

TABLE 1 Biological Factors[a] Associated with Various Routes of Drug
Delivery That Affect the Performance of Sustained Release Systems

Route	Factor
Oral	
1. Buccal/sublingual	Salivary dissolution and dilution
	Regional variations in keratinization and blood flow
	Generally lower permeability than other oral routes
2. Stomach	pH
3. Small intestine	Motility
4. Colon	Hepatic first-pass metabolism
	Luminal, membrane, and intracellular enzymes
	Active transport mechanisms (absorption windows)
	Bacteria
Transdermal	Low permeability
	Potential allergic responses
	Pathological states
	Potential binding in epidermis
Parenteral	Biocompatibility
	Involvement of reticuloendothelial system
	Systemic inactivation (metabolism)
	Vascular patency
	Potential lymphatic uptake

[a]Collectively, these constitute what is commonly referred to as "the
biological barrier" to drug delivery.

for this latter problem that infusion systems have had their greatest
impact and, indeed, that long-term implants and other parenteral forms
of drug administration are receiving increasing attention. It is obvious that with the appearance of more potent and specific drugs, many
of which will require unusual dosing patterns (e.g., peptides and proteins), greater attention to improved controlled delivery systems will
be necessary. That this is the case is evidenced by the substantial
increase in publications and oral presentations dealing with continuous
infusion and long-term implant systems.

II. DEFINITIONS AND FUNDAMENTALS

Over the past 30 years there has been a blizzard of descriptive terms associated with sustained and controlled release dosage forms. These terms, while serving to identify specific products, have tended to blur their performance characteristics. This blurring has obscured the capabilities of the products to the point where practitioners are often unclear about their advantages and limitations.

At the outset, it is helpful to distinguish *immediately* releasing from *sustaining* dosage forms. In immediately releasing delivery systems, the rate of appearance of drug in the body is controlled by the biological absorption process, whereas in sustaining systems this is controlled by the dosage form. According to this definition a substantial number of traditional dosage forms are sustaining systems. Thus, ointments, capsules, and tablets can be sustaining systems, depending on the drug at issue. Commonly, however, these traditional sustaining systems decrease the dosing frequency by less than a factor of 2 and/or, as in the case of ointments, the sustaining effect is inherent in the nature of the delivery system. More recently, sustained release products have been specifically developed to reduce dosing frequency by at least a factor of 2, and in most cases an attempt is being made for all routes of administration to prepare at least once-daily products.

Unfortunately, with increasing interest in sustained release drug delivery, a number of commercial products were advertised as *controlled release* systems, implying that controlled release is superior in performance to the more generally sustained or prolonged release drug delivery systems. Indeed there is a difference between sustained and controlled release products and, despite marketing claims for some products, we will restrict the use of the term "controlled release" to systems with which predictive control over the release pattern and subsequent tissue or blood levels can be achieved. With this definition, very few drug delivery systems, regardless of the route of administration, would be considered to be controlled release systems. Clearly, we would like all sustained release delivery systems to be controlled; that is, controlled delivery is a goal for all products.

The issue of what constitutes controlled release, as contrasted with sustained release, is not a trivial problem given the extent of intra- and intersubject variability that is typically associated with drugs and drug delivery systems. In some cases this variability, or "biological noise," has a coefficient of variation exceeding 100%, and on this basis even poor delivery systems could claim controlled release. It is hoped that in the future differentiation of sustained and controlled release systems will be based on objective criteria such as measurable improvement in toxicity or therapy, over and above the simple issue of patient compliance. For the remainder of this chapter we will employ the terms "sustained" and "extended" release and generally avoid the more difficult "controlled" release term.

To place the drug delivery issue in perspective, it is worthwhile to examine the criteria used to establish the desired rate of delivery for specific drugs. As will be clear from the following analysis, our understanding of the drug requirements necessary to optimize therapy is rather primitive.

The early oral sustained release products attempted either to incorporate multiple units of the single dose system into one dosage form or to maintain the maximum drug concentration in the plasma from a single dose for an extended period of time. In equation form [1]:

$$\text{Rate in} = \text{Rate out} \tag{1}$$

$$\text{Rate in} = k_{\text{elimination}} \times C_{\text{max}} \times V_d \tag{2}$$

where

$k_{\text{elimination}}$ = elimination constant from the blood
C_{max} = maximum drug level in the blood
V_d = volume of distribution for the drug

This elementary analysis, based on a simple one-compartment model, suggests that the oral dosage form should be equivalent to an intravenous infusion of drug, that is, zero-order input. Indeed, the units of Equation (2) (amount/time) show that a zero-order system is needed. This analysis assumes that blood-drug concentrations mirror pharmacological responses—that is, pharmacokinetics mimics pharmacodynamics— an assumption that is invalid for an increasing number of drugs, particularly peptide and protein drugs. Moreover, it assumes that the biological noise is small enough that zero-order delivery can be distinguished from other kinetic input functions.

It is becoming increasingly clear that the optimal rate of drug input may not necessarily be zero-order for all drugs and disease states. For example, it is known that circadian rhythm influences enzyme induction and inhibition [2] and that downregulation of receptors may modify drug response or metabolism [3-6]. In cases such as these, the optimal input of drug may be discrete (pulsatile) and noncontinuous, or perhaps of a mixed-order rate (gradient effect), both of which are difficult or, at present, impossible to include in traditional extended release delivery systems.

A final point regarding sustained release drug delivery systems pertains to mucosal versus parenteral routes of drug delivery. All mucosal routes of administration have inherent mucociliary clearance mechanisms that remove inserted or ingested material in, at most, a day or sometimes shorter periods of time. Occasionally, one can circumvent these normal clearance mechanisms, as for example with ocular drug delivery inserts, which can remain in place for several days. Nevertheless, mucosal routes will typically require frequent applications/installations to achieve long-term therapy. Moreover, these routes are so demanding that precise, controlled drug delivery over an extended period is difficult or, in some cases, presently impossible.

III. LIMITATIONS IN ROUTES OF DRUG DELIVERY

Every route of drug administration is capable of "processing" the drug and delivery system, and this naturally limits the capabilities of the route. These processing factors constitute a portion of the biological barrier that limits drug delivery. Consider the highlights of each route of administraiton.

A. Oral

Strictly speaking, the oral route of administration allows contact of drug with several anatomical areas of the gastrointestinal tract from which absorption may occur: the oral cavities inside the mouth (e.g., buccal and sublingual), the stomach, the small intestine, and the colon (large intestine). The rectal vault, the most distal region accessible by oral administration, is more commonly accessed by the use of suppositories and is not included in this discussion.

In general, a major characteristic of the gastrointestinal tract with regard to drugs is the exposure of these agents to potential destruction due to hepatic first-pass metabolism. Drugs that are absorbed from all the anatomical areas listed above, with the exception of the oral cavity, pass into the portal circulation and subsequently to the liver before entering the general circulation. For drugs that are sensitive to metabolic processes, first-pass metabolism can lead to a substantial loss of drug, thus limiting the effectiveness of the oral route for drug delivery. Nevertheless, the oral route represents the most common and acceptable way to deliver drugs. However, it is also the most difficult route for extended drug delivery. The four anatomical areas listed above are considered separately, since each offers a potential site for drug absorption and presents unique limitations to delivery.

Buccal/Sublingual

A drug or delivery system placed in the buccal cavity between the cheek and gingiva may contact two types of epithelium, the keratinized gingiva as well as the nonkeratinized tissue opposing the cheek and lip. The sublingual region generally consists of thinner, nonkeratinized epithelia [7]. Few examples of extended delivery specifically to these tissues can be cited. More commonly, these areas are used as platforms for oral ingestion and subsequent gastrointestinal processing of drug. The buccal and gingival routes are bathed by copious quantities of saliva, which can accelerate dissolution and dilution of drugs placed in this region. However, buccal delivery patches intended for systemic absorption (analogous to transdermal patches) can be made unidirectional, which helps to protect drug from salivary fluids. While the design of such patches is presently technologically feasible, various other aspects of their use, such as optimal location for placement and patient compliance with proper application, need to be addressed. Of some consequence is the fact that drug administration by the buccal route bypasses hepatic first-pass metabolism. Moreover, a number of studies suggest that buccal permeability to low molecular weight compounds appears to be a factor of 10 to 50 times greater than that of skin, in the absence of penetration enhancers for both routes. Given the accessibility of this route and its reasonable permeability, it is likely that it will receive increasing attention for drug delivery.

Stomach

During the longitudinal movement of the delivery system from the esophagus through the stomach, the product is exposed to a variable pH, ranging from approximately 1 to 4. It has been common for many traditional and even sustained delivery systems to use the stomach as an area of dosage form dissociation. Absorption from the stomach can and does occur for a great many drug entities, but absorption is limited in these cases to the residence time within the stomach. Gastrointestinal transit typically limits the duration of drug delivery to approximately 8 to 12 hr [8]. Motility is regulated primarily by the presence or absence of food (especially fats) in the stomach; the intestine seems to play a minor role in this regard. This factor is uncontrollable except in the hospital setting, where the diet can be well defined.

Many sustained release delivery systems act by slowing the release of the drug from the dosage form, and thus presenting it to the general circulation over a longer time interval than would be found from more traditional, immediate release systems. Of course, in the ever-changing environment of the stomach, the ability to reproduce absorption characteristics in actual practice is difficult to achieve due to inter- and intra-subject variability, as mentioned previously.

Because localizing the delivery systems in various regions of the gastrointestinal tract is very difficult, site-specific delivery is uncommon. Recent work on drug absorption in this region is attempting to understand the physiological processes well enough to permit drug delivery strategies to evolve from these processes. Examples include the insulin pump [9] and increased absorption of antigens by coadministration of vitamin B_{12} and certain sugars [10]. The antigens in this case are pinocytosed nonspecifically due to the specific uptake of vitamin B_{12} and the sugars.

In reality, we have this hostile environment to thank for our search for better drug delivery systems. Aside from the patient compliance issue favoring the oral route, the need to have better control over the delivery of drug to the site of action has prompted the search for other methods (i.e., implants and pumps, etc.).

Small Intestine

Since the optimal site of drug absorption is assumed to be the proximal and medial small intestine, if drug is continuously presented to this area over time, absorption will be extended relative to an immediate release product. In many instances there is an "absorption window," and if the drug passes this window before being released or before it is in the correct un-ionized form for absorption, the bioavailability will also be reduced [11].

Underlying the entire aspect of gastrointestinal absorption is the extensive inactivation that occurs, not only in the liver on first-pass as mentioned earlier, but throughout the entire system, from the point of introduciton of drug in the intestinal environment and the various membranes it must cross, to its entrance into the circulation and subsequent route to its receptor. Indeed, prodrugs and other entities that become active after metabolic conversion substantially address this issue [12]. However, as our level of sophistication grows, we find severe limitations to the oral route of drug delivery.

Colon

Since the colon is at the terminus of the gastrointestinal tract, it would seem that it would be relatively easy to target oral delivery systems there, for the purpose of systemic absorption as well as treatment of a number of local pathological conditions. However, unique environmental conditions, such as wide-ranging pH values of 6 to 8 [13] and the presence of high concentrations (10^{10}-10^{13}/ml) of bacteria [14], can substantially alter the rate of drug release from the delivery system. For a few drugs, these conditions can be advantageous. For example, the antimicrobial agent sulfasalazine, used for treatment of ulcerative colitis, relies on azoreduction by resident bacteria to be converted to 5-aminosalicylic acid and sulfpyridine. Similarly, steroid D-glycosides rely on local glycosidases for conversion. Most drugs, however, will not enjoy such benefits form the bacteria and instead are faced with potential degradation by them. This is particularly critical in the case of peptide and protein drugs. Furthermore, reliance on pH for colonic targeting with, for example, the use of high-pH-soluble polymer coatings is not foolproof, since the pH in the colon rarely fluctuates to such high levels and, in addition, may do so in the duodenum, depending on the type of food ingested [15].

B. Transdermal

Application of drugs to the skin for systemic absorption and action
is an approach that is rather old but has received increased attention
recently because of the success of the transdermal nitroglycerin products. Although there are only a few examples of commercially successful transdermal products, this route is being considered for a wide
variety of drugs and represents a viable alternative to the oral route
for a noninvasive means of delivering drugs.

There are some substantial limitations to the transdermal route
that must be considered. For example, it is a primary issue that most
drugs exhibit such low permeabilities that unless one covers a huge
surface area of the body with drug, some modification of the skin's
barrier properties must be undertaken to achieve therapeutic blood
levels. Assisting transdermal penetration through the use of iontophoresis [16] or with penetration enhancers [17,18] is possible and
can lead to substantial improvements in flux for some drugs. However,
aside from alcohol, propylene glycol, and other normal additives to
topical products, few penetration enhancers have been approved by
the U.S. Food and Drug Administration (FDA). Moreover, iontophoresis has yet to be applied in a commercial product.

It appears that application to the skin of many drugs, in patch
form, for more than a day leads to skin irritation/allergic reaction.
Thus, while in principle one can use the skin for prolonged drug delivery stretching to a week for a single patch and even longer if other
sites are used, other issues appear to limit effective time to a couple
of days.

Two additional issues need to be mentioned that present problems
in special circumstances: (a) a number of drugs appear to be bound
or retained in the skin, thus making the rate-limiting step for transdermal absorption flux through the skin rather than release of drug
from the delivery system [19-21] and (b) certain pathological conditions of the skin can substantially alter its permeability, thus yield-
ing unpredictable blood levels [22-24]. Neither issue should be overlooked when assessing the performance of transdermal devices.

C. Parenteral

In addition to direct placement of drug into the bloodstream via intravenous injection, it is possible to use subcutaneous, intramuscular,
and other routes such as intraperitoneal. The selection of one route
over another may be for practical therapeutic reasons such as quantity
of drug administered and duration of activity, or for more biochemical
reasons such as processing of drug at the site of injection and facility
for targeting from that site. Thus, one might argue that since insulin
naturally secreted from the pancreas is discharged into the liver before

entering the general circulation, an appropriate route for delivery of
exogenous insulin would be via intraperitoneal injection.

Substantial issues relative to the use of intravenous injection or
infusion of a drug substance are patency of the vascular bed, total
fluid load, and duration of therapy. External modulation of the rate
of drug input by the use of infusion pumps has made this the simplest
and most direct route of sustained release drug administration. Such
pump use has become routine for both hospital and home-use drug
therapy. It would be helpful if these pumps also contained a feedback
loop to monitor the steady state blood level, to avoid under- or overtreatment of the patient. For example, administration of insulin via
injection ports, implants, or injection into a muscle mass has been used
to evaluate a variety of monitoring devices for glucose or insulin [25].
These monitoring devices rely on mechanisms ranging from biochemical
(enzymatic) detection to more traditional analytic techniques such as
electrometry and spectrophotometry. Such feedback loops are generally at an exploratory stage, and development work in this area is continuing.

Placement of drugs subcutaneously, intramuscularly, intraperi-
toneally, intrathecally, and so on commonly raises several issues of
concern:

1. Is the delivery fluid or implant compatible with the tissue and,
    if not, will it alter drug delivery from the device, either by
    altering subsequent absorption or by macrophage inactivation
    of the drug?
2. As a result of the implant or formulation, will drug be seques-
    tered preferentially into the lymph or vascular bed?

The issue of biocompatibility of implanted or injected delivery systems is an extremely important issue that may influence the performance of some drugs. Not uncommonly, polymeric substances for implant purposes are not monodisperse relative to their molecular weight.
Such polydispersity can lead to tissue irritancy and subsequent events
associated with acute and chronic irritation. Unfortunately, the list
of polymers for extended drug delivery use is not extensive, and there
is a general reluctance to introduce new polymers, given the cost of
establishing their safety and lack of toxicity and the likelihood of greater time and cost for regulatory approval.

IV. DRUG DELIVERY FROM DEVICES

Given the relatively short duration of therapy and general inherent
variability associated with mucosal routes of administration, there is

substantial interest in a variety of nonmucosal routes for administration or placement of devices. These other routes offer a number of potential advantages, including increased duration of continuous drug delivery for as long as a year or two and the concomitant improvement in therapy or reduction in side effects.

Of some consequence for pump therapy is possible home use for certain drugs. The most successful example to date is the insulin infusion pump used to maintain more strict control over blood glucose levels. Naturally, an improved therapeutic profile of drug, while most desirable and necessary, must be weighed against the cost of such therapy. Not uncommonly, continuous or intermittent pump therapy can lead to a substantial cost reduction, particularly if there is a corresponding reduction in hospital inpatient costs.

Targeting of drugs remains a difficult challenge because of the normal physiological clearance mechanisms operating in the liver, spleen, and other components of the reticuloendothelial system. However, magnetic devices can theoretically be localized in many regions of the body, and even some modulation of drug release can occur with the assistance of externally applied magnetic fields [26]. Magnetic devices exemplify the type of nontraditional approaches that must be undertaken to target drugs to areas of the body unreachable by less sophisticated techniques.

V. SUMMARY

The purpose of this chapter has been to introduce the subject of extended release dosage forms and to place in perspective the need to improve drug delivery. Devices have been introduced into therapy for a variety of reasons, including long-term delivery of drugs, better control over the rate of drug delivery, lower cost, and greater convenience. It is very important to recognize that while the concept of extended drug delivery is centuries old, only in relatively recent times has there been substantial interest in understanding and improving drug delivery.

The concept of optimized drug therapy demands a thorough understanding of the biological barriers that commonly limit drug delivery. The technical issues of modulated drug delivery for both parenteral and nonparenteral forms, including approaches to minimize or circumvent biological barriers, are extensive. Some of these issues are not well understood and therefore not well controlled. It is therefore useful to consider drug delivery as an evolving discipline that is in its early stages of development.

REFERENCES

1. J. R. Robinson and S. P. Eriksen, *J. Pharm. Sci.*, 55:1254 (1966).
2. A. T. Florence and W. R. Vezin, in *Optimization of Drug Delivery*, Alfred Benzon Symposium 17 (H. Bundguaard, A. B. Hansen, and H. Kofod, eds.). Munksgaard, Copenhagen, 1982, pp. 93-113.
3. J. R. Gavin, J. Roth, D. M. Neville, P. deMeyts, and D. N. Buell, *Proc. Natl. Acad. Sci. USA*, 71:84 (1974).
4. A. J. W. Hsuen, H. L. Dufau, and K. J. Catt, *Biochem. Biophys. Res. Commun.*, 72:1145 (1976).
5. M. A. Lesniak and J. Roth, *J. Biol. Chem.*, 251:3720 (1976).
6. P. M. Hinkle and A. H. Tashjian, Jr., *Biochemistry*, 14:3845 (1975).
7. S.-Y. Chen and C. A. Squier, in *The Structure and Function of Oral Mucosa* (J. Meyer, C. A. Squier, and S. J. Gerson, eds.). Pergamon Press, Elmsford, NY, 1984, pp. 7-30.
8. P. Gruber, M. A. Longer, and J. R. Robinson, *Adv. Drug Delivery Rev.*, 1:1 (1987).
9. P. J. Blackshear, T. D. Rohde, J. D. Grotling, F. D. Dorman, P. R. Perkins, R. L. Varco, and H. Buchwald, *Diabetes*, 28:634 (1979).
10. P. J. Hoedemaeker, J. Ables, J. J. Wachters, A. Averds, and H. O. Nieweg, *Lab. Invest.*, 15:1163 (1966).
11. M. A. Longer, H. S. Ch'ng, and J. R. Robinson, *J. Pharm. Sci.*, 74:406 (1985).
12. D. Fleisher, B. H. Stewart, and G. L. Amidon, *Methods Enzymol.*, 112:360 (1985).
13. J. M. Rawlings and M. L. Lucas, *Gut*, 26:203 (1985).
14. B. E. Gustaffson, *Scand. J. Gastroenterol. Suppl.*, 77:117 (1982).
15. P. Gruber, A. Rubinstein, V. H. K. Li, P. Bass, and J. R. Robinson, *J. Pharm. Sci.*, 76:117 (1987).
16. R. R. Burnette and D. Marrero, *J. Pharm. Sci.*, 75:738 (1986).
17. R. E. Aroufhron, *Arch. Dermatol.*, 118:474 (1982).
18. R. E. Stoughton and W. O. McClure, *Drug Deve. Ind. Pharm.*, 9:725 (1983).
19. R. H. Guy and H. I. Maibach, *J. Pharm. Sci.*, 72:1375 (1983).
20. J. Wepierre and J.-P. Marty, *Trends Pharmacol. Sci.*, 1:23 (1979).
21. J. Wepierre, in *Actualites Pharmacologiques, 31e serie*, Masson, Paris, 1979, pp. 170-202.
22. R. L. Bronaugh and R. F. Stewart, *J. Pharm. Sci.*, 74:1062 (1985).
23. R. C. Scott and P. H. Dugard, *J. Pharm. Pharmacol.*, 34:35 (1982).

24. C. R. Behl, E. E. Linn, G. L. Flynn, N. F. H. Ho, W. I. Higuchi, and C. L. Pierson, *J. Pharm. Sci.*, 72:397 (1983).
25. R. Langer, *Pharmac. Ther.*, 21:35 (1983).
26. D. S. T. Hsieh and R. Langer, in, *Controlled Release Delivery Systems* (T. J. Roseman and S. Z. Mansdorf, eds.), Marcel Dekker, Inc., New York, 1983, Chap. 7.

2

Pharmacokinetic and Biopharmaceutical Aspects in Drug Delivery

WOLFGANG A. RITSCHEL / University of Cincinnati Medical Center, Cincinnati, Ohio

I. INTRODUCTION

The development of drug delivery devices is extremely complex and interwoven, and it requires a team approach. This chapter discusses only the general or basic pharmacokinetic and biopharmaceutical aspects of this endeavor. Specific information about the application of these principles is given in Section II; individual devices are mentioned where appropriate.

II. PHARMACOKINETIC CHARACTERIZATION OF DRUGS FOR SELECTION OF SUITABLE DELIVERY DEVICES

For practically all controlled release delivery devices, except those for immunostimulation and other immunological applications, a basic pharmacokinetic understanding of a given drug's disposition in the human (or animal) body is essential. Most devices are not intended just to release the drug at a delayed or prolonged rate, but are expected to reach and maintain a certain target concentration in blood, in plasma, or at specific sites or organs.

    Drug disposition is a composite of sequentially and simultaneously occurring processes, described by the LADMER (liberation, absorption, distribution, metabolism, elimination, response) system [1].

    For controlled delivery devices, the general absorbability must be established. The intrinsic rate of absorption is of minor importance, because the apparent rate of absorption will be dictated by the delivery device. In other words, ideally the liberation or drug release rate (therefore the term "controlled release delivery device") is the rate-limiting step for the absorption process. Controlled release delivery devices are multiple-dose devices designed to result in steady state concentrations, C_{ss}. The magnitude of C_{ss} depends on the dose rate R^0 (amount of drug per unit of time) and the total clearance CL (loss of drug from the volume of distribution per unit of time) of the drug. To understand the design and evaluation of controlled delivery devices, some basic principles are discussed here.

A. Compartment Model

A drug in the systemic circulation (blood), either directly introduced into the bloodstream by intravascular injection or reaching the blood by absorption after extravascular administration, is distributed not only within the bloodstream and the organs of immediate equilibrium but also to other organs and tissues; it is eventually eliminated by metabolism and/or excretion. Since the molecules entering first will have been distributed and perhaps eliminated before the last molecules are absorbed, the entire process is dynamic, that is, made up of simultaneously occurring individual kinetic processes. Since the blood is not only a means of drug transport but is also the only biological fluid that can be sampled easily and in well-defined series, the fate of a drug in the body can be characterized by a drug blood concentration-versus-time curve. In the case of controlled drug delivery devices, the absorption is not completed instantly as with an intravenous push (rapid i.v. injection). It is pertinent to discuss here the concentration-time curves only as they are observed upon extravascular or infusion administration.

Assuming first-order elimination, which is the case for most drugs, and plotting the concentration-time data semilogarithmically (concentration of drug in blood, plasma, or serum on the logarithmic ordinate and time on the numeric abscissa), the terminal slope is the elimination phase, characterized by a straight line.

One can now back-extrapolate this terminal phase to the origin. We wil find three possibilities as shown in Fig. 1.

1. If the drug is *rapidly absorbed* and *rapidly distributed* between the systemic circulation (including organs of instant equilibrium) and the tissues to which the drug eventually goes, the peak will be *below* the back-extrapolated terminal line (Fig. 1a).

2. If the drug is *rapidly absorbed* but *slowly distributed* between the systemic circulation (including organs of instant equilibrium = central compartment) and the tissues to which the drug eventually goes (peripheral compartment), the peak will be *above* the back-extrapolated terminal line (Fig. 1b).

3. If the drug is *slowly* absorbed but rapidly distributed between central and peripheral compartments, the peak will be *below* the back-extrapolated terminal line (Fig. 1c).

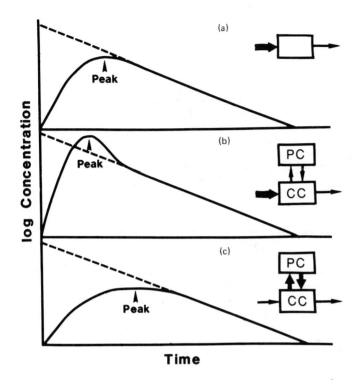

Time

Fig. 1 Schematic blood concentration-time curves after extravascular administration for one-compartment (a) and two-compartment (b and c) models: PC = peripheral compartment, CC = central compartment. For additional explanation see text. The thickness of the arrows indicates the relative magnitude of the corresponding rates of the process.

The concentration-time profile in Fig. 1c, having the peak below the terminal line, looks similar to that in Fig. 1a. The distribution phase in two-compartment models may vary from a few minutes to a few hours. Since in controlled drug delivery devices the drug liberation usually takes longer than the distribution phase, we can "collapse" the two-compartment model into a one-compartment model.

However, one has to be aware that in treating the case of Fig. 1c as a one-compartment model, the apparent absorption rate constant is overlapped by and approaches the distribution rate constant. Nevertheless, the one-compartment model is quite suitable and applicable for the design of drug delivery devices.

In Fig. 2 the collapsing of a two-compartment model to an "apparent" one-compartment model is shown as a function of the absorption rate constant k_a. However, for specific purposes, especially for

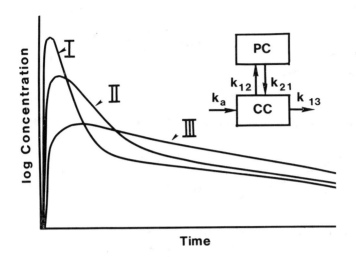

Fig. 2 Schematic diagram to demonstrate collapsing of a two-compartment model: $k_{12} = 0.8$ hr^{-1}; $k_{21} = 0.25$ hr^{-1}, $k_{13} = 0.2$ hr^{-1}. Only the absorption rate constant k_a is changed: for I it is 5.0 hr^{-1}, for II it is 1.25 hr^{-1}, and for III it is 0.7 hr^{-1}. The distribution rate constants are k_{12} and k_{21}, and the elimination rate constant is k_{13}.

targeting of tissues, special kinetics must be employed. In those cases it may be appropriate to use so-called physiological-pharmacokinetic models [2]. A discussion of those models is beyond the scope of this chapter.

> Rule of Thumb: In a one-compartment model distribution occurs instantly; in a two-compartment model the distribution process takes a measurable period of time. Because in controlled release delivery devices the rate of drug release is slower than the rate of distribution, one can "collapse" the concentration-time profile into a one-compartment model.

B. Elimination or Terminal Half-Life ($t_{1/2}$)

The elimination or terminal half-life (previously called biological half-life) is the time required to reduce the concentration in blood, plasma, or serum to one-half, after equilibrium has been reached.

The $t_{1/2}$ can be determined from the slope of the terminal line of a semilogarithmic plot by regression analysis.

> Rule of Thumb: The elimination half-life is an important parameter in selecting the category of drug delivery devices. The

shorter the $t_{1/2}$, the greater will be the amount of drug to be incorporated into the device. Only drugs whose $t_{1/2}$ can be correlated with the pharmacological response are candidates for controlled release drug delivery devices.

C. Area Under the Concentration-Time Curve (AUC)

The area under the curve (AUC) is a measure of the quantity of drug in the body. It is a "robust" pharmacokinetic parameter, which means that it is not very sensitive to small changes in the concentration-time data. If curve fitting is done, which assumes a specific model, the AUC can be determined from the coefficients and constants. However, most conveniently the AUC is determined by a compartment model-independent approach, using the linear trapezoidal rule.

The AUC is a very important parameter, permitting the estimation of total clearance, and consequently the apparent volume of distribution. The ratio of the AUCs between extravascular and intravascular administration is the absolute bioavailability F, and the ratio of AUCs between a test and standard product given by the same route of administration is the relative bioavailability.

Rule of Thumb: The area under the curve is the key parameter in determining absolute and relative bioavailability; it permits estimation of total clearance and apparent volume of distribution. The area under the curve determined by the linear trapezoidal rule is model independent.

D. Total Clearance (CL)

The total clearance (CL) is that hypothetical volume of distribution of unmetabolized drug that is cleared per unit of time by any pathway of drug removal.

The value of CL can be determined from the dose administered D, the absolute bioavailability F, and AUC:

$$CL = \frac{D \cdot F}{AUC} \tag{1}$$

In addition, CL, V_d, and $t_{1/2}$ are interrelated, whereby CL and V_d are the independent variables and $t_{1/2}$ is the dependent variable:

$$CL = \frac{0.693 V_d}{t_{1/2}} \tag{2}$$

Upon multiple dosing, once steady state is reached, CL is:

$$CL = \frac{D}{AUC(\tau_n \to \tau_{n+1})} \qquad (3)$$

where $AUC(\tau_n \to \tau_{n+1})$ is the AUC during any dosing interval.

The total clearance is the key to estimating the dose rate R^0 (= D/τ) for controlled release delivery devices and is related to the mean steady state concentration C_{ss}.

> Rule of Thumb: The total clearance is a measure of the volume of distribution cleared of drug per unit of time. It is the key parameter in estimating the required dose rate for controlled release drug delivery devices and for predicting the steady state concentration.

E. Apparent Volume of Distribution (V_d)

The apparent volume of distribution V_d is a hypothetical volume, indicating the volume of fluid that is required to dissolve the total amount of drug at the concentration that is found in blood. It is a proportionality constant relating the amount of drug in the body to the measured concentration in blood.

Using the model-independent approach, the V_d is calculated according to Equation (4):

$$V_d = \frac{D \cdot F}{AUC \cdot k_{el}} \qquad (4)$$

where k_{el} is the terminal elimination rate constant ($k_{el} = 0.693/t_{1/2}$).

F. Mean Steady State Concentration (C_{ss})

The mean steady state concentration C_{ss} is not the numeric mean between peak ($C_{ss\ max}$) and trough ($C_{ss\ min}$) at steady state but an integrated concentration. With constant rate infusion and in ideal controlled release delivery devices, no fluctuations occur at steady state, hence $C_{ss} = C_{ss\ max} = C_{ss\ min}$.

The value of C_{ss} can be estimated from the dose rate R^0 (= D/τ) and CL:

$$C_{ss} = \frac{R^0}{CL} \qquad (5)$$

or from AUC of any dosing interval at steady state:

$$C_{ss} = \frac{ACU(\tau_n \to \tau_{n+1})}{\tau} \qquad (6)$$

Rule of Thumb: The mean steady state concentration is usually the target concentration to be reached and maintained using controlled release delivery devices.

G. Mean Residence Time (MRT)

The mean residence time (MRT) is the mean time a drug molecule resides in the body; it is the time corresponding to 63.2% elimination from the body. It is calculated from AUC and AUMC (the area under the first-moment curve) [3].

$$MRT = \frac{AUMC}{AUC} \qquad (7)$$

Rule of Thumb: Controlled-release delivery devices should have an MRT significantly longer than is obtainable with conventional dosage forms.

H. First-Pass Effect (FPE); Presystemic Drug Loss

Presystemic loss of drug can occur regardless of whether the drug is administered systemically or locally, except when given intravascularly. It is that fraction of drug which is degraded, inactivated, or metabolized after its release from the dosage form. Tissue degradation should not be underestimated. For instance, kanamycin given intramuscularly has a systemic availability of only 70%. In cases of local administration a drug may be metabolized in the skin, or in the case of eye preparations, the drug may be lost in tear fluid, which is drained into the nasal cavity.

Most prominent is the presystemic loss of drug upon peroral administration, namely degradation by intestinal contents and enzymes, biotransformation by the intestinal microbial flora, and first-pass effect, the metabolism in the gut wall, mesenteric veins, portal vein, and liver.

In the case of FPE upon peroral administration, an estimate can be obtained from intravenous data of the drug:

$$f_{FPE} = 1 - \frac{D \; i.v.}{LBF \cdot AUC_{i.v.}} \qquad (8)$$

where f_{FPE} is the fraction of drug reaching the systemic circulation after peroral administration, LBF is the liver blood flow rate (1.5

liters/min or 90,000 ml/hr), and $D_{i.v.}$ and $AUC_{i.v.}$ are the dose and the total area under the curve after intravenous administration.

And since CL is the ratio of D and AUC, it can also be calculated from the total clearance:

$$f_{FPE} = 1 - \frac{CL}{LBF} \tag{9}$$

Rule of Thumb: Presystemic drug loss may be extensive. The finding of such loss suggests use of alternate routes of administration, such as bucally, nasally, or transdermally, if first-pass effect is extensive upon peroral administration.

I. Intrinsic Absorption Rate Constant (k_a)

The *intrinsic* absorption rate constant k_a is the rate constant for drug uptake into the systemic circulation under unrestricted conditions (i.e., when the drug is freely available in form of a true solution at the site of absorption). This is the case if the drug is administered in form of a solution and does not precipitate in the biological fluid (acidic compounds may precipitate in acid gastric fluid dependent on the drug's pK_a and the pH of gastric fluid), is not bound to other material present (e.g., to food or antacids present in the stomach, or to mucous material), and is not otherwise acted upon. The rate constant k_a can be calculated by selecting a proper model, by curve fitting and by pharmacokinetic analysis. Although k_a may be first, zero, or mixed-order, usually, it is assumed to be first-order.

There are several simple and fast methods that permit an estimate of k_a [4]:

1. First MRT method: from mean residence time after intravascular and extravascular administration:

$$k_a = (MRT_{e.v.} - MRT_{i.v.})^{-1} \tag{10}$$

2. Second MRT method: from extravascular mean residence time, assuming a one-compartment model:

$$k_a = (MRT_{e.v.} - \frac{1}{k_{el}})^{-1} \tag{11}$$

3. C_{max}-area method: knowing the peak concentration C_{max} and the AUC from time of peak to infinity $AUC(t_{max} \to \infty)$, k_a can be calculated:

$$k_a = \frac{C_{max}}{AUC(t_{max} \to \infty) - C_{max}/k_{el}} \quad (12)$$

4. *Absorption time method*: under the assumptions that at time zero upon extravascular administration 100% is unabsorbed and that at the point when the actual blood level-time curve after the peak is just distinguishable before entering the distribution phase or the terminal phase, only 1% is unabsorbed, k_a can be estimated from the absorption time t_a, assuming first-order kinetics. For graphically determining t_a see Fig. 3:

$$k_a = \frac{4.61}{t_a} \quad (13)$$

Controlled release delivery devices are usually designed so that the rate of drug release becomes the rate-limiting step in the absorption process, totally overriding the intrinsic k_a and providing in most cases a zero-order or near-zero-order release. For instance, in ideal transdermal drug delivery devices the release rate constant from the device should be the rate-limiting step in the drug absorption process and should be slower than the transport across the stratum corneum.

The intrinsic absorption rate does not play a role in certain devices or studies designed for specific tissue targeting and devices based on trigger mechanisms.

Rule of Thumb: For controlled release drug delivery devices based on a prolonged absorption process, the drug release rate constant from the device must be much smaller than the unrestricted, intrinsic absorption rate constant ($k_{release} <<< k_a$).

J. Relative Areas (RA)

The desired performance of a controlled release device has been achieved when the following conditions are obtained:

The dosing interval is much longer than with conventional dosage forms.
Fewer fluctuations are obtained between peak ($C_{ss\ max}$) and trough ($C_{ss\ min}$) concentrations.
The steady state concentration ideally results in $C_{ss} = C_{ss\ max} = C_{ss\ min}$.

We have already mentioned the mean residence time (MRT) as one possibility for evaluating controlled release. However, this parameter takes care of only the first of the three statements above.

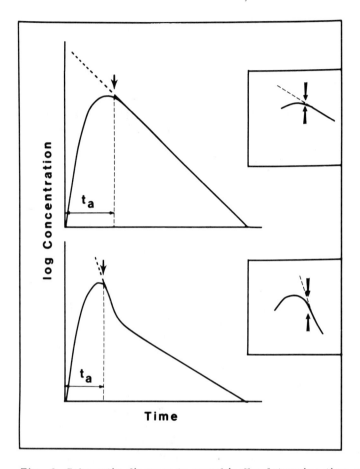

Fig. 3 Schematic diagram to graphically determine time of absorption t_a. The insets demonstrate that one should find the time when the actual blood level curve is still distinguishable from the terminal phase (top) or the distribution phase (bottom). (From W. A. Ritschel, *Handbook of Basic Pharmacokinetics*, 3rd ed. Drug Intelligence Publications, Hamilton, IL, 1986, p. 338.)

A method addressing the second statement, suggested by Boxenbaum [5], uses the absolute area *above* and *below* the horizontal mean steady state concentration, $C_{ss\ avg}$. The sum of both areas results in the relative area (RA) as shown in Fig. 4. The smaller the RA in comparison to a conventional dosage form whose RA is arbitrarily set at 100, the "better" the controlled release delivery device. The RA values should be calculated from individual subject data rather than from averaged (mean) blood level data.

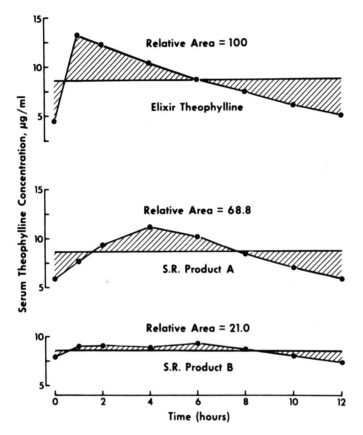

Fig. 4 Determination of "relative areas." Averaged steady state serum theophylline levels following 12 hourly peroral administrations of three dosage forms: Top, 250 mg elixir; middle, 250 mg sustained release (SR) capsule; bottom, 300 mg SR tablet. Serum levels in the top and center segments were multiplied by appropriate factors to produce values of $C_{ss\ avg}$ equivalent to the bottom figure (i.e., 8.63 µg/ml). Shaded regions are area deviations from the horizontal ideal. (From Ref. 5.)

Rule of Thumb: The "relative area" test is a useful tool in evaluating the performance of controlled release drug delivery devices. The smaller the RA value in comparison to conventional or other, competitive drug products, the fewer are the blood level fluctuations within a dosing interval.

K. Dosage Form Index (DI)

Addressing the third statement in Subsection J, Gibaldi and Perrier [6] used for evaluation of a constant plateau concentration the ratio between peak ($C_{ss\ max}$) and trough ($C_{ss\ min}$) values within a dosing interval. This ratio was termed the dosage form index, DI:

$$DI = \frac{C_{ss\ max}}{C_{ss\ min}} \tag{14}$$

If DI = 1, then $C_{ss} = C_{ss\ max} = C_{ss\ min}$.

Rule of Thumb: Ideally, a controlled release drug delivery device is capable of achieving a dosage form index as close to 1 as possible.

III. REASONS FOR CONTROLLED DRUG DELIVERY DESIGN

A. Short or Relatively Long Half-Life and Minimum Effective Concentration Required for Administration Every 7 Days or 2 Weeks

For very potent drugs, for which only small amounts give desired therapeutic concentrations and a therapy of 1 to 2 weeks is required with maintenance of a certain therapeutic level, it is feasible to administer the medications either transdermally, or by the intramuscular or subcutaneous route. Examples would be strong analgesics applied posttraumatically or postsurgically, antibiotics, hormones, and immunosuppressants administered before and after organ transplantation. Besides injection of suspended particles, solutions from which the drug precipitates after injection, also infusion devices are suitable. In case of acute illnesses, pre- and postoperative care, and transportation (sea and space travel), this area for therapeutic drug coverage of up to 2 weeks needs particular attention in the future and has a great potential for anti-infectives, antihypertensives, sedatives, analgesics, and so on.

B. Short or Long Half-Life and Minimum Effective Concentration Required for Several Weeks to One Year

With rising costs of health care services and the increase in geriatric population, there is a definite need for medication devices to guarantee long-time drug delivery for certain drugs that are usually administered over weeks, months, or years. These include analgesics for terminal cancer patients, insulin and other hormones, and anti-hypertensives. Implants and particularly infusion devices have already been developed.

Special aspects of products of greatly extended duration are the questions of retrieval of the device in case of emergency, termination of drug release (by inactivation of drug or device) and, particularly, changing of drug delivery rate. It should be possible to obtain changes in drug delivery rate externally—by resetting the release rate or alternating release rates within a period of time (e.g., day versus night, boosters at preset times, etc.)—and it should be possible to change release rate as response to the need is supplied via feedback [7-9]. For instance, microdevices cemented to teeth should be a possible route for some drugs.

C. Localizing of a Specific Tissue for Selective Drug Uptake and Distribution

Most of the drug products used today in conventional dosage forms contain many thousand times more drug than is needed at the receptor site. Most drugs are absorbed into the systemic circulation and carried to the receptor site by the circulation. However, the drug will first distribute within the circulation and the volume of distribution. It is generally accepted that the free drug concentration in plasma at steady state is identical with the drug concentration at the receptor site. The receptor site is often limited to a relatively small organ or tissue (e.g., brain for drugs that act on the central nervous system, heart muscle for cardiacs, eye for glaucoma drugs, tumor for cancerostatics, etc.). Although only a tiny fraction of the drug in the body is needed, the entire dose is necessary to "fill up" the volume of distribution, since the mass balance equation is applicable, saying that the product of concentration C and volume V equals the amount A:

$$C \times V = A \qquad (15)$$

In this case, to achieve a desired concentration at the receptor, the dose size D is given by the free drug concentraiton C_{free} in plasma plus the concentration of drug bound in blood to proteins and erythrocytes C_{bound} times the apparent volume of distribution V_d:

$$(C_{free} + C_{bound})V_d = D \qquad (16)$$

Although targeting of a specific organ or tissue would be ideal for many drugs, the application is limited at present time. Cases of successful application include the use of pilocarpine against glaucoma by using lamellae floating in the lacrimal fluid between the eye and the eyelid (duration one week), and the use of agents to deliver contraceptive drugs directly or close to the endometrium via intrauterine devices (duration one year) [10,11].

Such devices would be ideal for substitution therapy and in targeting of cancer tissue by making use of particular properties of those tissues such as minute changes in pH, presence of certain enzymes, and binding to certain structures [12-14]. Such devices by far exceed the physical means of barriers and matrices.

D. Targeting of a Specific Tissue by Implantation for Long-Term Release

Whereas the devices in Subsection C are administered to body cavities and are noninvasive, there are therapeutic needs for long-term delivery devices for substitution therapy, particularly hormones. It is foreseeable that the inplants used at present (usually subcutaneously applied) may be redesigned for direct implantation into target tissue.

E. Prevention of First-Pass Effect

Many drugs when given perorally or deep rectally undergo more or less extensive first-pass effect which is the biotransformation of the drug in the gut lumen prior to absorption and in the intestinal epithelium and/or liver after permeation of the intestinal mucosa (presystemic) but before entering systemic circulation. For such compounds the gastrointestinal tract is a poor choice for administration and other routes (transdermal, buccal, nasal) need to be used.

F. Improvement of Compliance

It is estimated that more than 60% of the U.S. patient population does not comply with prescribed dosage regimens regarding dose size, time of administration, or frequency of dosing. One possible way of improving compliance is to reduce the number of dosings from several times per day to once per day or once per week. Having dosage forms available for extended duration definitely would reduce personnel costs for drug distribution and administration in hospitals, care facilities for the handicapped and the elderly, nursing homes, and so on.

It has been stated that improved compliance is one of the advantages of controlled release delivery devices. However, so far no proof has been given that these devices actually improve compliance, nor has it been shown that it is more advantageous to forget to take one "once-a-dose" than to forget one out of three doses a day. It seems that the compliance argument has more rhetorical than scientific value.

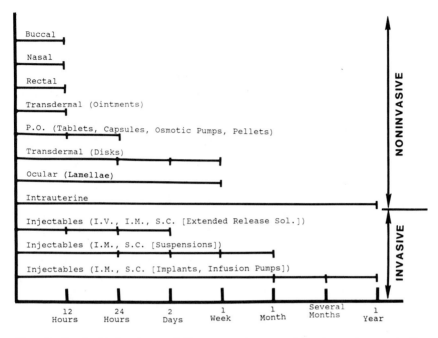

Fig. 5 Controlled release delivery systems and device: types available, routes of administration, and length of duration of action.

In summary, controlled drug delivery devices are available or being investigated for various routes of administration and various times of extension of duration. The devices may range in drug release from 12 hr to 1 year. Whereas for extent of duration up to about a week noninvasive devices are feasible and therefore usually preferred, most of the devices for longer duration (except intrauterine devices) are invasive. The drug delivery device types and their extent of duration are shown in Fig. 5.

IV. DESIRED BIOPHARMACEUTICAL CHARACTERISTICS OF DRUG PROPOSED FOR CONTROLLED DRUG DELIVERY DEVICES

Apart from pharmacological and pharmacokinetic considerations, the complex process of deciding on a feasible route of administration and appropriate type of drug delivery device involves a biopharmaceutical characterization of the drug under consideration. The biopharmaceutical evaluation is based on physicochemical parameters in conjunction with physiological aspects.

A. Molecular Weight (MW)

Convection

Small molecules may pass through pores of membranes by convective transport. The pore diameter varies between membranes (brain tissue < muscle tissue < capillaries < glomeruli < liver parenchymal cells < hepatic capillaries) and may be altered in certain disease states, particularly in inflammation, which increases pore diameter. Hence, only molecules with diameters smaller than that of a pore can pass through. In general, spherical compounds up to MW of 150 and chainlike compounds up to MW 400 are considered of being permeable by convective transport.

Diffusion

Most drugs are transported across membranes by passive diffusion. It may be assumed that more than 95% of all drugs follow this pathway of transport. Since in passive diffusion the drug outside and inside the aqueous compartment is in true solution, but dissolves in the lipid material of the membrane during the transport across the barrier, the compound must possess a minimal lipid solubility.

The transport stream Q depends on the diffusion constant of drug in lipid material D, the surface area of the membrane A, the partition coefficient K, the membrane thickness h, and the concentrations C_o and C_i on both sides of the membrane:

$$Q = D\frac{A}{h}K(C_o - C_i) \tag{17}$$

Under sink conditions, such as in unrestricted absorption, where the drug is immediately carried away by the blood after crossing the membrane and is diluted within the volume of distribution, one can use Fick's first law of diffusion:

$$dq = D \cdot A\frac{dc}{dx} dt \tag{18}$$

where dc/dx is the concentration gradient.

The flux and diffusion constant D decreases with increasing MW. The flux of some drugs and their molecular weights are listed in Table 1 [15].

The majority of drugs have relatively low molecular weights (MW 200-500). However, for some important drugs MW is between 500 and 1000, such as enkephalins (MW $\sim$ 600), digoxin (MW 781), amphotericin B (MW 924), and pyrvinium pamoate (MW 1151). In recent years increasing interest is being devoted to drugs of large MW (i.e.,

TABLE 1 Molecular Weights (MW) and Total Flux Across Skin of Some Selected Drugs

Drug	MW	Flux $(\mu g/cm^2/hr)$
Ephedrine	165	300
Diethylcarbamazine	199	100
Octanol	130	23
Nitroglycerin	227	13
Scopolamine	303	3.8
Ethanol	46	3.7
Chlorpheniramine	275	3.5
Fentanyl	337	2
Estradiol	272	0.016
Testosterone	288	0.014
Progesterone	315	0.011
Ouabain	585	0.008
Cortisone	402	0.0015
Hydrocortisone	362	0.00091
Digitoxin	765	0.00013
Dexamethasone	393	0.00012

Source: Ref. 15.

1000-30,000): the peptides such as insulin (MW 6000), growth hormone (MW 22,600), oxytocin (MW 1007), vasopressin (MW 1200), and antibodies (MW > 150,000).

Rule of Thumb: Usually the lower the MW, the faster and more complete is the transport.

B. pK_a: Ionization at Physiological pH

A large number of drugs belong to the group of weak electrolytes. The nonionized moiety is usually lipid soluble, hence may dissolve in the lipid material of a membrane and may be transported by passive diffusion, whereas the ionized moiety usually is not lipid soluble enough to permit permeation. The percent of ionization can be calculated from the Henderson-Hasselbalch equation:

$$\% \text{ ionized (for acidic compounds)} = \frac{100}{1 + \text{antilog}(pK_a - pH)} \qquad (19)$$

$$\% \text{ ionized (for basic compounds)} = \frac{100}{1 + \text{antilog}(pH - pK_a)} \qquad (20)$$

Considerable change in degree of ionization can be expected with change of pH for acidic drugs having a pK_a between 3 and 7.5, and for basic drugs having a pK_a between 7 and 11.

It seems that drugs are well absorbed by passive diffusion from the small intestine upon peroral administration if at least 0.1 to 1% is in nonionized form, and from the rectum upon administration if 1 to 5% is in nonionized form [16].

In drug delivery design it is important to calculate the degree of ionization and the percentage of drug nonionized to obtain an indication of whether absorption from a particular site or transport can be assumed to be unrestricted in case of passive diffusion. Table 2 gives a survey of pH values of body fluids and anatomical units [17,18].

Rule of Thumb: To cross or to reach membranes or regions by passive diffusion within the body, the percentage of drug nonionized at that site should be between at least 0.1 and 5%.

C. Isoelectric Point (IP)

The isoelectric point is that pH or hydrogen ion concentration at which the zwitterion concentration of protein or peptide is at a maximum and the net movement of the molecules is negligible.

A compound's solubility is at its minimum at the isoelectric point. Contrary to what one may expect, also the permeation across the membranes is at its minimum at the isoelectric point. This has been shown for permeation across the intestinal membrane upon rectal administration of insulin [19] and for permeation across skin upon topical administration of vasopressin [20]. The relationship of isoelectric point and extent of absorption is shown in Fig. 6.

Rule of Thumb: For absorption of peptides, select a pH for the vehicle away from the isoelectric point in a range most compatible with the physiological pH at the site of absorption.

TABLE 2 Body pH Values

Anatomical or physiological unit	Mean	Range
Bile	6.9	5.6-8.0
Blood, arterial	7.40	7.35-7.45
Blood, venous	7.37	7.32-7.42
Cerebrospinal fluid	7.34	7.32-7.37
Feces		
infants	4.9	4.6-5.2
adults	7.15	5.85-8.45
Gastric fluid		
newborns	2.52	1.2-7.4
children	3.27	0.9-7.7
adult men	1.92	1.0-2.5
adult women	2.59	1.5-3.5
aged	3.0	2.5-5.0
Gastrointestinal tract (adult)		
stomach	1.5	1.0-3.5
duodenum	6.9	6.5-7.6
jejunum	6.9	6.3-7.3
ileum	7.6	6.9-7.9
cecum	7.7	7.5-8.0
colon	7.95	7.9-8.0
rectum	7.7	7.5-8.0
Milk	6.6	6.6-7.0
Pancreatic fluid	8.0	7.5-8.8
Plasma	7.4	7.38-7.42
Saliva		
mixed	6.4	5.8-7.1
parotid	5.7	5.1-6.25
submandibular	6.4	5.9-7.3
Semen	7.19	6.9-7.36
Urine		
newborns	6.2	—
infants	6.0	5.1-6.8
children	6.2	5.3-7.2
adults	5.7	4.8-7.5

Source: Refs. 17 and 18.

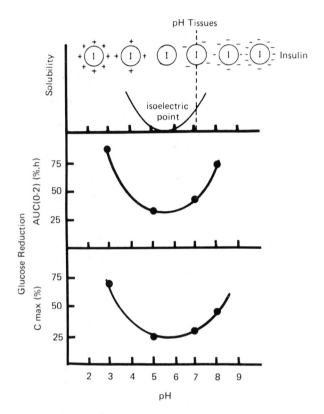

Fig. 6 Schematic presentation of the relationship between isoelectric point and extent of absorption across the intestinal (rectal) mucosa. (Data from Ref. 17 for the top portion and Ref. 15 for the middle and bottom.)

D. Solubility

Except for the limited case of pinocytosis, a subgroup of endocytosis, which might be useful in some special cases of drug delivery devices, for all other mechanisms of absorption the drug to be absorbed must be present at the site of absorption in the form of a true solution.

During the preformulation phase it is necessary to determine a drug's solubility not only in water but also at various pH values, depending on the anticipated route of administration. Usually the pH-solubility profile will cover the pH values of 1.5 (stomach), 3 (stomach), 4.5 (acid mantle of skin, sweat), 5.5 (acidic urine), 6.5 (duodenum, bile, jejunum, saliva), 7.4 (plasma, ileum, cerebrospinal fluid), and 7.8 (colon, rectum). (See the survey of physiological pH values in Table 2.)

The aqueous and pH-dependent solubility is of importance for drug release. When considering delivery devices by diffusion whereby the drug is present in the liquid compartment, one would select the limit of solubility in order to utilize the concentration gradient as the driving force for drug release.

The pH-dependent aqueous solubility and the solubility of the drug in various solvents other than water are frequently used for incorporation of the drug into devices. In this case, the drug release will be due to partitioning between the drug in the nonaqueous and the aqueous (of certain pH) medium (see also Section IV.E—Apparent Partition Coefficient).

The pH differences between various anatomical regions are being investigated for "targeting" devices that release the drug at specific pH values. This area is being studied as a means of attacking tumors because some neoplastic tissues possess a pH different from the surrounding healthy tissue. The mechanism of drug release from a specified device could be that the polymer dissolves or becomes permeable at a certain pH, as is known for enteric coated tablets and controlled release tablets and capsules using substances such as the Eudragit polymers (see Fig. 7 [21]), by enzymatic reaction of enzymes incorporated into devices [22], breakup of liposomes [23], and so on.

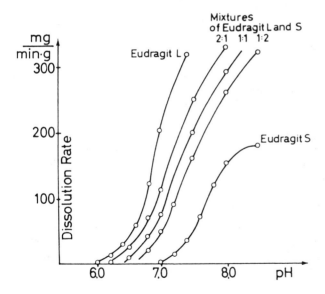

Fig. 7 Dissolution rate of different copolymers of methacrylic acid methacrylate esters (Eudragit S and Eudragit L) along and in combination. (From Ref. 21.)

pH-Dependent Precipitation

A special case of application of solubility to the design of drug delivery devices is the precipitation of the drug as a function of pH change. The classical example is dilantin, where the injection solution has a pH of 10 to 12.3. Thus when administered by slow intravenous injection dilantin does not precipitate in the systemic circulation due to immediate dilution in blood of the central compartment (the velocity of blood in the veins is 0.3 to 5 cm/sec and the venous volume is 2200 ml). However, when administered intramuscularly, dilantin precipitates in the muscle tissue, forming a depot of solid particles in a saturated solution of the injected volume. From this site the drug slowly dissolves in the interstitial fluid and the dissolved drug permeates into the capillaries to be carried away by the systemic circulation. In muscle tissue the blood flow rate is between 9.6 and 11.6 ml/min per 100 g of tissue. Hence, dilantin given intravenously is of immediate onset, whereas when given intramuscularly sustained release is observed, as shown in Fig. 8 [24].

Most drugs are weak electrolytes. Hence, one can calculate the pH required for a drug to precipitate from aqueous solution, pH_{precip}.
Acid compounds:

$$pH_{precip\ acidic} = pK_a + log\left(\frac{S - S_0}{S_0}\right) \tag{21}$$

Basic compounds:

$$pH_{precip\ basic} = pK_a + log\left(\frac{S_0}{S - S_0}\right) \tag{22}$$

where $pH_{precip\ acid}$ is the pH of an acidic compound *below* which the drug precipitates, $pH_{precip\ basic}$ is the pH *above* which the free base precipitates, S is the total solubility, and S_0 is the solubility of the undissociated moiety.

Solvent Change-Dependent Precipitation

A drug dissolved in a nonaqueous, nonirritant solvent may precipitate in the aqueous tissue upon subcutaneous or intramuscular administration due to dilution of the nonaqueous solvent. This principle was once used for obtaining a sustained action of parenteral anesthetics [25,26].

Rule of Thumb: Solubility is a prerequisite for a drug to be absorbed and transported in the body. For weak electrolytes,

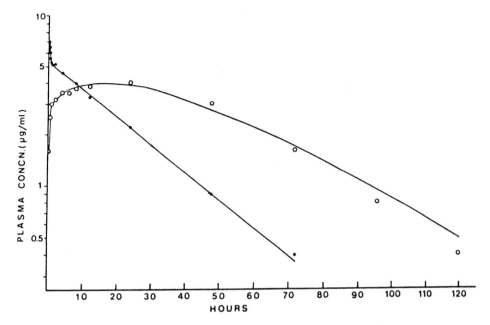

Fig. 8 Dilantin (sodium phenytoin) injected intravenously (250 mg) in normal subjects (n = 12) results in immediate onset (solid circles), whereas when given (500 mg) intramuscularly, sustained release (open circles) results due to precipitation in muscle tissue. (From Ref. 24.)

solubility is a function of pH. Many polymers exhibit solubility and permeability as a function of pH. Thus a change of pH or of solvents can result in desired precipitation of drug in tissue.

E. Apparent Partition Coefficient (APC)

The lipid/water partition coefficient APC denotes the ratio of the concentrations of drug in two (practically) immiscible phases. Whereas the "true" partition coefficient applies only to completely immiscible, nonassociating or dissociating species in either fluid, at low concentration and slight solubility in either phase, in biopharmaceutics the *apparent* partition coefficient is used, since mostly nonideal conditions are found. Usually APC is determined between n-octanol and a buffer solution of certain pH at 37°C according to Equation (23):

$$ APC = \frac{(C_2^0 - C_2')\, a}{C_2'\, b} \qquad (23) $$

where C_2^0 is the drug concentration in the aqueous phase before equilibration, C_2' is the drug concentration in the aqueous phase after equilibration, a is the volume of the aqueous phase, and b is the volume of the lipid phase. The APC can be considered as a measure of the relative affinity of a drug for two immiscible phases, as well as an index of comparative solubilities in solvents and as a parameter of the relative rate of partitioning from one phase into another.

Drugs being absorbed by passive diffusion must have a certain minimal APC. With increasing APC the drug will increasingly enter the brain tissue (CNS drugs) due to the high lipid content of the myelin sheath surrounding the nerve fibers in the gray matter. Also, with increasing APC the volume of distribution may increase due to partitioning into fat tissue.

The partitioning of nitroglycerin between n-octanol and buffer of varying pH is shown in Fig. 9 [27]. The time scale on the abscissa indicates the approximate transit times at varying pH in the human gastrointestinal tract. One can derive from Fig. 9 that at gastric pH of 1.5 to 2, about 15% partitions into the lipid phase and partitioning increases with pH.

Drugs of high APC exhibit pronounced characteristics of models having two or more compartments. This is explained physiologically by noting that the blood flow rate in aqueous tissue (muscle, 9.6-11.6; heart and liver, 85; kidney, 350; and lungs, 400 ml/min per 100 g of tissue) is much higher than in fat tissue (adipose tissue, 3 ml/min per 100 g of tissue).

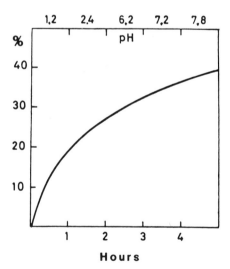

Fig. 9 Partitioning of nitroglycerin between n-octanol and buffer of varying pH values. (From Ref. 27.)

A survey on blood flow rates is given in Table 3 [28].

The apparent partition coefficient must also be applied for partitioning of the drug between the tissue fluid and the delivery device in case of certain devices. For instance, the partitioning (release) of a drug of high APC from a fat-based device or lipophilic matrix will be slow and may be incomplete. On the other hand, this very principle is the basis of several controlled release drug delivery devices.

Rule of Thumb: Rate and extent of absorption of drugs usually increase with increasing APC. Drugs with high APC usually exhibit characteristics of models having two or more compartments. Increasing affinity of the drug for the device decreases rate and extent of drug release.

F. Extent of Protein Binding (EPB)

Many drugs are bound to plasma proteins, particularly to albumin (MW 67,500). The basic groups of the amino acids (arginine, histidine, lysine) bind acid drugs, and the acidic groups of the amino acids (aspartic acid, glutamic acid, tyrosine) bind basic drugs. Only the unbound fraction is free to equilibrate in the body and is responsible for the drug-receptor interaction. Protein binding may occur particularly in plasma (180 g of plasma proteins in the adult) or in tissue (10 kg of tissue proteins in the adult), or in both. Proteins and other colloidal carriers have a transport function in the body, which at present is being investigated for possible use in drug targeting [29].

One has to be aware that extent of protein binding is not constant; rather, it depends on concentration and on temperature. Moreover, displacement form protein binding occurs with drugs (or endogenous substances such as free fatty acids) of higher affinity for the proteins. Also, the extent of protein binding may change due to disease (liver and/or renal impairment may cause reduced EPB); some conditions (burns, cancer, cardiac failure, liver impairment, malabsorption, nephrotic syndrome, renal failure, sepsis, trauma) may cause *hypo*albuminemia, and others (benign tumors, myalgia, neuroses, psychoses, schizophrenia, paranoia) may cause *hyper*albuminemia [30]. Hypoalbuminemia is found in geriatric patients, during pregnancy and under conditions of prolonged immobilizaiton and with prolonged stress and smoking [30].

Rule of Thumb: Extent of binding to plasma and tissue proteins is not constant and may change due to physiological and pathological factors, or displacement. The transport function of proteins may be utilized for drug targeting.

TABLE 3 Blood Flow Rates in Humans

Organ or unit	Percent of cardiac output	Percent of body weight	Flow rate per 100 g of tissue (ml/min)	Average flow rate in organ (ml/min)	Range between rest and maximum exercise (ml/min)
Lungs	100	1.5	400	4200	4000–6100
Kidneys	20	0.5	350	1225	1100–1400
Liver	24	2.8	85	1666	500–3000
Heart	4	0.5	84	294	200–1000
Brain	12	2.0	55	770	750–2100
Gastrointestinal tract	24	2.8	72	1400	700–5500
Skeletal muscle	23	40.0	5	1400	750–18000
Muscle, deltoid			11.6		
Muscle, vastus			10.8		
Muscle, gluteus			9.6		
Forearm			1.9		
Skin	6	10.0	5	350	200–3800
Adipose tissue	10	19.0	3	399	

Source: Ref. 28.

G. Extent of α_1-Acid Glycoprotein Binding (EAAGB)

The globulin α_1-acid glycoprotein (AAG; MW 41,000-45,000) binds basic drugs. Drugs found to be bound significantly to AAG are listed in Table 4 [30]. The AAG concentration in plasma is usually only 0.6 to 0.8%. However, under pathological conditions (fever, surgery, inflammation) the AAG concentration may increase up to 10-fold the normal value.

To the author's knowledge no attempts have been made to employ AAG for drug targeting. It is conceivable that for certain basic drugs and in certain diseases AAG could be utilized as drug carrier.

H. Erythrocyte Uptake (EU)

Erythrocytes may take up drugs to an appreciable amount in the order of magnitude of plasma protein binding. The phenomenon of erythrocyte uptake (EU) may occur by several mechanisms: (a) lipophilic molecules dissolving in the erythrocyte membrane, (b) anions being attracted and entering the positively charged pores of the erythrocyte, (c) adsorption to the erythrocyte membrane, and (d) binding within erythrocytes to carbonic anhydrase [acetazolamide], oxyhemoglobin [phenothiazines], or nucleoside transport system [benzodiazepines].

Drugs found to be significantly taken up by erythrocytes are listed in Table 5.

TABLE 4 Drugs Showing Significant Binding to α_1-Acid Glycoprotein

Alprenolol	Imipramine
Amitriptyline	Lidocaine
Bupivacaine	Meperidine
Chlorpromazine	Perphenazine
Diazepam	Pindolol
Dipyridamole	Prazosin
Disopyramide	Quinidine
Erythromycin	Thioridazine
Fentanyl	Timolol
Haloperidol	Zimelidine

Source: Ref. 30.

TABLE 5 Drugs Showing Significant Uptake by Erythrocytes

Acetazolamide	Cyclosporin	Mefloquine
Alfentanyl	Desmethylchlorpromazine	Myotrisin
Amantadine	Desmethyldiazepam	Oxazepam
Amobarbital	Diazepam	Pentazocine
Artenesinine	Dilantin	Pentobarbital
Auranofin	Fentanyl	Perphenazine
Bepridil	Flurazepam	Prochlorperazine
Bupivacaine	Hydromorphone	Promazine
Chlorambucil	Imipramine	Quinidine
Chloroquanide	Lidocaine	Quinine
Chloroquine	Lithium	Sufentanyl
Chlorpromazine	Lofentanyl	Trifluperazine
Clonazepam	Lorazepam	Triflupromazine

The EU is being investigated for the possible use of drug delivery [31,32].

A physiological aspect has to be considered if EU is being envisioned for drug delivery: highlanders (>4000 m above sea level) may have a red blood cell count of 8 million to 10 million per cubic millimeter, versus lowlanders of about 5 million RBC/mm^3.

Rule of Thumb: Erythrocytes are capable of drug uptake whereby drug loading is feasible intra- and extracorporally.

I. General Absorbability

The parameters molecular weight, pK$_a$, solubility, and APC may give reasonable information on the potential for absorption from a given site, and this information may be sufficient for some routes of administration and delivery devices, such as intramuscular and subcutaneous administration. The mechanisms of absorption from the nasal cavity, the mouth cavity and the rectum, and across the skin are by passive diffusion and, to some extent, convective transport. Hence, drugs absorbed by carrier-mediated transport (active transport, facilitated active transport) are not suitable for these routes. Also for drugs given orally and perorally and for which absorption throughout the entire length of the alimentary tract is required, active transport limits this route. The absorption mechanisms present in various segments of the alimentary canal are listed in Table 6 [33]. Therefore, a test is required to differentiate a drug's transport mechanism between passive diffusion and active transport.

Additionally, for drugs intended for peroral controlled-release delivery devices, general absorbability throughout the entire tract must be established.

Passive Diffusion /Active Transport Test

The Wilson-Wiseman test [34] for testing of active transport uses the guinea pig ileum sac and the everted guinea pig ileum sac. The normal ileum bag tied on both sides is filled with a drug solution and immersed into oxygenated, thermostatically controlled Ringer's solution. In the case of passive diffusion, the drug will diffuse into the outside liquid (C_s = concentration at serosa side) until equilibrium is obtained. In the case of active transport, most of the drug will be transported to the outside solution. If the everted ileum bag is used (serosa is inside, mucosa is outside), passive diffusion will commence as before; however, the drug transported by active transport will stay in the bag. A schematic diagram of the procedure and the differentiation curves between passive diffusion and active transport is given in Fig. 10 [35].

Buccal Absorption Test

The buccal absorption test, introduced by Beckett and co-workers [36,37] and later modified [27], is carried out by first rinsing the buccal cavity for 10 sec with a buffer solution of the same pH as the test solution. Then the drug solution is swirled in the mouth cavity for 5 min, followed by rinsing the mouth cavity twice with a buffer solution of same pH, and determining the amount of drug recovered from the drug solution and the two rinsings by spitting the solutions into a beaker. Using nitroglycerin as a test compound, the buccal absorption is shown in Fig. 11 [27]. As Fig. 11 indicates, the nitroglycerin uptake ranges from more than 90% to 30% between pH 2 and 8.

However, one has to realize that the buccal absorption test is an *indirect* test not really measuring the extent of absorption but rather the loss of drug from the solution. The drug is not necessarily absorbed by the buccal mucosa but may be adsorbed or bound to the epithelial cells. Of course, a stability test is required to determine that the drug does not decompose at the pH values studied.

General Absorbability

The test for general absorbability is carried out by in situ perfusion of intestinal segments of the rat. Under general anesthesia an intesti-

TABLE 6 Biopharmaceutical Data of the Human Alimentary Tract

Anatomical unit	Average length (cm)	Diameter (cm)	Villi present	Absorption mechanism	pH	Enzymes and other secretions	Amount of secretion (ml/day)	Transit time
Mouth cavity	15-20	10	-	Passive diffusion Convective transport	6.4	Ptyalin Maltase Mucin	Saliva: 500-1500	Instant
Esophagus	25	2.5	-	-	5-6	-	-	1-5 min
Stomach	20	15	-	Passive diffusion Convective transport Active transport(?)	1-3.5	Pepsin Lipase Rennin Hydrochloric acid	Gastric fluid: 2000-3000	1-4 hr
Duodenum	25	5	+	Passive diffusion Convective transport Active transport Facilitated transport Ion pair Pinocytosis	6.5-7.6	Bile Trypsin Chymotrypsin Amylase Maltase Nuclease	Bile: 250-1100 Pancreatic juice: 300-1500	5 min

Region				Transport mechanisms	pH	Enzymes	Intestinal fluid: 3000	
Jejunum	300	5	++	Passive diffusion Convective transport Active transport Facilitated transport	6.3-7.3	Erepsin Amylase Maltase Lactase Sucrase	3000	2 hr
Ileum	300	2.5-5	++	Passive diffusion Convective transport Active transport Facilitated transport Ion pair Pinocytosis	7.6-7.9	Lipase Nuclease Nucleotidase Enterokinase	–	3-6 hr
Cecum	10-30	7	+	Passive diffusion Convective transport Active transport Pinocytosis	7.5-8.0	–	–	0.5-1 hr
Colon	150	5	–	Passive diffusion Convective transport	7.9-8.0	–	–	6-12 hr
Rectum	15-19	2.5	–	Passive diffusion Convective transport Pinocytosis	7.5-8.0	–	–	6-12 hr

Source: Modified after Ref. 33.

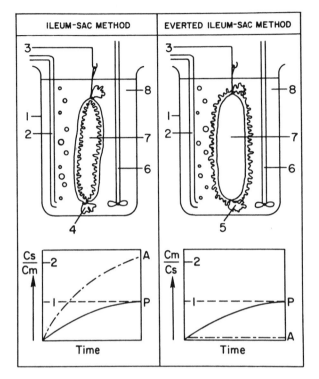

Fig. 10 Schematic diagram of experimental setup and resulting concentration ratio versus time curve for testing transport mechanism by passive diffusion and active transport using the living, isolated guinea pig ileum in a perfusion chamber: 1 = beaker, 2 = oxygen supply, 3 = hook, 4 = guinea pig ileum sac, 5 = everted guinea pig ileum sac, 6 = stirrer, 7 = drug solution, 8 = Ringer's solution, C_s = concentration at serosa side, C_m = concentration at mucosa side, P = passive diffusion, A = active transport. (From Ref. 35.)

nal segment is ligated and rinsed with saline solution at 37°C until the effluent is clear. Then the jejunal vein, draining all intestinal segments, is cannulated for blood collection in 5 min intervals. Blood flow is maintained by blood infusion via the jugular vein using blood from donor rats. In principle there are four commonly used techniques: single-pass perfusion [38-41], recirculating perfusion [42-45], oscillating perfusion [46], and the closed-loop method [47,48]. In a recent study the four methods were compared and constant values for absorption and similar coefficients of variation were obtained with the first three methods listed above [49]. The absorption process

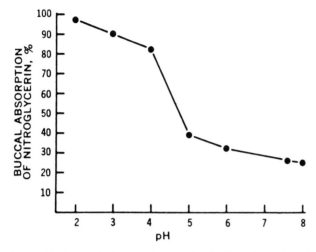

Fig. 11 Buccal absorption test of nitroglycerin at varying pH values.
(From Ref. 27.)

seems to be highly dependent on the hydrodynamics in the gastrointestinal lumen. The principle of the four methods is shown in the schematic diagram of Fig. 12 [49].

In a recent study the closed-loop method was used to study allopurinol absorption from different sites of the intestine [50]. The
results (Table 7) show that allopurinol is well absorbed from the small
intestine but poorly absorbed from the large intestine [50]. Hence,
a peroral controlled release preparation with a release time exceeding
the transit time of the small intestine would not be feasible. Also,
the rectal route of administration is not applicable.

Regarding intestinal transit time, the data listed in Table 8 can
be used as guideline [51].

Rule of Thumb: When a controlled release drug delivery device is considered, verify the absorbability of the drug from
the site of administration, or throughout the gastrointestinal
tract in case of peroral administration, to ensure drug uptake
throughout the length of exposure of the device or its transit
time. The tests include those for passive diffusion/active
transport, pH dependence, and general absorbability from
specific segments.

J. Biopharmaecutical Aspects for Routes of Administration

The major routes of administration of controlled release drug delivery
devices at present are peroral (to be swallowed), intramuscular (in-

(a)   (b)   (c)   (d)

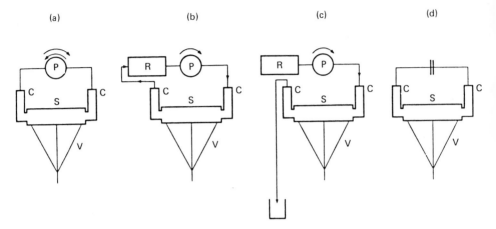

Fig. 12 Schematic drawings of the different perfusion methods: (a) oscillating perfusion, (b) recirculating perfusion, (c) single-pass perfusion, and (d) closed loop. Key: S = perfused intestinal segment, C = cannula, V = jejunal veins, P = pump, and R = reservoir. (From Ref. 49.)

jection, implantation), and percutaneous (transdermal). Several other routes have recently gained increased attention, and some products have already been marketed or are under clinical testing or experimental study, such as for oral (buccal), intranasal, intrauterine, intravenous, ophthalmic, and rectal administration.

The route of administration is usually dictated by the dose size, the duration of the extended delivery time (see Fig. 5), the physicochemical drug properties, drug stability, and absorption characteristics. Also, the route of administration will often determine the possible (at this time) type of drug delivery device. A general classification of these devices and the most appropriate manipulation techniques has been given by Olsen and Sadek [52].

Peroral

The peroral route is the one most preferred, but it has several limitations. First, the desired duration is ideally for 12 to a maximum of 24 hr. Based on human gastrointestinal tract transit time, the drug needs to be released within about a maximum of 14 hr. Second, as the delivery device passes through the gastrointestinal tract, environmental conditions change; these include pH, enzyme content, fluidity (viscosity), surface characteristics (smooth lining, macrovilli, microvilli), and pathways of absorption (transport mechanisms) (see Tables 2 and 6). These differences show wide variability across individuals

TABLE 7 Absorption Rate of Allopurinol from Different Segments of the Rat Gastrointestinal Tract

Segment of gastrointestinal tract	Normal segment dimension in adult rats: area/unit length (cm^2/cm ± SD)	Allopurinol absorption		
		Rate (μg/min/cm ± SD)	Normalized rate (μg/min/cm^2 ± SD)	Relative rate (%)
Duodenum	8.2 ± 0.8	0.559 ± 0.10	0.068 ± 0.01	100.0
Midgut	6.3 ± 0.7	0.478 ± 0.12	0.070 ± 0.01	85.3
Ileum	4.4 ± 0.8	0.325 ± 0.14	0.071 ± 0.04	58.1
Upper colon	2.2	0.027 ± 0.06	0.012 ± 0.03	4.9
Lower colon	2.2	0.056 ± 0.08	0.025 ± 0.05	9.9

Source: Modified after Ref. 50.

TABLE 8 Gastrointestinal Transit Times of Pellets and Intact
Tablets in Humans

Formulation	Gastric emptying time (min ± SEM)	Small intestine transit time (min ± SEM)	Colonic arrival time (min ± SEM)
Pellets[a]	79 ± 20	277 ± 82	305 ± 100
Tablets	164 ± 92	188 ± 23	265 ± 59

[a]For pellets the transit time is for 50% of the particles to leave or
arrive at the particular site.
Source: Ref. 51.

(vegetarians have a 20% longer intestinal tract; food and diseases
may markedly influence transit time).

Drugs given perorally in form of controlled release delivery devices must show a general absorbability throughout the entire gastrointestinal tract.

Many attempts have been made to keep the delivery device at a
certain site for an extended time: tablets that adhere or stick to the
stomach wall, tablets or capsules that float in the gastric fluid, devices
of a size calculated to delay gastric emptying, or devices (or a portion
of the dosage form) coated to prevent release of drug in acid environment (enteric coating). However, lodging of a one-unit matrix-type
delivery device at the pylorus or cecum might be undesirable, particularly if the drug exhibits irritant properties. Another problem associated with peroral administration is the sometimes low bioavailability
due to presystemic loss of drug resulting from instability (pH dependent), hydrolytic degradation in the contents of the gastrointestinal
tract, microbial inactivation by the gastrointestinal flora, and metabolism in the gut wall, mesenteric veins, portal vein, and liver (see Section II.H: First-Pass Effect).

For many drugs, however, the peroral route is feasible, and rather
large amounts, up to about 500 mg, can be incorporated into some devices. Even though that first-order release can result in highly effective delivery devices [6], it is widely believed that the ultimate goal
is a zero-order release profile. One must keep in mind that zero-order
in vitro release will produce zero-order in vivo release and zero-order
(in vivo) absorption only if: (a) the entire gastrointestinal tract be-
haves as a one-compartment model (i.e., the various segments throughout the tract are homogeneous with respect to absorption) and (b)
drug release rate is the rate-limiting step in the absorption process
[5].

Constant delivery rate over some period of time is not universally applicable to all drugs. For instance, it is believed that constant rate of delivery of nitroglycerin is undesirable because blood vessels lose their capability of constriction/dilation; or, gonadotropin releasing hormone (GnRH) administered in spaced intervals stimulates ovaries and testes, whereas when given continuously the opposite effect is obtained: the function of ovaries or testes is inhibited (chemical sterilization).

With first-order release, on the other hand, smaller and smaller amounts are released per unit of time with increasing time. Assuming that the rate of absorption gets lower past the small intestine due to to increased viscosity, decreased mixing (peristalis), and decreased intestinal surface area, less drug is absorbed, when in fact the opposite should occur, namely larger amounts should be released toward the latter part of the duration of the delivery device.

Intramuscular and Subcutaneous

The intramuscular and subcutaneous routes are capable of providing prolonged drug delivery. Aqueous and oleaginous solutions and suspensions, emulsions, and implants are employed. The advantage is that the duration may be from 24 hr to a year, limited by the amount of drug that can feasibly be incorporated (about 2 ml or 2 g). The most important consideration must be given to the vehicle regarding tissue compatibility (tissue damage, pain). The use of biodegradable materials is increasingly sought. The major factors influencing drug release are the drug's pK_a, its molecular weight and diffusion coefficient, the type of delivery device, and the blood flow rate at the site of administration.

The rate-limiting step for drug release from such devices is the contact surface area between delivery device and surrounding tissue. In case of suspensions, having a larger contact area than solid implants, the release is faster due to the faster change in surface area. The declining order of release in general terms is: aqueous solution, oleaginous solution, aqueous suspension, oleaginous suspension, implant.

There are other disadvangages of intramuscular and subcutaneous delivery devices beside the limited amount of drug to be possibly incorporated. For example, in case of emergency or toxic effect, solutions and suspensions cannot be removed from the body, and implants cannot be removed except by surgery. All these products, moreover, must be sterile.

Transdermal

Transdermal delivery devices are of increasing interest for numerous drugs, particularly those exhibiting first-pass effect upon peroral administration. A disadvantage is the relatively small amount of drug that can be incorporated, usually in the range of a few milligrams, although recently therapeutic levels have been achieved with 120 mg doses in 11 cm^2 transdermal disks [53].

The rate-limiting step in transdermal absorption is the stratum corneum. Skin permeability is a passive process of dissolution and molecular diffusion. The rate and extent of transdermal absorption depends on many factors, such as drug concentration in the device, type of device, surface area of contact, occlusion, anatomical region of application, skin condition, age, metabolism in the skin, and skin blood perfusion rate.

Transdermal devices have the following advantages: they need not to be sterile, and they can be removed instantly.

Intravenous

The intravenous route, except for the conventional constant rate infusion by intravenous drip or infusion pump, is another area of recent activity and promising application. In principle, a differentiation can be made between controlled delivery devices and controlled delivery systems, although, these may be combined.

Controlled delivery intravenous devices are the mobile infusion pumps and implantable (refillable) infusion pumps. Controlled delivery systems are injectable liposomes, nanoparticles, or polymer solutions. The latter ones may not primarily be controlled delivery systems but rather, specific delivery systems for organ targeting for diagnostic, therapeutic, and immunological purposes.

The disadvantage of intravenous devices is that with certain exceptions (the mobile infusion pumps, and the surgical removal of the implantable pumps, or their emptying by external fluid aspiration from the reservoir using a syringe), they cannot be removed.

Other Routes

Several devices such as buccal, vaginal, ocular, nasal, and rectal delivery devices are under investigation. In principle, their release mechanisms are similar to those for the other routes, being based on dissolution, diffusion, or erosion. Specific consideration for these devices is given to anatomical and physiological sites of application (such as pH, fluid volume, enzymes present), and to adhesive problems [54].

Rule of Thumb: For selecting a route of administration for controlled delivery devices, consideration must be given to required dose size, desired duration of device, the drug's physicochemical characteristics, and general absorbability from the application site.

V. SORPTION PROMOTERS

Sorption promoters are of particular interest for transdermal absorption but may also be employed for peroral, buccal, nasal, rectal, intramuscular, and subcutaneous routes of administration. Sorption promoters may increase the amount absorbed by several orders of magnitude. In other words, they are intended to increase the absolute bioavailability of a drug for a given route of administration.

Sorption promoters or sorption enhancers are not drugs but compounds of supposedly pharmacological inertness in the amount used for a given dosage form. Their mechanisms differ widely:

To increase solubility (cosolvents)
To increase wettability by reducing surface tension (surface active agents, tensides)
To increase spreadability (increase contact surface area)
To increase miscibility with epithelial (mucus) and skin cover (skin lipids)
To increase permeability of membrane by interacting with phospholipids (tensides)
To increase peremability of membrane by binding surface Ca^{2+} and Mg^{2+} (chelating agents)
To change hydrostatic pressure to act on water-filled pores (sugars, glycols)

Regarding wettability, only relatively hydrophobic drugs show improvement in the presence of surfactants, whereas for hydrophilic drugs contact angles are unchanged or even increased [55]. However, sorption promotion may be observed for both hydrophobic and hydrophilic drugs if the mechanism is based on change of membrane permeability.

A listing of sorption promoters is given in Table 9 [55,56]. These will be important in future development of subcutaneous devices like infusion pumps.

Rule of Thumb: For drugs not completely absorbed from a given site, the incorporation of a sorption promoter into the drug delivery device may be considered to improve the permeability across a membrane (by increasing the interaction of the drug with the membrane) or to directly influence the membrane permeability.

VI. CLINICAL PHARMACOLOGY

The clinical pharmacologist must supply pertinent information on the desired interaction between the drug molecules and the receptor:

TABLE 9 Commonly Used Sorption Promoters

Group/representatives

Organic solvent

Dimethylacetamide
Dimethylformamide
Dimethylsulfoxide
Ethanol
Ethyleneglycol
N,N-Dimethyl tolumaide
Polyethylene glycol
Propylene glycol
Tetrahydrofurfuryl alcohol

Fatty alcohols and esters of fatty acids

Decyl oleate
Diisopropyl adipate
Hexyl laurate
Isopropyl myristate
Isopropyl palmitate
Mixtures of triglycerides C_8-C_{12}
Mixtures of esters of aliphatic
  dicarboxylic acids

Salts

Calcium lactate
Sodium oleate
Sodium salicylate
Homovanillate
Methoxysalicylate

Bile salts/acids

Chenodeoxycholic acid
Cholic acid
Deoxycholic acid
Glycocholic acid
Sodium Cholate
Sodium taurocholate

Saponins

Saponin
Sapogenins

Phospholipids

Lecithin

Surface active agents

Nonionics
  Polyoxyethylene esters
  Polyoxyethylene ethers
  Sorbitan esters
  Saccharose esters

Anionics

  Sodium cetyl sterate
  Sodium diethylsulfosuccinate
  Sodium dioctylsulfosuccinate
  Sodium lauryl sulfate

Cationics

  Cetylpyridinium chloride
  Cetyltrimethylammonium
    bromide
  Benzalkonium chloride
  Benzethonium chloride
  Lauryl dimethylamino acid
    betaine
  Stearyl trimethylammonium
    chloride

Complexing agents

Citric acid
EDTA
Sodium metaphosphate

Source: Modified after Refs. 55 and 56.

whether a local effect, a general systemic concentration, or a specific target (tissue) shall be chosen, what the desired or required concentration at the site of action shall be, and its acceptable range and toxic limitation. Furthermore, the usual therapeutic dose will be a decisive factor regarding the types of delivery devices that are feasible.

A. Local Effect, Systemic Distribution, and Target Organ

Local Effect

For some drugs, such as antiviral substances and fungistatics, therapy may be done by systemic application when in fact the site of desired drug-causative agent (such as herpes virus, fungus, etc.) is very much localized. Only a fraction of the systemically administered drug will reach the site of action. If the drug concentration required at the local site is known and the drug is able to reach that site by local application, a local delivery device would be advantageous because the body burden by the drug could be reduced. For instance, as shown in Fig. 13, using a proper sorption promoter, skin levels of the fungistatic griseofulvin were at least equal to those obtained at steady state upon peroral administration [57].

Nevertheless, if a drug passes across the skin barrier (stratum corneum), there is no hindrance to its entering the systemic circulation, being distributed throughout the volume of distribution, and undergoing metabolism and elimination. The differences from systemic administration are that the drug reaches the receptor site first and pre-

Fungal Invasion	Skin Anatomy	Skin Depth (um)	Topical Conc. (ug/ml)	P.O. Conc. (ug/ml)	MIC (ug/ml)
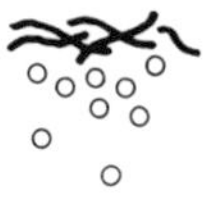	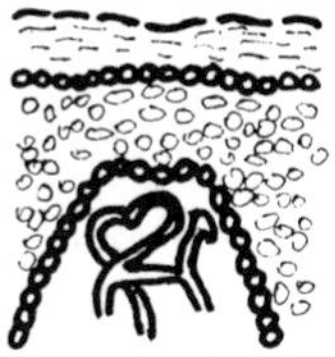	25	304	58 22 19	14-46 [a]
		75	74		
		150	22		

Fig. 13 Griseofulvin skin levels upon peroral administration (500 mg every 12 hr for 7 days) and application of transdermal ointment (64 mg per square centimeter of ointment = 160 µg of griseofulvin per square centimeter of skin) in the presence of a sorption promoter. The wavy lines represent hyphae, the circles spores, and it should be noted that the minimum inhibitory concentration (MIC) includes a "safety factor" of 100 (a). (From Ref. 57.)

dominantly before being distributed and that the total systemic body burden is much lower. This is demonstrated in Fig. 14.

Examples of applications of local drug delivery devices are for the skin, the eyes, and the body cavities.

Classical commercial examples are the antiglaucoma product Ocusert and the contraceptive delivery device Progestasert. In the latter case the drug is delivered to the endometrium, thus reducing the dose that would be needed by the systemic approach to achieve the same endometrial drug level.

Systemic Distribution

For many drugs the present therapeutic approach is based on reaching and maintaining a certain concentration or concentration range in blood. To achieve this, a certain dose size has to be given in appropriate dosing intervals (dosage regimen) such that after distribution of the drug within its volume of distribution, the desired concentration is obtained at steady state. In case of an immediate effect, an appropriate loading dose may be given to "fill up" the volume of distribution. Drugs for which the systemic approach applies are the analgesics, antiasthmatics, antiepileptics, and antibiotics. The reaching and maintenance of the desired drug concentrations is often verified and adjusted by blood level drug monitoring.

Target Organ

Similar to the local effect, a desired drug concentration is often required only in a specific organ or tissue. The concept of targeting an organ is only a few years old, but it has a tremendous potential for future application.

In case of drug targeting the delivery device may be administered intra- or extravascularly. However, the drug is either in form of a prodrug, which is activated at the target organ only, or is somehow entrapped and released at the target organ. *Note*: For such devices special pharmacokinetic treatment is required to encounter for the entrapped and the "available" drug.

The rationale for organ targeting is to reach a therapeutic drug concentration at the receptor site with minimal systemic body burden.

B. Dose Size

Consideration must be given to *usual* (non-controlled-release) dose size and the dose rate. Drugs that act systemically and are therapeutically effective only in relatively large doses do not qualify a priori for controlled release devices. A controlled release drug delivery device is essentially a multiple-dose unit. Even though the dose is *not* exactly the amount of a single dose multiplied by the number of dosing

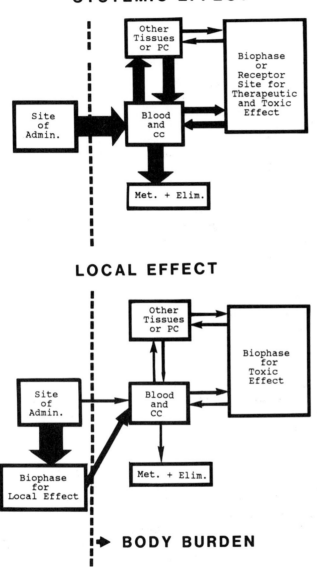

Fig. 14 Schematic diagram of body burden by drugs administered for local or systemic effect. The thickness of the arrows indicates the relative magnitude of body burden.

intervals, for usual doses equivalent to the duration of a controlled delivery device, the total amount per unit is much higher than that of a single dose.

C. Concentrations (MEC and C_{max}) and Limited Fluctuation

Theoretically and desirably, a controlled release delivery device, unless programmed for trigger mechanism, should release the drug by a zero-order process, which would result in a blood level-time profile similar to that after intravenous constant rate infusion.

However, zero-order release is rarely achieved and if so, the resulting steady state concentration probably will not be a straight line parallel to the abscissa but more likely will be a "soft" wave due to many factors such as circadian rhythm, body activity, stress, and food intake. Nevertheless, in the design of most controlled release delivery devices it is necessary to select a desired (or required) target concentration or concentration range.

The types of dosage regimen pattern for conventional dosage forms can be classified as shown in Table 10 [58].

For controlled release delivery devices the target concentration should usually be the same as for conventional dosage forms. The difference will be that the fluctuations of drug concentration in blood will be much smaller for the duration of the device as observed within each dosing interval of a conventional drug product (see Fig. 15).

D. Therapeutic Range

Ideally, candidates for controlled release drug delivery devices will be drugs of such wide therapeutic range that neither batch-to-batch variations in release rate nor individual physiological variations exceed the therapeutic range.

E. Toxic Concentration

Ideally, the toxic concentration of a candidate for a controlled release drug delivery device should be much higher than the therapeutic range. This is of particular consideration in cases of the accidental destruciton of the device, rupture, or malfunction. Peroral controlled delivery devices ought not to be chewed or masticated, but even if this is done accidentally, the drug dose should not be dumped, with resulting toxic blood levels.

Another consideration is the question of whether the drug is metabolized to pharmacologically highly potent structures or to toxic metabolites. Because the delivery devices control only the release of the parent compound but not its biotransformation, and since the rate

TABLE 10 Types of Dosage Regimen Patterns for Multiple Dose Therapy with Conventional Dosage Forms

Number	Pattern	Desired target drug concentration in blood	Examples
1	Log dose-response (LDR)	$C_{ss\ avg}$	Digoxin, theophylline
2	Therapeutic window (TW)	$C_{ss\ avg}$	Tricyclic antidepressants
3	Minimum effective (MEC) or minimum inhibitory (MIC) concentration	$C_{ss\ min}$	Bacteriostatic antibiotics and chemotherapeutics
4	Peak concentration (PC)	$C_{ss\ max}$	Some antibiotics
5	Limited fluctuation	$C_{ss\ min} - C_{ss\ max}$	Gentamicin

Source: Modified after Ref. 58.

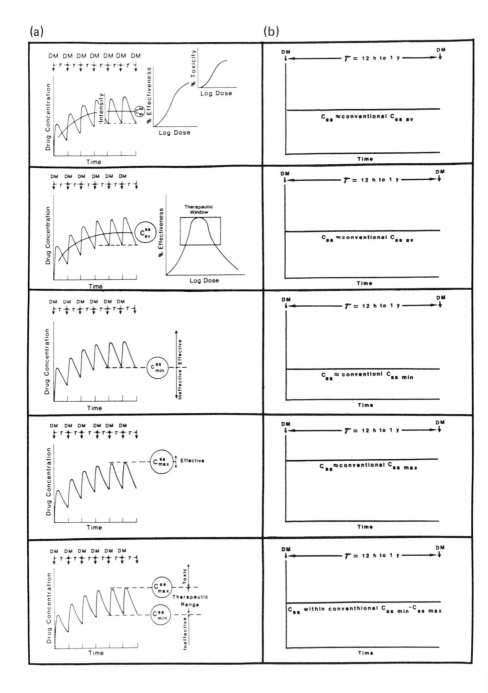

Figure 15 Schematic diagram of desired drug concentrations in blood
for (a) conventional dosage forms and (b) target concentrations for
controlled release delivery devices or systems.

of metabolism may vary widely among individuals and in the same individual, long-range predictions are difficult to make.

Regarding safety, the transdermal drug delivery devices seem to pose the fewest problems because they can easily and instantly be removed. Nevertheless, toxicity from transdermal disks was reported when a disk accidentally was lost and "picked up" by the partner [59, 60].

Rule of Thumb: A requirement during the preformulation stage is knowledge about the clinical pharmacological properties of the drug to be used in a controlled delivery device. It must be decided whether the drug shall act locally or systemically or shall target an organ. The dose size of conventional dosage forms is a guide to the route of administration and the type of delivery device. The desired or required target concentration must be established, and consideration must be given to the therapeutic range and toxic concentration.

VII. COMPUTATION OF DESIRED RELEASE RATE (R^0) AND DESIRED DOSE (DM) FOR CONTROLLED RELEASE DRUG DELIVERY

A. Input Rate (R^0)

Controlled release drug delivery devices are in fact multiple-dose products and usually are comparable to intravenous constant rate infusions. Infusions deliver specific amounts of drug in extremely short dosing intervals, τ. In drip infusions, for instance, with an infusion rate of 20 drops per minute, x mg of drug is delivered every 0.05 hr. Using an infusion pump of constant delivery, τ becomes infinitely small. The delivery rate R^0 is:

$$R^0 = \frac{D}{\tau} \qquad (24)$$

The desired release rate R^0 of controlled release delivery devices can therefore be treated according to intravenous constant rate infusion model, assuming that a constant, desired target steady state concentration, C_{ss}, is maintained. If the drug's elimination follows a first-order process and the drug release from the delivery device follows a zero-order process, the rate of drug release or rate of drug input, R^0 must be equal to the rate of elimination or rate of drug output, R_{output}:

$$R^0 = R_{output} \qquad (25)$$

The rate of drug output is the product of the maintenance dose DM and the elimination rate constant k_{el}:

$$R_{output} = DM \cdot k_{el} \tag{26}$$

Since k_{el} is:

$$k_{el} = \frac{0.693}{t_{1/2}} \tag{27}$$

Equation (26) can be rewritten:

$$R_{output} = \frac{DM0.693}{t_{1/2}} \tag{28}$$

and because amount is equal to concentration times volume, the rate of output is also:

$$R_{output} = k_{el} \, C_{ss} \, V_d \tag{29}$$

and since the product of k_{el} and V_d is the total clearance CL:

$$CL = k_{el} \, V_d \tag{30}$$

Equation (29) can be rewritten:

$$R_{output} = C_{ss} \, CL \tag{31}$$

Substituting equation (30) in (25), one obtains the input rate:

$$R^0 = C_{ss} \, CL \tag{32}$$

However, controlled release drug delivery devices do not quantitatively release all the drug that is incorporated and, additionally, presystemic drug loss may occur. Hence, the input rate must be corrected for the absolute bioavailability F:

$$R^0 = \frac{F \cdot DM}{\tau} \tag{33}$$

Transdermal Input

In case of transdermal controlled delivery devices, the input rate R^0 is corrected for the surface area A of the delivery device:

$$R^0 = \frac{C_{ss} CL}{A} \qquad (34)$$

The transdermal route is often used to bypass hepatic metabolism. Let us assume that the active moiety M_1 is systemically metabolized to M_2 (for instance estradiol to estrone). The steady state concentration of the active moiety C_{ss} can be described by the following equation [61]:

$$C_{ss} = \frac{R^0_{M_1} (1 - P_{12})}{CL} \qquad (35)$$

where $R^0_{M_1}$ is the required input rate and P_{12} is the ratio of the rate of conversion of M_1 to M_2 to the input rate. At steady state P_{12} is a constant and is referred to as the metabolic transfer coefficient. The input rate $R^0_{M_1}$ is thus:

$$R^0_{M_1} = C_{ss} \frac{CL}{(1 - P_{12})} \qquad (36)$$

If for instance the active moiety is also endogenously available (such as estradiol), then ΔC_{ss} is used instead of C_{ss}, where ΔC_{ss} is the incremental plasma concentration required above the endogeneous blood level [61].

B. Dose Size (DM)

Substituting Equation (33) to (32) and solving for DM, the required dose size for the controlled release drug delivery device is obtained:

$$DM = \frac{C_{ss} CL \cdot \tau}{F} \qquad (37)$$

If a conventional dosage form $(DM \cdot F)_{conventional}$ at steady state results in a desired concentration, the amount of drug needed in the controlled release component of the dosage form is:

$$DM_{controlled\ release} = \frac{(DM \cdot F)_{conventional} 0.693\tau}{t_{1/2}} \quad (39)$$

assuming that F is equal for conventional and controlled release delivery devices.

In Table 11 a listing is given for percentages of conventional maintenance doses needed in a controlled release device as a function of intended dosing intervals [62].

Often controlled release drug delivery devices contain two or more dose components regarding release: an immediately available dose d_i, resulting in a blood level with a fast peak (considered as a type of loading dose) and one or more controlled release doses d_{cr}, resulting in a kind of flat plateau. The total dose DM is then:

$$DM = d_i + d_{cr} \quad (39)$$

The quantity of d_{cr} can be estimated from Equation (40):

$$d_{cr} = \frac{0.693DM_{conventional} F \cdot f \cdot \tau}{t_{1/2}} \quad (40)$$

where f is the fraction AUC_{cr} of $(AUC_{cr} + AUC_i)$.

TABLE 11 Percentage of Usual Maintenance Dose Needed in the Sustained Release Component as a Function of Intended Dosing Interval

Elimination half-life (hr)	Percent usual maintenance dose for dosing intervals at:				
	6 hr	12 hr	24 hr	36 hr	48 hr
1	416	832	1663	2495	3326
2	208	416	832	1247	1663
3	139	277	554	831	1109
4	104	208	416	624	832
5	83	166	333	499	666
6	69	139	277	416	554

Source: Ref. 62.

C. Zero-Order with Input Time (t_i) Being Shorter than Dosing Interval (τ)

Let us envision a controlled release delivery device from which 90% of the drug is released (P = 0.9) within 8 hr (Q = 8), selection 12 hr as the dosing interval. The release rate R^0 is then [63]:

$$R^0 = \frac{DM_{test} P}{Q} \tag{41}$$

For experimental purposes for DM_{test} a given amount, say 100 mg, is selected. One can now estimate the peak after the first dose, $C_{max\ 1}$, and the trough after the first dose, $C_{min\ 1}$:

$$C_{max\ 1} = \frac{R^0 [1 - \exp(-k_{el} t_i)]}{V_d \cdot k_{el}} \tag{42}$$

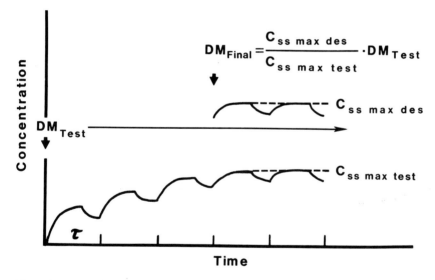

Fig. 16 Selecting a test dose DM_{test}, percent of drug released by zero-order kinetics P, over a period of time Q, the release rate R^0, is estimated. Employing population pharmacokinetic parameters for V_d and k_{el}, the concentration-time profile for the first test dose is established. Using the superposition method, the expected steady state concentration-time profile for the test dose upon multiple dosing is generated. The final dose required, DM_{final}, is calculated from the ratio of $C_{ss\ max\ des}$ and $C_{ss\ max\ test}$. The chosen dosing interval is τ.

$$C_{min\ 1} = \frac{R^0\ [(1 - \exp(-k_{el}\ t_i)]\ \{\exp[-k_{el}(t - t_1)]\}}{V_d \cdot k_{el}} \qquad (43)$$

Applying the superposition method, one can predict the steady state concentration-time profile.

The actual dose size required, DM_{final}, to achieve a desired $C_{ss\ max\ des}$ is then a simple ratio:

$$DM_{final} = \frac{C_{ss\ max\ des}}{C_{ss\ max\ test}} \qquad (44)$$

as shown in Fig. 16.

D. First-Order Release from Two-Component Delivery Device

The concentration-time profile after a single dose of a two-component, controlled-release delivery device can be predicted form the model given in Fig. 17 [64]:

$$C(t) = \frac{DFf_s k_a k_r}{V_d\ (k_a - k_r)\ [(k_m + k_{el}) - k_r]} \{\exp[-\ (k_m + k_{el})t]$$

$$[-\exp(-k_r't)]\}$$

$$+ \frac{DFf_i k_a - [(DFf_s - k_a k_r)/(k_a - k_r')]}{V_d\ [(k_m + k_{el}) - k_a]}$$

$$\{\exp[-(k_m + k_{el})t] - [\exp(-k_a t)]\} \qquad (45)$$

This model assumes identical k_a for the immediate and slow fraction (f_i and f_s), and identical bioavailability F for both fractions. The first-order release rate constant k_r' may be taken from in vitro experiments, and k_a is the intrinsic absorption rate.

For optimizaiton of f_i and f_s see Subsection F.

E. First-Order Release form Three-Component Delivery Device

Using three components in a controlled release delivery device with one fraction of immediate release (f_i), one for slower release (f_s), and one for very slow release (f_{vs}), where the absorption rate for

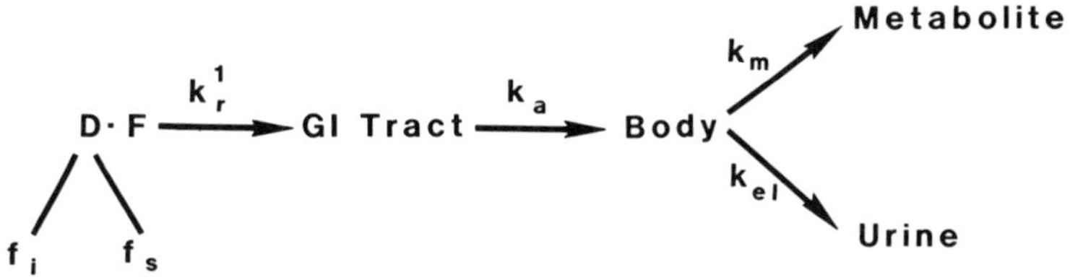

Fig. 17 Model for controlled drug release dosage form with two components, instant and slow release by first-order kinetics. (From Ref. 64.)

f_i is k_a, for f_s is k_s and for f_{cs} is k_{vs}, the concentration-time profiles for each component, $C(t)_i$, $C(t)_s$, and $C(t)_{vs}$ can be predicted [65]:

$$C(t)_i = \frac{DFk_a f_i}{V_d (k_a - k_{el})} \left[\exp(-k_{el}t) - \exp(-k_a t) \right] \tag{46}$$

$$C(t)_s = \frac{DFk_a k_s f_s}{V_d} \left[\frac{\exp(-k_s t)}{(k_a - k_s)(k_{el} - k_s)} + \frac{\exp(-k_a t)}{(k_s - k_a)(k_{el} - k_a)} \right.$$

$$\left. + \frac{\exp(-k_{el}t)}{(k_s - k_{el})(k_a - k_{el})} \right] \tag{47}$$

$$C(t)_{vs} = \frac{DFk_a k_{vs} f_{vs}}{V_d} \left[\frac{\exp(-k_{vs}t)}{(k_a - k_{vs})(k_{el} - k_{vs})} \right.$$

$$\left. + \frac{\exp(-k_a t)}{(k_{vs} - k_a)(k_{el} - k_a)} + \frac{\exp(-k_{el}t)}{(k_{vs} - k_{el})(k_a - k_{el})} \right] \tag{48}$$

By first superimposing the concentration-time profiles of the three fractions, a composite concentration-time curve is obtained which, by the superposition method, will result in a steady state concentration-time profile for each dosing interval. For optimization see next subsection.

F. First-Order Release from Four-Component Delivery Device to Mimic Zero-Order Release

Boxenbaum [5] suggested a two-stage procedure for the development of controlled release devices for drugs with first-order release from

several (four) fractions showing different first-order release characteristics. For the four fractions—for instance, beads with different
coat thickness—concentration-time profiles are generated in which each
fraction contains the same dose size as a hypothetical zero-order release dosage form, as seen in Fig. 18 [5]. State I involves an empirical mixing of different proportions of the four types of release preparation to match the theoretical zero-order absorption curve. This is
done by superposition of the individual fractions and graphic iteration.
Figure 19 (top) shows such a single-dose concentration-time profile.
In stage II superposition is done to steady state, and again graphic
iteration is used to obtain a dosage form index as close to 1 as possible,
as shown in Fig. 19 (bottom). If one uses now the selected composition and predicts a single-dose concentration-time profile, as in Fig.
19 (middle), it differs from the stage I optimization. However, at
steady state, the apparently slower absorption during the first 12 hr
is counterbalanced by the continued absorption.

VIII. PHARMACOKINETIC EVALUATION OF CONTROLLED RELEASE IN VIVO

The in vivo evaluation of controlled release delivery devices involves
two basic questions [66]:

1. Is the desired rate-time profile of release as shown in vitro
   actually obtained in vivo?
2. Is the desired response-time profile obtained in vivo?

In case the pharmacological or clinical response can be quantitated
directly (blood pressure, dilatation of pupils, intraocular pressure,
urinary output, electrolyte excretion, blood glucose levels, etc.),
the second question can be answered by direct measurement. Otherwise, long-range clinical double-blind, parallel design studies are required.

To answer the first question, in principle four approaches are
available [66]:

1. Assay of unreleased drug in the delivery device
2. Assay of parent drug and/or metabolite in blood, plasma, or
   serum
3. Assay of parent drug and/or metabolite in excreta
4. Quantitation of response intensity

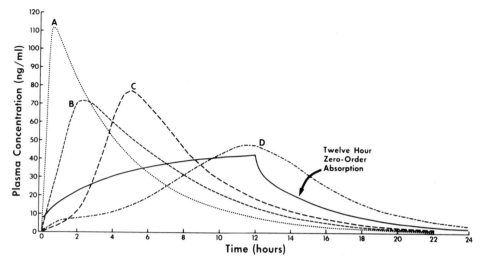

Fig. 18 Smoothed plasma concentration-time curves resulting from administration of four bead types (A-D) of a hypothetical drug at 12 mg doses to a panel of subjects. Also illustrated is a theoretical curve for 12 hr zero-order absorption. (From Ref. 5.)

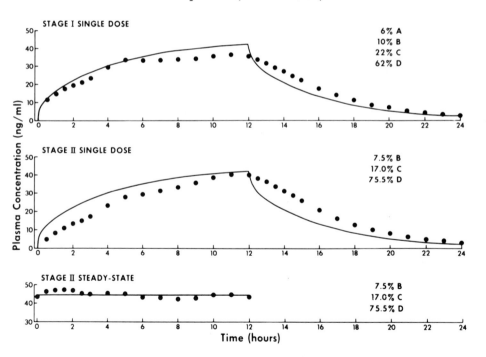

Fig. 19 Stage I and II plasma level-time profiles for 12 mg doses of a hypothetical drug. Solid lines represent theoretical curves for the perfect 12 hr zero-order absorption product. Data points are from mixtures of the indicated bead types. See text for discussion. (From Ref. 5.)

A. Assay of Unreleased Drug in the Delivery Device as a Function of Time

The procedure for the assay of unreleased drug requires the recovery or removal of the device from the body at a specified time after administration and analysis of drug content. The amount remaining in the delivery device or the log of that quantity is plotted versus time t, square root of time $t^{1/2}$, or cube root of time $t^{1/3}$. Each device recovered from a subject becomes one data point in such a plot. By regression analysis an overall release rate-time profile of the study population is obtained. Such an approach, although important from a population point of view, may show large standard deviations due to differences in the release characteristics between individual devices, as well as interindividual subject differences.

This approach can be used only for devices applied to the skin or body cavities, for excisable implants, and for accessible pump devices.

B. Assay of Parent Drug and/or Metabolite in Blood, Plasma, or Serum as a Function of Time

The Loo-Riegelman method [67-69] is usually employed to assess the rate of drug input, which in addition requires the concentration-time profile after intravenous administration and assumes absence of dose dependency and consistency of pharmacokinetic parameters between intravenous and nonintravenous administration. An advantage of the Loo-Riegelman method is that it is applicable independent of the type of kinetic processes involved in the absorption.

Another approach is by numeric devonvoluation [70], which also requires intravenous administration of the drug and assumes that the disposition of the drug is linear. An advantage is that this method does not require a specific pharmacokinetic model.

The Wagner-Nelson method [71] is similar to the Loo-Riegelman method but does not require intravenous administration. The method postulates that the terminal position of the curve is a measure of rate of elimination. Since in controlled release delivery devices the rate of release, hence of apparent absorption, is often slower than the elimination rate, the method is not applicable in those cases.

C. Assay of Parent Drug and/or Metabolite in Excreta

Assay as a function of time of drug or metabolite(s) excreted into urine, feces, or expired air assumes that the measured elimination rate is representative for the drug release from the device, which necessitates another assumption, namely absence of any presystemic loss of drug. Problems arise if the drug is presystemically biotransformed and the metabolites are absorbed. In such cases additionally,

TABLE 12 Summary of Characteristics of Alternative Pharmacokinetic Methods for Evaluating Controlled Release in Vivo

Method	Advantages	Disadvantages	Cautions
Assay of unreleased drug	Assay of biological media not required Amount remaining measured directly Does not require radioactive drug	One data point per subject; need many subjects together to characterize an average release rate-time profile Difficult to check for presystemic drug loss Average release rate obtained for entire time period if calculated for an individual subject	Assay interference from delivery system components or adhering biological material
Assay of metabolized and excreted drug	Radioactivity assay	Complete collection of excreta necessary Influence of retention of radioactivity in feces Very difficult to check for presystemic drug loss	Equating elimination rates with release rates should not be done unless complete recovery of dose is obtained
Assay of drug concentrations in plasma	Does not require radioactive drug Does not require collection of excreta Presystemic drug loss can be evaluated by dose-recovery determination	Assay of plasma necessary Requires i.v. push dose determination of drug pharmacokinetics Requires assumption of constancy of pharmacokinetic parameters in subjects	Check for adequate specificity and sensitivity No systemic deviation in fit of the i.v. push plasma drug level-time curve Adequate sampling times
Quantitation of response intensity	No drug assay required Response to drug may be quantitated directly	Limited to drugs that elicit a quantifiable response that is a graded function of dose Several i.v. push doses required for calibration	Must demonstrate reproducibility of response measurement Time-dependent phenomena such as tolerance

Source: Ref. 66.

intravenous constant rate infusion may be used. By "matching" the excretion rates after intravenous and extravascular administration, the rate of systemic availability can be estimated [72].

D. Quantitation of Response Intensity

For those situations in which the pharmacological response can be quantitated on a graded scale (not applicable for simple yes or no response), Smolen [73-76] has demonstrated that the drug input into the body can be estimated from the response measurements. The drug disposition should be linear, the change in response must be very fast in relation to change in blood levels, and the change in intensity of effect must follow a linear or nonlinear pattern as a function of dose or concentration. The method requires intravenous administration of the drug to establish a calibration curve of the maximum response versus dose.

Table 12 summarizes the methods employed for pharmacokinetic evaluation of controlled release delivery devices [66].

REFERENCES

1. W. A. Ritschel, *Handbook of Basic Pharmacokinetics*, 3rd ed. Drug Intelligence Publications, Hamilton, IL, 1986, p. 18.
2. W. A. Ritschel and P. Banerjee, *Methods Findings Exp. Clin. Pharmacol.*, 8:603 (1986).
3. K. Yamaoka, T. Nakagawa, and T. Uno, *J. Pharmacokinet. Biopharm.* 6:547 (1978).
4. W. A. Ritschel, *Handbook of Basic Pharmacokinetics*, 3rd ed. Drug Intelligence Publications, Hamilton, IL, 1986, p. 337.
5. H. Boxenbaum, *Pharm. Res.*, 1:82 (1984).
6. M. Gibaldi and D. Perrier, *Pharmacokinetics*, 2nd ed. Dekker, New York, 1982, p. 188.
7. Anonymous, *Med. Trib.*, No. 24, June 13, 1980, through: *Oesterr. Apoth. Ztg.*, 34:815 (1980).
8. R. K. Campbell, *Am. Pharm.*, 22:22 (1982).
9. B. J. Kennedy, D. Covell, and W. J. M. Hrushesky, Implantable and extracorporeal programmable drug delivery devices: What to Program. In: *Annual Review of Chronopharmacology* (A. Reinberg, M. Smolensky, and G. Labrecque, eds.). Pergamon Press, Oxford, 1984, p. 193.
10. C. H. Dohlman, D. Pavan-Langton, and J. Rose, *Ann. Ophthalmol.*, 4:823 (1972).
11. H. J. Tatum, *Am. J. Obstet. Gynecol.*, 112:1000 (1972).
12. C. G. Pitt, *Pharm. Int.*, 7:88 (1986).
13. J. Heller, *Med. Device Diagnost. Ind.*, 7(9):32 (1985).

14. W. Cushley, *Pharm. Int.*, 6:33 (1985).
15. A. S. Michaels, S. K. Chandrasekaran, and J. E. Shaw, *AIChE*, 27:985 (1975).
16. W. A. Ritschel, *Handbook of Basic Pharmacokinetics*, 3rd ed. Drug Intelligence Publications, Hamilton, IL, 1986, p. 62.
17. W. A. Ritschel, *Handbook of Basic Pharmacokinetics*, 3rd ed. Drug Intelligence Publications, Hamilton, IL, 1986, p. 71.
18. K. Diem and C. Lentner, eds., *Documenta Geigy: Scientific Tables*, 7th ed. J. R. Geigy, Basle, Switzerland, 1970, pp. 643, 647, 657, 662, 682.
19. K. Ichikawa, I. Ohata, M. Mitomi, S. Kawamura, H. Maeno, and H. Kawata, *J. Pharm. Pharmacol.*, 32:314 (1980).
20. P. S. Banerjee and W. A. Ritschel, "Effect of pH on in vitro skin permeation of vasopressin. American Association of Pharmaceutical Scientists Symposium, Washington, DC, Nov. 5, 1986.
21. K. Lehmann, *Drugs Made Ger.*, 11:34 (1968).
22. J. Heller and P. V. Trescony, *J. Pharm. Sci.* 68:919 (1979).
23. K. Seki and D. A. Tirrell, *Macromolecules*, 17:1692 (1984).
24. H. B. Kostenbauder, R. P. Rapp, J. P. McGovren, T. S. Foster, D. G. Perrier, H. M. Blaker, W. C. Hulon, and A. W. Kinkel, *Clin. Pharmacol. Ther.*, 18:449 (1976).
25. G. Weis-Fogh, *Arch. Pharm. Chem.*, 61:455 (1954).
26. W. Mannheimer, P. Pizzoloto, and J. Adriani, *JAMA*, 154:29 (1954).
27. W. A. Ritschel and R. Clotten, *Arzneimittel-Forschung*, 20:1180 (1970).
28. W. A. Ritschel, *Handbook of Basic Pharmacokinetics*, 3rd ed. Drug Intelligence Publications, Hamilton, IL, 1986, p. 125.
29. S. S. Davis and L. Illum, *Acta Pharm. Technol.*, 32:4 (1986).
30. W. A. Ritschel, *Handbook of Basic Pharmacokinetics*, 3rd ed. Drug Intelligence Publications, Hamilton, IL, 1986, p. 127.
31. G. Gregoriadis, ed., *Liposome Technology*. CRC Press, Boca Raton, FL, 1984.
32. G. A. Ihler, in *Drug Carriers in Biology and Medicine* (G. Gregoriadis, ed.). Academic Press, London, 1979, p. 129.
33. W. A. Ritschel, *Handbook of Basic Pharmacokinetics*, 3rd ed. Drug Intelligence Publications, Hamilton, IL, 1986, p. 98.
34. T. H. Wilson, *Intestinal Absorption*. Saunders, Philadelphia, 1962.
35. W. A. Ritschel, *Laboratory Manual of Biopharmaceutics and Pharmacokinetics*. Drug Intelligence Publications, Hamilton, IL, 1974, p. 121.
36. A. H. Beckett and G. T. Tucker, *J. Pharm. Pharmacol.*, 19:31 (1967).
37. A. H. Beckett, R. N. Boyes, and E. J. Triggs, *J. Pharm. Pharmacol.*, 20:92 (1968).

38. D. Winne, *Naunyn-Schmiedebergs Arch. Pharmacol.*, 304:175 (1978).
39. I. Komiya, J. Y. Park, A. Yamani, N. F. H. Ho, and W. I. Higuchi, *Int. J. Pharm.*, 4:249 (1980).
40. P. M. Savina, A. E. Staubus, T. S. Gaginella, and D. F. Smith, *J. Pharm. Sci.*, 70:239 (1980).
41. A. G. Amidon, N. F. H. Ho, A. B. French, and W. I. Higuchi, *J. Theor. Biol.*, 89:195 (1981).
42. H. Van Rees, F. A. De Wolff, and E. L. Noach, *Eur. J. Pharmacol.*, 28:310 (1974).
43. C. D. Lewis and J. S. Fordtran, *Gastroenterology*, 68:1509 (1975).
44. A. Tsuji, E. Miyamoto, N. Hashimoto, and T. Yamana, *J. Pharm. Sci.*, 67:1705 (1978).
45. N. Schurgers and C. J. DeBlaey, *Pharm. Res.*, 1:23 (1984).
46. N. Schurgers and C. J. DeBlaey, *Int. J. Pharm.*, 19:283 (1984).
47. J. T. Doluisio, N. F. Billups, L. W. Dittert, E. T. Sugita, and J. V. Swintosky, *J. Pharm. Sci.*, 58:1196 (1969).
48. R. M. Levine, M. R. Blair, and B. B. Clark, *J. Pharmacol. Exp. Ther.*, 114:78 (1955).
49. N. Schurgers, J. Bijdendijk, J. J. Tukker, and D. J. A. Crommelin, *J. Pharm. Sci.*, 75:117 (1986).
50. V. S. Patel and W. G. Kramer, *J. Pharm. Sci.*, 75:275 (1986).
51. S. S. Davis, J. G. Hardy, M. J. Taylor, D. R. Whalley, and C. G. Wilson, *Int. J. Pharm.*, 21:167 (1984).
52. J. L. Olsen and H. M. Sadek, *The Biopolymeric Controlled-Release Devices*, Vol. I (D. L. Wise, ed.). CRC Press, Boca Raton, FL, 1984, p. 193.
53. W. A. Ritschel and P. M. Nayak. Evaluation in vitro and in vivo of silicone elastomer transdermal therapeutic devices. Paper presented at the 133rd annual American Pharmaceutical Association Meeting, San Francisco, March 19, 1986.
54. M. A. Longer and J. R. Robinson, *Pharm. Int.*, 7:114 (1986).
55. W. A. Ritschel, *Angew. Chem. Int. Ed. Engl.*, 8:699 (1969).
56. W. A. Ritschel and G. B. Ritschel, *Methods Findings Exp. Clin. Pharmacol.*, 6:513 (1984).
57. W. A. Ritschel and A. S. Hussain. Influence of selected solvents on skin penetration of griseofulvin. American Association of Pharmaceutical Scientists Symposium, Washington, DC, Nov. 5, 1986.
58. W. A. Ritschel, in *Clinical Chemistry: Theory, Analysis, and Correlation* (L. A. Kaplan and A. J. Pesce, eds). Mosby, St. Louis, 1984, p. 962.
59. M. T. Reed and E. L. Hamburg, *New Engl. J. Med.*, 314:1120 (1986).
60. J. D. Talley and I. Sylvia, *Ann. Intern. Med.*, 103:804 (1985).
61. W. A. Ritschel, *J. Pharm. Sci.*, 60:1683 (1971).

62. P. L. Madan, *Pharm. Manuft.*, April 1985, p. 39.
63. W. A. Ritschel and B. Gangadharan, Design, development and evaluation of a controlled-release p.o. unit dosage form for theophylline, American Association of Pharmaceutical Scientists Symposium, Washington, DC, Nov. 5, 1986.
64. W. A. Ritschel, in *Problems of Clinical Pharmacology in Therapeutic Research: Phase I* (H. P. Kuemmerle, T. K. Shibuya, and E. Kimura, eds.), Urban and Schwarzenberg, Munich, 1977, p. 212.
65. L. J. Leeson, *Pharm. Ind.*, 48:519 (1986).
66. R. H. Reuning, in *Biopolymer Controlled Release Devices*, Vol. I (D. L. Wise, ed.). CRC Press, Boca Raton, FL, 1984, p. 93.
67. J. C. K. Loo and S. Riegelman, *J. Pharm. Sci.*, 57:918 (1968).
68. J. G. Wagner, *J. Pharmacokinet. Biopharm.*, 3:51 (1975).
69. W. G. Kramer, R. P. Lewis, T. C. Cobb, W. F. Forester, J. A. Visconti, L. A. Wanke, H. G. Boxenbaum, and R. H. Reuning, *J. Pharmacokinet. Biopharm.*, 2:299 (1974).
70. D. J. Cutler, *J. Pharmacokinet. Biopharm.*, 6:265 (1978).
71. J. G. Wagner and E. Nelson, *J. Pharm. Sci.*, 52:610 (1963).
72. H. Shaw and J. Urguhart, *Trends Pharmacol. Sci.*, 1:208 (1980).
73. V. F. Smolen, *J. Pharmacokinet. Biopharm.*, 4:355 (1976).
74. V. F. Smolen, *J. Pharmacokinet. Biopharm.*, 4:337 (1976).
75. V. F. Smolen and W. A. Weigand, *J. Pharmacokinet. Biopharm.*, 1:329 (1973).
76. V. F. Smolen and R. D. Schoenewald, *J. Pharm. Sci.*, 60:96 (1971).

3

The Regulation of Drug Delivery Devices

JOHN F. STIGI / Division of Small Manufacturers Assistance, Food and Drug Administation, Washington, D.C.

I. HISTORY OF MEDICAL DEVICE REGULATION

With the passage of the federal Food, Drug, and Cosmetic (FD&C) Act of 1938, the Food and Drug Administration (FDA) was authorized for the first time to regulate medical devices to assure their safety. This legislation defined a medical device as "any instrument, apparatus, or contrivance, including any of its components or parts, intended for use in the diagnosis, cure, treatment, or prevention of disease in man or other animals."

The act provided for regulation of adulterated or misbranded medical devices that were entered into interstate commerce. Devices were considered to be adulterated if they included any filthy, putrid, or decomposed substance, or if they were prepared, packed, or held under unsanitary conditions. They were held to be misbranded if their labeling was false or misleading or if it failed to identify the manufacturer, packer, or distributor or to disclose the quantity of its contents.

When a device was determined to be in violation of the act, FDA was empowered to seize the product; request an injunction against its production, distribution, or use; and/or recommend criminal prosecution of the manufacturer or other persons responsible for its manufacture or distribution.

The 1938 act, however, was limited in its effectiveness because it did not require any form of premarket approval for devices entered into interstate commerce. As a result, any device could be marketed without having undergone federally approved testing procedures like those that applied to drugs. Most of FDA's device-related actions and litigations during this early period concentrated on assuring proper labeling and on removing fraudulent devices from the market place.

Following World War II, much of the military technology that had been developed was redirected toward medicine. Medical technology rapidly improved; devices became more complicated and more critical to patient care. Technological advance in electronics, plastics, metallurgy, ceramics, and engineering design affected all aspects of medicine and led to development of such devices as cardiac and renal catheters, surgical implants, artificial vessels and heart valves, intensive care monitoring units, intrauterine devices, replacement joints, and other diagnostic and therapeutic products. With the growth of clinical laboratories, the ability to diagnose increased enormously.

By the early 1960s, it became clear that the provisions of the 1938 act were not adequate to regulate these new, more complex devices. For example, anyone with an understanding of engineering and the concepts involved could design, produce, and market a programmable implantable medication system without any standardized testing. The device might then be implanted before any problems associated with its use were encountered. Problems with critical devices underscored the need for new device legislation.

Before passage of the Medical Device Amendments in May 1976, the courts filled this regulatory gap by ruling that some medical devices were, in fact, drugs and could be regulated as such. Examples of products that were regulated as drugs include soft contact lenses, bone cements, and some in vitro diagnostic products.

In 1969 a study group headed by Dr. Theodore Cooper was formed to examine problems associated with medical devices and to develop concepts for new legislation. This group, known as the Cooper Committee, reported that over a 10 year period, problems associated with medical devices had resulted in 10,000 injuries, 751 of them resulting in death [1].

The committee recommended that device legislation be enacted to create a three-tiered regulatory system in which devices would be classified according to the extent of regulatory control necessary to assure safety and effectiveness. The three classes recommended by the committee were:

A class for devices that would be exempt from premarket clearance and performance standards

A class for devices that could be marketed without premarket clearance (provided adequate safety and effectiveness standards or data were available, with which they would have to comply)

A third class, intended particularly for critical or life-supporting devices, that would be required to undergo a premarket clearance process because adequate performance standards to assure their safety or effectiveness did not exist

On May 28, 1976, President Gerald R. Ford signed into law the Medical Device Amendments to the Food, Drug, and Cosmetic Act. The purpose of the amendments is to ensure that medical devices are safe and effective. To accomplish this mandate, the amendments provide FDA with authority to regulate devices during most phases of their development, testing, production, distribution, and use.

FDA has identified approximately 1700 types of medical devices that are regulated under the legislation. The range of devices is broad and diverse, including hypodermic syringes, thermometers, ECG electrodes, infusion pumps, cardiac pacemakers, and hemodialysis machines. In addition to the three regulatory classes, these devices fall into five nonmutually exclusive categories defined on the basis of procedures and utilization:

Over-the-counter devices: those that can be purchased by the consumer without a prescription

Prescription devices: those for which adequate directions for use cannot be devised to permit lay persons to use the device safely and effectively unless under the supervision and direction of a practitioner

Investigational devices: Those still in developmental stages and used on human subjects only for purposes of developing safety and effectiveness data

Custom devices: those ordered from manufacturers by physicians or dentists to conform to their special needs or those of individual patients and not generally available to or generally used by other practitioners

Critical devices: those, as defined in the Good Manufacturing Practice Regulation, that are life-sustaining, life-supporting, or intended to be implanted into the human body and whose failure can be reasonably expected to result in a significant injury.

The term "medical device" describes a large and diverse set of products. Regulation of these products is a difficult and complicated process, not only because of sheer volume and variety, but also because of their increasing importance in the delivery of patient health care.

II. DRUG VERSUS MEDICAL DEVICE

For the first time, the 1976 amendments clearly distinguished devices from drugs. Thus articles to which the term *drug* applies include [2]:

Articles recognized in the official United States Pharmacopeia, the official Homeopathic Pharmacopeia of the United States, or official National Formulary, or any supplement to any of them

Articles intended for use in the diagnosis, cure, mitigation, treatment, or prevention of disease in man or other animals

Articles (other than food) intended to affect the structure of any function of the body of man or other animals

Articles intended for use as a component of any articles specified in the three previous clauses; but does not include devices or their components, parts, or accessories

The term *device* is defined as follows [3]:

any instrument, apparatus, implement, machine, contrivance, implant, in vitro reagent, or other similar or related article including any component, part, or accessory, which is:

recognized in the official National Formulary, or the United States Pharmacopeia, or any supplement of them;

intended for use in the diagnosis of disease or other conditions, or in the cure, mitigation, treatment, or prevention of disease, in man or other animals; or

intended to affect the structure or any function of the body of man or other animals; and

does not achieve any of its principal intended purposes through chemical action within or on the body of man or other animals and which is not dependent upon being metabolized for the achievement of any of its principal intended purposes.

A major distinction between drugs and devices is made in the final portion of the definition of a device. Products that satisfy any of the first three criteria and are not metabolized or are not dependent on being metabolized to achieve their principal intended purpose are to be regulated as devices and not drugs. The FD&C Act is mute as to how a drug achieves its principal intended effect.

The definition of a medical device includes products intended for use on humans and those intended for use on animals. To date, none of the requirements authorized and implemented under the Medical Device Amendments have encompassed devices for veterinary use.

However, the FD&C Act prohibits the adulteration or misbranding of veterinary devices. If a veterinary device is promoted for a therapeutic purpose, credible scientific evidence must exist to demonstrate that the device is effective for the labeled claim. If the FDA judges the available evidence lacking, the device will be deemed misbranded under Section 502(a) of the act.

The definition of a "device" also includes in vitro diagnostic products—devices that aid in the diagnosis of disease by using human or animal components to cause chemical reactions, fermentation, and the like. In these instances, except for some specimen collection devices, the device is not placed in or permanently attached to the body.

Finally, a medical device also can be any article intended for use in the diagnosis of conditions other than disease. An example of this would be a device used to diagnose pregnancy.

In a drug delivery system a product that satisfies the definition of a device is used in conjunction with a product that satisfies the definition of a drug. In this situation the drug/device distinction is less apparent.

The FDA regulations applicable to devices that contain or deliver a drug depend on:

1. Whether the delivery system is marketed empty or filled. Generally, products that are intended to deliver drugs to the patient and are *not* prefilled by the manufacturer will be regulated as devices. An example is an empty implantable infusion pump.

2. If prefilled, whether the drug component is intended to improve the safe use of the device, in which case the product will be regulated as a device. An example is a surgical drape impregnated with antimicrobial agents. If, on the other hand, the drug component is intended to have a therapeutic effect on the patient, the product will be regulated as a drug. An example of a product that many people might consider a medical device but is actually regulated as a drug is an intrauterine contraceptive device that functions by release of progesterone contained in a reservoir within the device.

3. Whether the device is intended to administer a drug that is the subject of an approved new drug application (NDA) versus a drug that has not yet undergone approval. For a drug with an approved NDA, a manufacturer must document that the drug delivery device will not have a deleterious effect on the drug nor the drug on the device. However, if the drug does not have an approved NDA, an approved NDA must be granted that demonstrates that the drug is safe and effective under the prescribed conditions before the device could be cleared for marketing.

Let's use the example of a mythical firm, New Technology, Inc., which wishes to market a programmable implantable medication system called the Lifepump. Is the product regulated by FDA as a drug or as a device?

If the Lifepump is marketed empty for filling by medical personnel, FDA would consider it to be a medical device. The product would be evaluated, primarily, by the FDA's Center for Devices and Radiological Health (CDRH). Since no similar product was marketed prior to the enactment date of the Medical Device Amendments (May 28, 1976), a premarket approval (PMA) application would have to be approved before the device could be marketed. If the labeling on the empty Lifepump recommends the use of particular drugs that are already approved for intravenous administraiton or other similar routes of administration, the PMA must include information showing compatibility between those drug dosage forms and the Lifepump. However, if the indicated drug is not approved for human use or if the device would be delivering the drug by a route of administration not approved for that drug, the device could not be marketed until an approved NDA had been granted.

If the Lifepump is to be marketed prefilled with the drug, FDA would consider it to be a drug. The product would be evaluated, primarily, by the FDA's Center for Drugs and Biologics. If the Lifepump is prefilled with a drug that is already the subject of an approved NDA, an amended application would be required. If the delivery system is prefilled with a drug that does not have an approved NDA, an acceptable investigational new drug (IND) application would be required for the sponsor to develop safety and effectiveness data. Prior to commercial distribution, an approved NDA would be required. (See Section VII: New Drug Application Versus Premarket Approval Application for the specific contents of these submissions.)

Of the approximately 1700 generic medical devices identified by FDA, approximately 70 generic types of device could be referred to as "Drug-Related Devices" (see Table 1). These devices can be subdivided into three categories.

1. The primary intended use* is for the delivery of a drug to the patient.

---

*The reader should be aware of the distinction between "functional use" and "intended use". "Intended use" has a well-established meaning for purposes of the FD&C Act. It evolves from regulations, agency policies, and case law. "Intended use" is the use intended by the person who placed the product in commercial distribution, as illustrated by labeling claims, advertising matter, or oral or written statements. Functional use, however, is often determined by the user. Be aware, however, that a manufacturer who knows a device introduced into interstate commerce by him is to be used for conditions, purposes, or uses other than the ones for which he offers it is required to provide for such a device adequate labeling that addresses the other uses to which the article is to be put (21 CFR 801.4).

TABLE 1 Drug-Related Devices

Classification regulation	Device	Section[a]	Class
Anesthesiology	Bourdon gauge flowmeter	868.2300*	II
	Uncompensated Thrope tube flowmeter[b]	868.2320*	II
	Compensated Thrope tube flowmeter	868.2340*	II
	Anesthesia conduction catheter	868.5120*	II
	Anesthesia conduction filter	868.5130*	II
	Anesthesia conduction needle gas machines for anesthesia or analgesia	868.5150*	II
	Laryngotracheal topical anesthesia applicator	868.5170*	II
	Anesthesia breathing circuit	868.5240*	II
	Nasal oxygen cannula	868.5340*	I
	Nasal oxygen catheter	868.5350*	I
	Nonrebreathing mask	868.5570*	II
	Oxygen mask	868.5580*	II
	Scavenging mask	868.5590*	II
	Venturi mask	868.5600*	II
	Medical nonventilatory nebulizer (atomizer)[c]	868.5640*	I
	Portable liquid oxygen unit	868.5655*	II
	Nonpowered oxygen tent	868.5700*	II
	Electric powered oxygen tent	868.5710*	II
	Anesthetic vaporizer[d]	868.5880*	II
	Manual emergency ventilator[e]	868.5915**	II
	Powered emergency ventilator	868.5925**	II
Cardiovascular	Continuous flush catheter[f]	870.1210***	II
	Percutaneous catheter	870.1250**	II
	Programmable diagnostic computer[g]	870.1425***	II
	Single-function, preprogrammed diagnostic computer	870.1435***	I
	Withdrawal-infusion pump	870.1800*	II
	Cardiopulmonary bypass vascular catheter, cannula, or tubing[h]	870.4210**	II
	Cardiopulmonary bypass fitting, manifold, stopcock, and adaptor	870.4290**	II

TABLE 1 (*continued*)

Classification regulation	Device	Section[a]	Class
	Cardiopulmonary bypass oxygenator	870.4350**	II
	Cariopulmonary bypass blood reservoir[i]	870.4400***	II
Dental (proposed)	Dental injection needle	872.4730*	II
	Cartridge syringe	872.7770*	II
	Periodontic or endodontic irrigating syringe	872.6800**	I
	Manual toothbrush[j]	872.6855**	I
	Powered toothbrush	872.6865**	II
Ear, nose, and throat	Nasopharyngeal catheter	874.4175**	I
	Ear, nose, and throat drug administration set	874.5220*	I
General hospital and personal use	Intravenous container	880.5025**	II
	Intravascular catheter	880.5200**	II
	Intravascular administration set	880.5440**	II
	Hypodermic single-lumen needle	880.5570**	II
	Infusion pump	880.5725*	II
	Piston syringe	880.5860**	II
	Irrigating syringe	880.6960**	I
General and plastic surgery (proposed)	Inflatable breast prosthesis[k]	878.3530**	II
	Nonabsorbable gauze, surgical sponge, and wound dressing for external use[l]	878.4060**	I
	Introduction/drainage catheter and accessories	878.4200*	II
	Surgical drape and accessories[m]	878.4370***	II
Gastroenterology/ urology	Biliary catheter and accessories[n]	876.5010**	II
	Urological catheter and accessories	876.5130**	II
	Enema kit	876.5210**	I
	Colonic irrigation system, blood access device, and	876.5220**	II, III
	accessories	876.5540**	II, III
	Peritoneal dialysis system and accessories	876.5630**	II

TABLE 1 (continued)

Classification regulation	Device	Section[a]	Class
	Gastrointestinal tube and accessories	876.5980**	II
Obstetrical/ gynecological	Uterotubal carbon dioxide insufflator and accessories[o]	884.1300***	II
	Obstetric-gynecological general manual instrument-vaginal applicator	884.4520**	I
	Obstetric anesthesia set	884.5100*	II
	Contraceptive diaphragm and accessories	884.5350***	II
	Therapeutic vaginal douche apparatus	884.5900*	II
	Vaginal insufflator	884.5920*	I
Ophthalmic (proposed)	Vitreous aspiration and cutting instrument	886.4150***	III
	Ocular surgery irrigation device	886.4360**	I
	Eye pad	886.4650**	I
	Ophthalmic sponge	886.4790**	II
Orthopedic	Polymethylmethacrylate (bone cement) with antibiotic[p]	888.3027***	III
Physical medicine	Ultrasonic diathermy	890.5300**	II, III
	Iontophoresis device	890.5525*	II, III

[a]Asterisks following a numbered section of 21 CFR have the following meanings:

* = primary intended use is for delivery of a drug to the patient

** = primary intended use is not drug delivery, but device can be functionally used for that purpose

*** = drug is essential to the safe and effective use of the device and may be delivered to the patient during its use

[b]Anesthetic gases and oxygen are passed through this device before entering the patient to control flow rate.

[c]Drugs, primarily bronchodilators, are administered to patients with this device in aerosol form.

[d]Liquid anesthetic such as Halothane or Flurane is administered to patient in vapor form with this device.

[e]At times oxygen (a drug) is delivered to patients during emergency respiratory support.

TABLE 1 (*continued*)

[f]Device utilizes saline solution for flushing of a catheter transducer
system to prevent clotting before blood is returned to patient.
[g]One function is to measure cardiac output. A cold saline solution is
injected into the patient to enable device to measure this activity.
[h]System is used to connect the patient to an oxygenator through which
drugs such as heparin and protomene are administered during surgery.
[i]Heparin is introduced into the reservoir to prevent clotting before
blood is returned to the patient.
[j]Many toothpastes contain fluoride (a drug).
[k]Some surgeons will inject steroids and antibiotics with the saline
solution to inflate the prosthesis to reduce fibrous capsular contrac-
tion.
[l]Drugs, primarily antiseptics, are typically administered with this
device.
[m]Antimicrobial agents are impregnated into the drape to create a
barrier to microbes.
[n]Drug for the dissolution of gallstones may be administered to the
biliary tract with this device.
[o]Carbon dioxide is administered to the patient to test the patency of
the fallopian tube.
[p]Transitional devices were previously regulated as drugs and are
automatically classified into class III.

  2. The primary intended use[*] (see page 87) is not drug de-
     livery; however, it can be functionally used for that purpose.
  3. A drug is essential to the safe and effective use of the device
     and may be delivered to the patient during the use of the
     device.

This chapter addresses the regulatory requirements for categories
1 and 2.

III. CLASSIFICATION OF MEDICAL DEVICES

Essentially, the FDA's regulatory responsibility for devices is to assure
that all devices intended for human use that are manufactured, imported, or distributed in the United States are reasonably safe and
effective. Because of the wide range of devices, from the simple to
the complex, some devices will require more regulatory control than
others to achieve safety and effectiveness.
     Under Section 513 of the FD&C Act, the FDA is required to classify
all devices intended for human use into one of three regulatory classes

according to the extent of control necessary to assure device safety and effectiveness. Classification is the cornerstone for all medical device regulations. It matches levels of regulatory control to individual or generic groups of devices.

The three regulatory categories or classes are defined as follows.

Class I, "General Controls." The first category regulates devices for which controls other than performance standards or premarket approval are sufficient to assure safety and effectiveness. Such controls include regulations that (a) prohibit adulterated or misbranded devices, (b) require domestic device manufacturers and initial distributors to register their establishments and list their devices, (c) grant FDA authority to ban certain devices, (d) provide for notification of risks and of repair, replacement, or refund, (e) restrict the sale, distribution, or use of certain devices, and (f) govern Good Manufacturing Practices, records and reports, and inspections. These minimum requirements apply also to class II and class III devices. Approximately 35% of all devices fall into class I. Examples of class I drug delivery devices are nasal oxygen catheters, ear, nose, and throat drug administration sets, irrigating syringes, and nonabsorbable wound dressings (medicated).

Class II, "Performance Standards." The second category regulates devices for which general controls alone are insufficient to assure safety and effectiveness and for which existing information is sufficient to establish a performance standard that provides this assurance. Class II devices must comply not only with general controls but also with an applicable standard developed under Section 514 of the FD&C Act. Until performance standards have been established by regulation, only general controls apply. Approximately 55% of all devices fall into class II. Examples of class II drug delivery devices are gas machines for anesthesia, oxygen tents, infusion pumps, and obstetric anesthesia sets.

Class III, "Premarket Approval." The final category regulates devices for which insufficient information exists to assure that general controls and performance standards provide reasonable assurance of safety and effectiveness. Generally, class III devices are those represented to be life sustaining or life supporting, those implanted in the body, or those presenting potential unreasonable risk of illness or injury. Class III devices must eventually undergo premarket approval. Until FDA calls for PMAs by regulation, however, preamendment class III devices (and postamendment devices substantially equivalent to them) are subject only to general controls. Approximately 10% of all devices fall into class III. However, due to advances in metallurgy, electronics, and computer sciences, coupled with the increase in technology transfer from the aerospace to the medical industry, FDA is seeing a wealth of drug delivery devices that require class III controls. We list three examples of class III drug delivery devices.

1. The sensor-actuated medication system (SAMS), an implantable device that releases antihypertensive medication in accordance with signals received from a blood pressure sensing component. This represents closed-loop control of hypertension through a sensor-activated, microprocessor-controlled medication infusion system. The medication is continuously available and is administered in direct response to the needs of the body.

2. Iontophoresis devices intended to use a direct current to introduce ions of soluble salts or other drugs into the body for medical purposes.

3. Implanted blood access devices consisting of various flexible or rigid tubes, which are surgically implanted in appropriate blood vessels, may extend through the skin, and are intended to remain in the body for 30 days or more. This generic type of device includes various shunts and connectors specifically designed to provide access to blood, such as the arteriovenous (A-V) shunt cannula and vessel tip.

A. The Classification Process

There are several aspects to the classification process. Panels of experts were established to provide FDA with advice and recommendations on device classification. Their function will continue until final rules have been issued to classify all devices. (At this writing some device classifications are in the proposal state; see Table 2.)

FDA receives the panel recommendations, determines which class is appropriate, and classifies the device by regulation. Before issuing a final order, however, FDA publishes the classification as a proposal in the *Federal Register* (FR) for comment.

At present, there are 16 operating classification panels:

Anesthesiology and Respiratory Therapy Devices
Circulatory System Devices
Clinical Chemistry and Clinical Toxicology Devices
Dental Devices
Ear, Nose, and Throat Devices
Gastroenterology-Urology Devices
General and Plastic Surgery Devices
General Hospital and Personal Use Devices
Hematology and Pathology Devices
Immunology Devices
Microbiology Devices
Neurological Devices
Obstetrics and Gynecology Devices
Ophthalmic Devices

Orthopedic and Rehabilitation Devices
Radiological Devices

(See Table 2 for the current status of these classification regulations.)
Each panel consists of eight members, six voting and two nonvoting.
Voting members are appointed from the research and medical communi-
ties. One nonvoting member represents industry and the other represents consumer interest. The panel review process considers the
following factors:

Persons for whose use the device is intended
Conditions of use for the device
Probable benefit to health from use of the device weighed against
    any probable injury or illness from such use
Reliability of the device

To aid panel review of devices, CDRH has developed a classification
scheme that consists of two questionnaires—one for devices and the
other for in vitro diagnostic products—to determine and identify characteristics of individual devices. Questions seek to elicit baseline information on each device. In addition to the classification scheme, panel
members must complete a supplemental data sheet for each device they
review. Once a panel has completed its review of a device, it must
submit, along with its classification recommendation, the following documentation:

A summary of reasons for the recommendation
A summary of data on which its recommendation is based
An identification of any unreasonable risks to health presented by
    the device
Exemption recommendations for class I devices
Priority recommendations for class II and class III devices

FDA reviews a panel's recommended classification for each device and
decides whether to accept it. If the agency assigns the device to a
different class, FDA must document its reasons.
    The panel recommendation and the proposed FDA classification
are both published in the *Federal Register* (FR) as a proposed classification regulation. All interested parties are allowed 60 days in which
to comment. After comments have been received and evaluated, a
final notice classifying the device is published in the FR. Usually 30
days after publication of the FR notice, this final regulation becomes
effective, and the device is legally classified.

TABLE 2 Proposed and Final Rule Listing of Classified Devices Under the Federal Food, Drug, and Cosmetic Act as of November 1986

Device section	Date of proposal	Date of final rule	Class I	Class II	Class III	Exemptions GMP	Exemptions 510(k)
Neurology	11/78	9/79	23	66	11	4	0
Cardiovascular	3/79	2/80	3	108	24	0	0
Obstetrical/ gynecological	4/79	2/80	5	48	16	0	0
Hematology/ pathology	9/79	9/80	42	57	5	4	0
General hospital	8/79	01/80	53	43	2	33	30
Anesthesiology	11/79	7/82	21	105	7	10	0
Microbiology/ immunology	4/80	11/82	93	64	2	5	7
Gastroenterology/ urology	1/81	11/83	9	32	9	4	0
Physical medicine	8/79	11/83	32	42	2	24	19
Ear, nose and throat	1/82	11/86	15	28	6	0	1
Clinical chemistry/ toxicology	2/82						
Dental	12/80						
General and plastic surgery	1/82						
Radiology	1/82						
Ophthalmology	1/82						
Orthopedic	7/82						

B. Transitional Devices

Under the expanded (1976) definition of "device," certain items previously regulated as new drugs became devices. Under transitional provision of Section 520(1) of the FD&C Act, these devices were automatically placed in class III, but are regulated in a way consistent with their former status as drugs.

As a result, medical devices that were subject to approved NDAs are regarded as class III devices with approved PMAs.

On December 16, 1977, FDA published (see *Federal Register*, Vol. 42, pp. 63472-63476) two lists of devices previously regulated as drugs. One list contains those devices for which premarket approval is needed; the other names those for which premarket approval is not needed [4].

C. Changes in Device Classification

The Medical Device Amendments contain provisions for changing the classification of a device, based on new information about the device. FDA may, on its own initiative or in response to a petition by an interested party (including manufacturers), change a device's classification by regulation. The agency may also revoke any regulation or requirement under Section 514 (performance standards) or Section 515 (premarket approval) that pertains to the device. Sections of the FD&C Act that apply to changing classification are 513(e), 513(f), 514(b), 515(b), and 520(1)(1).

A manufacturer who wishes to have a device reclassified to a lower class must convince CDRH that the less stringent class requirements will be sufficient. For example, a manufacturer might petition for a device to be moved from class III to class II. The firm's petition must include information to prove that sufficient data exist for developing a performance standard to assure FDA that the device is reasonably safe and effective for its intended use(s).

First, FDA determined whether a reclassification petition contains deficiencies that would preclude reaching a decision on it. Second, FDA refers the petition to an appropriate classification panel for review and solicits a recommendation to approve or deny. Third, the panel's recommendation and a proposed FDA reclassification order are published in the *Federal Register* for comment.

After completing its review of comments, FDA notifies the petitioner by letter whether the petition has been denied or approved. For an approved petition, an order classifying the device into class I or II will be published in the *Federal Register*.

Petitions for reclassification should be sent directly to the Food and Drug Administration, CDRH, HFZ-401, 8757 Georgia Avenue, Silver Spring, Maryland 20910. The outside of the envelope should be clearly marked with the section of the law under which the petition is being submitted: for example, "513(e) Petition" or other applicable section. The petition and five copies should be submitted on standard size paper.

IV. REGISTRATION OF FIRMS AND LISTING OF DEVICES

The FD&C Act requires manufacturers to register their establishments with FDA and to list their devices. Repackers and relabelers, as well as initial distributors of imported devices, must also register with FDA. Form FDA 2891 is used to register an establishment. Form FDA 2892 is used to list a device.

Manufacturers of raw materials or components used in manufacturing a finished device are exempted from registration if (a) they also market the same material or components to nondevice manufacturers and (b) they are not providing the device manufacturer with a "finished" device. Examples of other establishments exempt from registration are as follows [5]:

Licensed practitioners, including physicians, dentists, and optometrists, who manufacture or alter devices solely for use in their practice.

Pharmacies and other retail outlets that dispense or sell devices in the normal course of business.

Persons who manufacture devices solely for use in research, teaching, or analysis and do not distribute such devices in commerce.

Warehousers and wholesalers who do not revise devices or their containers.

Carriers who receive, carry, hold, or deliver devices in their normal conduct of business.

Persons who dispense devices to the user or render a service necessary to provide the user with a device or its benefits, that is, hearing aid dispenser, optician, clinical laboratory, X-ray assembler, dental laboratory, orthotic or prosthetic retailer, and others whose primary responsibility to the user is to dispense or provide a service through the use of a previously manufactured device.

The following are also required to list their devices on form FDA 2892: domestic firms (except contract manufacturers) with a registration obligation with FDA; manufacturers, relabelers and repackers, and specifications developers and initial distributors, if either is a specification developer or repacker and/or relabeler of an imported device; and foreign establishments that export devices into the United States. Initial distributors of foreign-manufactured devices do not submit an FDA form 2892; they comply with their device listing obligation by identifying to FDA the foreign firms whose devices they import into this country.

V. PREMARKET NOTIFICATION

Section 510(k) of the FD&C Act requires device manufacturers who must register to notify FDA, at least 90 days in advance, of their intent to market a device. This filing, known as premarket notification, allows FDA to determine whether the device is equivalent to a device already placed into one of the three classification categories. Thus, "new" devices (i.e., those that were not in commercial distribution prior to May 28, 1976) that have not been classified can be properly identified.

Medical device manufacturers must submit a premarket notification if they intend to (a) introduce a device into commercial distribution for the first time or (b) introduce, or reintroduce, a device so significantly changed or modified that its safety or effectiveness could be affected. Such change or modification could relate to design, material, chemical composition, energy source, manufacturing process, or intended use. In brief, the premarket notification program aims to do the following.

Identify new devices that must be placed automatically into class III and undergo premarket approval or reclassification before they are marketed

Classify new devices—a not substantially equivalent (NSE) new device is in class III, and a substantially equivalent (SE) new device is in the same regulatory class as the device to which it is found equivalent

Achieve marketing equity by allowing manufacturers of new devices that are substantially equivalent to preamendments devices to market their device without facing any greater regulatory burdens than faced by manufacturers of the preamendments device

The FD&C Act specifies how a "new" device (a postamendments device) is to be classified. A postamendments device is automatically in class III and must undergo premarket approval or reclassification before it can be marketed, unless it is within a type of device that was in commercial distribution prior to May 28, 1976, and is substantially

equivalent to another device within such type; or, it is within a type
or device introduced after May 28, 1976, that has been reclassified
into class I or II and is substantially equivalent to another device
within such type. A substantially equivalent device is in the same
class, and is subject to the same requirements, as the device to which
it is substantially equivalent.

Premarket notifications should be securely bound, if necessary,
and should be submitted in duplicate. They should contain the following information:

All names of the device, including trade (proprietary) name, common (usual) name, and classification name as defined by the
classification panel.
Registration number of the notifying establishment (if applicable).
Class of the device and the appropriate classification panel. If
the device has not yet been classified, include a statement
to that effect.
Actions taken to comply with performance standards if the device
is a class II device and a final FDA standard exists for that
device.
Samples of proposed labels, labeling, and advertisements sufficient
to describe the device, its intended uses, and directions for
use.
Statement of how the device is either similar to or different from
other devices on the market, plus data to support the statement.
Information describing a significant change or modification, if any
occurred, that could affect the device's safety or effectiveness.

The amendments provide that a new device can be substantially equivalent to one of two types of devices (from here on referred to as a
"predicate device"). A predicate device is one that was in distribution prior to enactment of the amendments, or it is a postamendments
device that was subject to reclassification from class III to class I or
II. The Center for Devices and Radiological Health does not routinely
require that manufacturers perform research to determine what specific
predicate devices were available in 1976 or were available at the time
a postamendments device was reclassified form class III to class I or
II; nor does CDRH routinely require that all submissions under Section 510(k) of the FD&C Act initially provide information on a predicate
device. Instead, CDRH requires submitters to provide information
that compares the new device to a marketed device of a similar type,
regardless of whether that marketed device was marketed before or
after enactment of the amendments, or before or after a type of postamendments device was reclassified.

This means that the manufacturer can make a submission under Section 510(k) comparing a new device to a device that has been found to be substantially equivalent. It does not mean, however, that CDRH finds new devices substantially equivalent to devices that have been previously found substantially equivalent. It only reflects the FDA's position that the similarity of a new device to a marketed device is evidence that can be considered in determining that the new device is, as is the marketed device to which it is compared, substantially equivalent to a predicate device. Nevertheless, the ultimate burden of demonstrating the substantial equivalence of a new device to a predicate device remains with the 510(k) submitter, and when the center is unfamiliar with certain aspects of the predicate device, the submitter will be required to provide information that substantiates a claim of substantial equivalence.

[Note: The guidance that follows assumes that documentation submitted to comply with Section 510(k) of the FD&C Act provides comparisons with marketed devices.]

A. General Points Considered by the Center for Devices and Radiological Health During Review of Submissions Under Section 510(k)

CDRH normally approaches the review of 510(k)s by considering the following.

Does the new device have the same intended use as a predicate device?

Does the new device have the same technological characteristics (i.e., same materials, design, or energy source)?

If it has new technological characteristics, could they affect safety or effectiveness?

If the new device has a new intended use (we discuss below what constitutes a new intended use), it is considered not substantially equivalent. If the new device has the same intended use as a predicate device and the same technological characteristics related to safety and effectiveness, the new device is considered substantially equivalent. If the new device has the same intended use as a predicate device, but it has new technological features that could affect safety or effectiveness, additional issues must be considered:

Do the new technological features pose the same type of questions about safety or effectiveness as are posed by the predicate device with the same intended use?

Are there accepted scientific methods for evaluating whether safety or effectiveness has been adversely affected as a result of the use of new technological characteristics?

Is there information to demonstrate that the new technological features have not diminished safety and effectiveness?

If the answer to any of these questions is "no," the device is generally not substantially equivalent.

Thus, as a matter of practice, CDRH generally considers a device to be substantially equivalent to a predicate device if, in comparison to the predicate device, the new device has the same technological characteristics (i.e., the same materials, design, energy source), or, it has new technological characteristics that could not affect safety or effectiveness; or, it has new technological characteristics that could affect safety or effectiveness and:

It generates the same type of questions about safety or effectiveness.

There are accepted scientific methods for evaluating whether safety or effectiveness has been adversely affected as a result of the use of new technological characteristics.

There are data to demonstrate that the new technological features have not diminished safety or effectiveness.

Premarket notification submissions should be designed to answer the foregoing questions.

For the purposes of determining whether the new device has the same intended use as a predicate device, CDRH assesses any differences in label indications in terms of the safety and effectiveness questions they may raise. CDRH considers such points as physiological purpose (e.g., removes water from blood, transports blood, cuts tissue), condition or disease to be treated or diagnosed, professional or lay use, parts of the body or types of tissue involved, and frequency of use. If a new device is determined to have the same intended use, CDRH may then proceed to determine whether it is substantially equivalent. (Devices that do not have the same intended use cannot be substantially equivalent.) The following examples illustrate this point.

Nonimplanted Blood Access Device: This type of preamendments class II device is intended to provide access to a patient's blood so that blood can, for example, be subjected to hemodialysis. Pre-1976 devices are labeled for insertion into the femoral vein. New devices that are labeled for insertion into the subclavian vein may have the same intended use to the extent that labeling for the new and predicate devices indicates that both are intended to provide access to a patient's blood for similar purposes. The differences in labeling described above do not undercut the fact that the new and predicate devices have the same intended use. CDRH was further able to conclude that the new device was substantially equivalent, because (a) the differences in labeling related only to a method of use not relevant to the effect that the insertion is to achieve (and therefore did not pose new safety or effectiveness questions) and (b) there was no other significant change (in technology, design, etc.) [6].

The labeling difference relating to the subclavian catheter is not significant enough to require a finding that the device is for a different intended use. Moreover, the specific use associated with the labeling modification does not present issues of safety and effectiveness different from those posed by the use of the predicate device and therefore, the device can be found substantially equivalent in terms of intended use. On the other hand, for some new devices, modifications in label indications will not be found to represent the same intended use as a predicate device, even though the intended effect of the new device is very similar to that of the predicate device. This is because slight modification in intended use can be significant to the claimed effect or purpose of the predicate device. If a device has a different intended use, there is no reason to proceed further to decide whether the devices are substantially equivalent. (Obviously, however, some of the same issues relevant to substantial equivalence determinations may arise in assessing whether devices are for the same intended use, i.e., differences in labeling are judged in terms of any safety and effectiveness questions they may raise.) For example, consider:

Long-term Precutaneous Intravascular Catheter: This pre-amendments, unclassified device consists of a slender tube labeled for insertion into the vascular system for extended periods in order to sample blood, monitor blood pressure, or administer drugs. A similarly designed device has been found not substantially equivalent because it is labeled for use as a spinal canal access catheter. The new device was intended to deliver drugs over an extended period of time to the spinal canal. While both devices deliver drugs into the human body, they relate to different body systems. The concern raised by this difference led to the conclusion that the intended uses of the devices are not the same. Inserting the device into, and maintaining it in, the spinal canal raises significantly different safety issues compared to the issues posed by intravascular insertion; namely, the new device potentially posed risks to the spinal cord, whereas the predicate device did not [6].

As the examples above show, for a device to be found substantially equivalent, it is important that the documents submitted to comply with Section 510(k) demonstrate that (a) the intended use of the device does not differ form the intended use of marketed devices within the same type, and (b) any changes in labeling are immaterial in terms of safety and effectiveness issues.

B. Devices with New Technological Features

If a new device has the same intended use as a predicate device and if there is no technological difference between the new and a predicate device, the new device is substantially equivalent. If the device has the same intended use and a technological difference, but the technological difference could not affect safety or effectiveness, it is substantially equivalent. Technological differences may include modifications in design, materials, or energy sources; examples are changes in the power supply of electronic infusion pumps, the use of new materials in implantable devices, and the use of new battery designs in implanted pacemakers and infusion pumps. Devices are not substantially equivalent when the new technological feature could adversely affect safety or effectiveness in a way that is consequential under the conditions of intended use. In taking this approach, CDRH focuses on the technological differences that are medically and scientifically significant. It avoids difficulties of a mechanical application of rigid, formal criteria to the wide variety of substantial equivalence questions posed by new devices proposed for marking under Seciton 510(k). Substantial equivalence determinations require CDRH to exercise reasonable scientific judgment. For example, a rule that would make all devices not substantially equivalent if they have a new material would be inappropriate for such devices as bed pans. For other devices (e.g., for implants), a "materials rule" may seem more appropriate. Even for implants, however, such a rule would be too strict if applied to substitute materials known to be, or easily shown to be, equivalent or superior. An example is a new postamendments hip made of titanium, which is generally known to be, and can easily be shown to be, stronger and less corrosive than some stainless steels that were used in preamendments hips.

Thus, from a scientific perspective, to determine consequential technological changes, CDRH considers the following conditions. Whether:

The new device poses the same type of questions about safety or effectiveness as a predicate device.

There are accepted scientific methods for evaluating whether safety or effectiveness has been adversely affected as a result of the use of new technological characteristics.

There are data to demonstrate that new technological characteristics have not diminished safety or effectiveness.

For a device to be found substantially equivalent, it is important that submissions under Section 510(k) either demonstrate that the technology of the device does not differ from the technology of marketed devices within the same type or, to the extent that the technology does differ, explain why the device does not present new questions about safety or effectiveness, describe what accepted methods exist to test comparability of performance, and present data, generated from such tests, that demonstrate comparability.

C. Data Requirements for Submissions Under Section 510(k)

The requirements of Section 510(k) of the FD&C Act enable FDA to determine whether a device is substantially equivalent to one already in commercial distribution. To do this, CDRH requires that a submission include descriptive data needed to understand a new device's intended use, physical composition, method of operation, specifications, and performance claims. Similar information may also be required about the device to which the new device is being compared. In addition, CDRH may require performance testing information (i.e., data from bench, animal, or clinical tests) to determine that a device performs according to its description. While CDRH has concluded that it should sometimes require performance testing data to confirm that a new device is substantially equivalent, the review process under Section 510(k) is not a substitute for premarket approval. CDRH does not attempt to address all the issues that would be answered in a PMA in its review of these materials. Data submitted should show *comparability* of a new device to a predicate device. Demonstration, in an absolute sense, of a device's safety and effectiveness is reserved for PMAs.

VI. EXEMPTION OF DEVICES FOR INVESTIGATIONAL USE

To encourage discovery and development of useful medical devices, the amendments created a key exemption from premarket notification, premarket approval, and other controls of the FD&C Act: the investigational device exemption (IDE) permits devices to be shipped in interstate commerce for clinical investigation to determine their safety and effectiveness. The exemption requires safeguards for humans who are subjects of investigations, maintenance of sound ethical standards, and establishment of procedures to assure development of reliable scientific data.

Section 520(g) of the act authorizes the FDA to grant an IDE in cases of studies undertaken to develop safety, effectiveness, and other data for medical devices that involve the use of human subjects.

Sponsors of clinical studies that have an approved IDE are not required to comply during the period of their investigations with certain sections of the FD&C Act—for example, registration, listing, premarket notification, premarket approval, good manufacturing practices, performance standards, restricted device, banned device, and color additive requirements.

All devices slated for clinical investigation must have an approved IDE or must be exempt from the IDE regulation. For device investigations that are not exempt from the IDE regulation, procedures for obtaining an approved IDE depend on whether the risk is significant or nonsignificant. (These two risk categories will be discussed later.)

The following device investigations are exempt from the IDE regulation:

Preamendments devices (i.e., devices in commercial distribution before the Medical Device Amendments of May 28, 1976), and substantially equivalent devices if used or investigated in accord with the labeling in effect at the time. For class II and III devices, this exemption expires at the time premarket approval applications (PMAs) are required or an FDA mandatory standard takes effect. This exemption does not apply to transitional devices.

Postamendments devices (i.e., devices in commercial distribution after May 28, 1976, if determined to be substantially equivalent and used in accordance with labeling reviewed at the time equivalence was determined). For class II and III devices, this exemption expires under the same circumstance specified under "Preamendments devices," above. This exemption does not apply to transitional devices.

Diagnostic devices that comply with all the applicable federal requirements [21 CFR 809.10(c)] and if the testing (a) is noninvasive, (b) does not require an invasive sampling procedure that presents significant risk, (c) does not by design or intention introduce energy into a subject, and (d) is not used as a diagnostic procedure without confirmation by another medically established diagnostic product or procedure.

Devices undergoing consumer preference testing, testing of a modification, or testing of a combination of devices in commercial distribution, if the testing is not to determine safety or effectiveness.

Devices intended solely for veterinary use or for research with laboratory animals and so designated in the labeling.

Custom devices [as defined in 21 CFR 812.3(b)], unless used to determine safety or effectiveness for commercial distribution.

Intraocular lenses (IOLs), which are covered under 21 CFR part 13. All clinical investigations of IOLs are subject to FDA approval of an IDE application [7].

A. Significant Risk Versus Nonsignificant Risk Devices

The IDE regulation distinguishes between significant and nonsignificant risk. Procedures for obtaining an IDE differ for the two types of devices.

A significant risk device is one that presents a potential for seriour risk to the health, safety, or welfare of a subject and is:

An implant
Used in supporting or sustaining human life
Substantially important in diagnosing, curing, mitigating, or treating disease or in preventing impairment of human health

All implanted drug delivery devices would be considered significant risk. However, external closed-loop infusion pumps would also be considered significant risk if the drug being administered is life supporting/life sustaining or if the immediate failure of the pump could likely result in death or serious injury.

The sponsor initially determines if a device presents nonsignificant or significant risk. The proposed study is then submitted to an institutional review board (IRB) for review. IRBs may ask for and obtain certain information prior to determining the risk status of the device. A risk assessment determination and the rationale of the sponsor's decision should be provided to the IRB by the sponsor.

In deciding whether a device presents significant or nonsignificant risks, the sponsor and, ultimately, the IRB should consider the device's total risks, not the risks compared with those of alternative devices or procedures. If the device is used in conjunction with a procedure involving risk, the IRB should consider the risks of the procedure in conjunction with the risks of the device. The IRB may choose to agree or disagree with the sponsor's initial determination of degree of risk. Sponsors must notify FDA when an IRB determines that a device, judged by the sponsor to present a nonsignificant risk, is, in fact, a significant risk device. On rare occasions, FDA may differ from the IRB's conclusion and overrule the board's decision that a device presents a nonsignificant risk.

B. Requirements for Investigation of Nonsignificant Risk Devices

Sponsors of studies involving nonsignificant risk devices must submit IDE applications to FDA only if FDA notifies them that submission is required. FDA considers a nonsignificant risk device investigation to have an approved IDE application if the sponsor (a) obtains a nonsignificant risk determination from the IRB, after presenting the IRB with a brief explanation of why the device does not pose a significant risk, and (b) obtains IRB approval for the study.

To maintain consideration of the study as having an approved IDE application, the sponsor must:

Label the device in accordance with the IDE regulation.
Maintain IRB approval throughout the investigation.
Ensure that investigators obtain and document informed consent under 21 CFR Part 50 for each subject under their care unless, in accordance with 21 CFR 56.109(c), documentation is waived by an IRB.
Comply with IDE requirements, as specified, for monitoring investigations, maintaining records, and making reports.
Ensure that participating investigators maintain records and make reports as required.
Comply with prohibitions on promotion, test marketing, and commercialization of investigational devices, and on unduly prolonging an investigation.

C. Requirements for Investigation of Significant Risk Devices

A sponsor of a significant risk device investigation must obtain approval from both FDA and an IRB before beginning an investigation. Under the IDE, sponsors are required to have an approved IDE application to conduct clinical investigations on the safety and effectiveness of significant risk devices.

To obtain IDE approval for a significant risk device investigation, a sponsor must do the following.

Develop an investigational plan and assemble reports of prior investigations.
Select qualified investigators, provide them with all necessary information on the plan and on reports of prior investigations, and obtain signed agreements from them.
Submit the investigational plan and reports of prior investigations to the IRB for review and approval.
Submit a complete IDE application to FDA for review and obtain FDA approval of the IDE.

An IDE application is considered approved 30 days after a complete IDE application has been received by FDA unless FDA otherwise informs the sponsor.

D. Content of Applications

Original Application

There is no preprinted form for IDE applications, but the Code of Federal Regulations [21 CFR 812.20(b)] details the kinds of information they must contain, including the following items.

1. Name and address of sponsor
2. Complete reports of prior investigation, including:

    (a) Results of all prior clinical, animal, and laboratory testing
    (b) Bibliography of relevant unpublished information, whether adverse or supportive
    (c) Summary of relevant unpublished information, whether adverse or supportive
    (d) Statement of extent of compliance with the Good Laboratory Practices regulation

3. Complete investigational plan, or an accurate summary, in the following order:

    (a) Name and intended use of the device and objectives and duration of the investigation
    (b) Written protocol describing the methodology and scientific soundness of the investigation
    (c) Risk analysis
    (d) Description of the device, important components, and principles of operation
    (e) Monitoring procedures and names and addresses of monitors

4. Description of methods, facilities, and controls used for manufacture, processing, packing, storage, and installation of the device
5. Example of the agreement to be signed by investigators and a list of names and addresses of investigators
6. Certification that all investigators have signed the agreement
7. List of name, address, and chairperson of each IRB that reviews the investigation and certification of IRB action concerning the investigation
8. Name and address of any institution (other than those above) at which a part of the investigation may be conducted
9. The amount, if any, charged for the device and an explanation of why sale does not constitute commercialization
10. A claim for categorical exclusion or an environmental assessment, under 21 CFR 25—the Environmental Impact Consideration regulation
11. All labeling for the device
12. Copies of all informed consent forms and all related informational materials to be provided to subjects
13. Any other relevant information that FDA requests for review

E. Responsibilities

The IDE regulation specifies basic requirements for conducting investigations and identifies the responsibilities of participants. Sponsors are required to do the following.

Submit an IDE application (or supplemental application) to FDA.

Ensure that both FDA and an IRB have approved the application (or supplemental application) before beginning an investigation (or part of an investigation).

Select investigators qualified by training and experience to investigate the device and obtain signed investigator agreements as well as curricula vitae.

Ensure proper monitoring of the investigation directly or through qualified monitors, including immediate evaluation of unanticipated adverse device effects and termination of investigations that present unreasonable risks to the subject.

Provide investigators with copies of the investigational plan and reports of prior investigations.

Secure compliance, or discontinue shipment of device if an investigator is not complying with the signed agreement, investigational plan, or stipulation of approval by FDA or an IRB.

Ship the devices only to qualified investigators.

Ensure that the IRBs and FDA are informed of significant new information about the investigation.

Secure IRB and FDA approval for resumption of terminated investigations.

Maintain accurate, complete, and current records on the investigation, including correspondence, records of shipment or disposition, signed investigator agreements, and records of adverse effects.

Prepare and submit complete, accurate, and timely reports, including unanticipated adverse device effects, withdrawal of IRB or FDA approval, investigator lists, progress and final reports, recall and device dispositions, reports of emergency protocol deviations, and reports of device use without informed consent.

Avoid commercialization or testing marketing of the device under investigation.

Avoid representing the investigational device to be safe and effective for its investigated use.

Ensure that the investigation is not unduly prolonged.

Permit FDA inspection.

Investigators are required to do the following.

Obtain IRB and FDA approval before allowing a subject to participate in the investigation.

Conduct investigations according to signed agreements, the investigational plan, applicable FDA regulations, and any other conditions of approval imposed by an IRB or FDA.

Ensure that informed consent has been properly obtained and documented in accordance with 21 CFR Part 50.

Supervise the use of devices on subjects who are in the investigator's area of supervision.

Maintain records relating to investigations, including correspondence, shipment records, subjects' case histories and exposure to the device, informed consent, adverse device effects, and protocol deviations.

Prepare and submit reports including unanticipated adverse device effects, withdrawal of IRB approval, progress and final reports, deviations from investigational plan, and device use without informed consent.

Permit FDA inspection.

IRBs must comply with all applicable requirements of the IRB, informed consent, and the IDE regulations (21 CFR Parts 50, 56, and 812) in reviewing and approving investigations. IRBs are required to:

Be composed of qualified members as specified in the regulation.

Adopt and follow written review procedures.

Ensure that IRB business is conducted with a majority of members present and that members with conflicts of interest do not participate in the review of investigations.

Review all research activities.

Evaluate risks and benefits to subjects, knowledge to be gained, and the adequacy of informed consent.

Review proposed investigations in a timely manner.

Notify investigators, officials of the institutions, and sponsors, if appropriate, of IRB decisions and the basis for them.

Maintain certain records in accordance with 21 CFR Part 56.

Permit authorized FDA employees to inspect records.

VII. NEW DRUG APPLICATION VERSUS PREMARKET APPROVAL APPLICATION

Under the conditions described in Section II, a drug delivery system may be regulated as a drug or as a device. This section describes the two primary premarketing approval processes: the new drug application (NDA); for "new" drugs and the premarket approval application (PMA) for "new" devices (Tables 3 and 4).

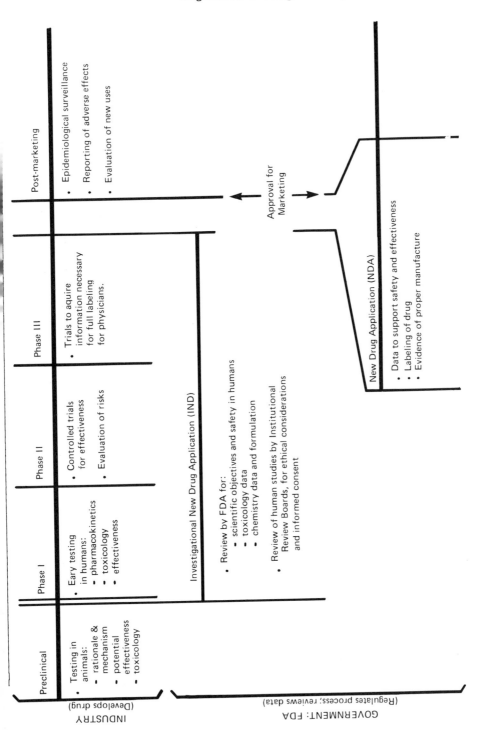

112

TABLE 4 Bringing Devices to Market

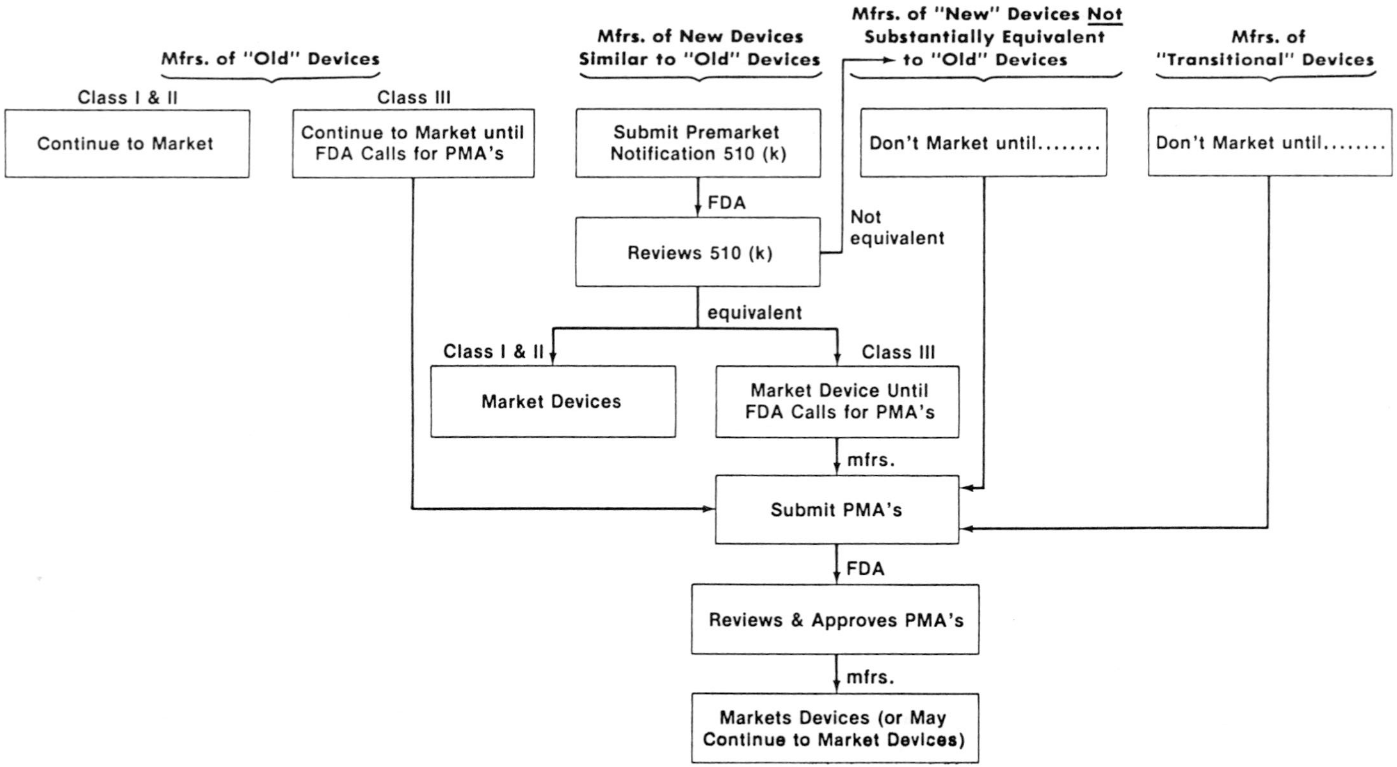

Mfrs. of "Old" Devices

Class I & II
Continue to Market

Class III
Continue to Market until
FDA Calls for PMA's

Mfrs. of New Devices
Similar to "Old" Devices

Submit Premarket
Notification 510 (k)

FDA

Reviews 510 (k)

Not equivalent

equivalent

Class I & II
Market Devices

Class III
Market Device Until
FDA Calls for PMA's

mfrs.

Submit PMA's

FDA

Reviews & Approves PMA's

mfrs.

Markets Devices (or May
Continue to Market Devices)

Mfrs. of "New" Devices Not
Substantially Equivalent
to "Old" Devices

Don't Market until........

Mfrs. of
"Transitional" Devices

Don't Market until........

A. New Drug Application

The Center for Drugs and Biologics (CDB) is the FDA element responsible for ensuring that human drugs and biologics are safe and effective and that product labeling is truthful and informative. CDB reviews NDAs. Headquarters of the Center are at 5600 Fishers Lane,
Rockville, Maryland 20857. Laboratory facilities are located on the
National Institutes of Health campus, Bethesda, Maryland; in Washington, DC; and in St. Louis, Missouri.

CDB evaluates and approves new drugs for marketing on the basis
of safety and effectiveness and also assures that these drugs are properly labeled. Human drug regulation involves two different processes
called the IND (investigational new drug) and the NDA (new drug application) review processes.

Before the center permits a new drug to be tested on humans,
the drug's sponsor must file an IND—a "Notice of Claimed Investigational Exemption for a New Drug." The IND contains the drug's structural formula, results of animal testing, proposed protocol for clinical
testing on humans, patient consent forms, and other data. The center
reviews the IND to determine whether the data are complete and sufficient to permit initiating clinical trials. Investigations may begin 30
days after a sponsor files an application unless FDA advises to the
contrary. The center monitors the clinical trials performed under the
IND.

Before marketing a drug that it believes has demonstrated safety
and efficacy, the sponsor must file an NDA, which contains full information about the proposed product, including results of the clinical
testing. Under the law FDA can approve the NDA only if it finds substantial evidence that the drug is effective. Clinical trials demonstrating this must be adequate and well controlled. In addition, the
drug must be found to be safe; that is, the risks and side effects of
the drug must be acceptable in relation to the benefits of the drug.

An applicant may incorporate by reference [21 CFR 314.50(g)]
information that has previously been submitted to the agency in drug
master files, INDs, and other new drug applications. The identity of
the reference file should be fully described, such as the file name,
the reference number, the date of the submission, and the volume number. If the reference document was submitted by a party other than
the applicant, a "letter of authorization" from such party must be
filed.

To facilitate drug approval, the applicant is required to submit
to copies of an application: an archival copy and a review copy.

Archival Copy [21 CFR 314.50(h)(1)]

The archival copy of an NDA is a complete application; it will be retained as the sole postapproval file copy. Format of the archival copy

includes: (a) an application form, (b) an index, (c) a summary, (d) five technical sections (six for anti-infectives), (e) drug samples and labeling, and (f) case report forms and tabulations. These sections are described below.

Application Form [CFR 314.50(a)]

The application form serves as a cover sheet and contains basic identifying information on the applicant and the proposed drug product. Examples of information to be provided are name and address of the applicant, date of the application, name of the drug product, and a checklist identifying the enclosures filed.

Index [CFR 314.50(b)]

A comprehensive index is required. It must indicate the volume number and page numbers at which the summary, the technical sections, and other supporting information can be located.

Summary [CFR 314.50(c)]

The archival copy must contain an overall summary of the entire application. Each segmented copy of the review copy must also contain this overall summary. The summary is to contain an annotated copy of the proposed labeling, discussion of the benefits and risks of the drug product, a brief description of any marketing history of the drug outside the United States, and a synopsis of each technical section.

Length of the summary depends on the nature of the drug and on the degree of information available. It should be written in the same detail and should meet the editorial standards required for publication in refereed scientific and medical journals. Since FDA uses the overall summary to prepare the summary basis for approval document, updated summaries should be filed with major resubmissions.

Technical Sections [CFR 314.50(d)]

The five technical sections (six with anti-infectives) of the application must contain all specific information needed by the review of the proposed drug product.

The required technical sections for a new drug application are:

1. Chemistry, Manufacturing, and Controls Section[*]
2. Nonclinical Pharmacology and Toxicology Section

---

[*]This section is described in detail under the discussion of the review copy, below.

3. Human Pharmacokinetics and Bioavailability Section
4. Microbiology Section (anti-infective drugs only)
5. Clinical Data Section
6. Statistical Section

Samples and Labeling [CFR 314.50(e)]

When requested, the applicant is required to provide samples of the drug substance, the drug product, and the reference standards directly to FDA laboratories to determine the regulatory suitability of the proposed analytical methods. The review chemist may also request additional samples to perform a visual examination of the container/closure system and placement of the immediate container label. This section of the application must also include copies of the proposed labels and all other labeling for the drug product.

Case Report Forms and Tabulations [CFR 314.50(f)]

The last section of the archival copy contains the case report tabulations for each adequate and well-controlled study and the case report forms for each patient who died during a clinical study and for each who did not complete the study due to adverse events. Additional case report forms may be requested by the agency, should ancillary data be necessary to conduct a proper review of the application. Applicants are encouraged to meet with the agency prior to submitting an application to discuss the extent of the information that this section requires.

Review Copy [21 CFR 314.50(h)(2)]

The second copy of an application filed with the agency is the reveiw copy. This submission is to have the five or six detailed technical sections, each containing an overall summary and a copy of the application form.

These separately bound sections contain the technical and scientific information required for approval by each of the various review disciplines: clinical, pharmacology, chemistry, statistics, biopharmaceutics, and microbiology (anti-infective drugs only). Filing of this segmented review copy will enable the various scientific reviewers of the agency to evaluate the application *concurrently*, thereby expediting the approval process. Guidelines are available from FDA setting forth the extent and nature of information that should be provided in each technical section.

The chemistry technical section should fully describe the composition, synthesis, manufacture, and stability, as well as the specifications and control procedures for the drug substance, the drug product, and the components used in preparing the drug product. The require-

ments that should be addressed, using the same or similar format to
expedite review, are outlined next.

Drug Substance (active ingredient)

1. *Description.* This material is to include physical properties,
ties, chemical properties, and stability data.

 (a) *Names.* A listing of the names used for the drug substance should be provided, including, where appropriate, the established name, the proprietary name, and
 the chemical name.

 (b) *Formulas.* The chemical structural formula, the molecular
 molecular formula, and the molecular weight should be
 indicated.

 (c) *Physical and chemical properties.* The pertinent physio-
 cochemical characteristics should be described, including
 appearance, odor, density, solubility properties, pH and
 pK_a values, melting and boiling points, isomeric and polymorphic forms, and chemical stability (e.g., potential
 degradation products).

 (d) *Proof of structure.* A full technical description and
 interpretation of the data obtained and the reference
 standards employed in the structure elucidation of the
 drug substance should be provided.

 (e) *Stability.* A complete description and interpretation of
 the studies performed and of the data collected should
 be submitted, including validation data demonstrating
 suitability of the analytical methods utilized. Stability
 samples should be evaluated in containers that approximate
 the containers in which the drug substance is to be stored
 and shipped.

2. *Manufacturers.* The name and address of each manufacturer
that will perform any part of the synthesis, extraction, isolation, and/or purification of the drug substance should be
stated and the responsibilities of each such party described.

3. *Methods of manufacture.* A full description should be provided of the acceptance tests and specifications for the raw
materials, as well as of the methods and components used in
the synthesis, preparation, and purification of the drug substances. This description should be equivalent in detail to
that used in scientific journals. If the drug substance is
prepared by fermentation or by extraction from natural
sources (plant or animal), a full description of each step of
the process should be provided.

4. *Process controls.* A full description of the control procedures
   performed at each stage of the manufacturing, processing, and
   packaging of the drug substance should be provided, including
   the specification and test procedures for pivotal and key/critical
   intermediates.
5. *Specifications and analytical methods.* A full description of
   the acceptance specifications and the analytical methods used
   to assure the identity, strength, quality, and purity of the
   drug substance should be provided. Actual and potential
   impurities should be indicated, such as by-products, degradation products, isomeric and polymorphic components, heavy
   metal contaminants, and residual solvents.

Drug Product (finished dosage form)

1. *Components.* A list of all components used in the manufacture
   of the drug product, regardless of whether they undergo
   chemical change or are removed during manufacture, should
   be included. Each component should be identified by its
   established name, if any, or by its complete chemical name,
   using structural formulas when necessary for specific identification. If any proprietary preparation or other mixtures are
   used as components, their identity should be fully described,
   including a complete statement of composition and of any other
   information that will properly identify the material. Proposed
   alternatives for any listed component should be fully justified.
2. *Composition.* A statement of the quantitative composition
   of the drug product should be provided, specifying the name
   and amount of each active and inactive ingredient contained
   in a stated quantity of the drug product. A batch formula
   should be included which represents the one to be employed
   in the manufacture of the finished dosage form. Any calculated
   excess for an ingredient over the label declaration should be
   designated as such, and the percent excess shown.
3. *Specifications and analytical methods for components.* A full
   description should be provided of the acceptance specifications
   and the test methods used to assure the identity, strength,
   quality, and purity of each inactive ingredient.
4. *Manufacturers.* The name and address of each manufacturer
   that performs the manufacturing, processing, packaging,
   labeling, or control operations of the drug product should
   be listed and the responsibilities of each such party described.
5. *Methods of manufacture, packaging procedures, and in-process
   controls.* A detailed description of the manufacturing and
   packaging procedures should be included. The facilities, the
   materials flow plan, the equipment used, and the various

sampling points should be specified. Submission of a schematic diagram of the production process may be of value. A description of the in-process controls, including analytical tests and appropriate data to support the specifications, should be included.

6. *Specifications and analytical methods for drug product.* A full description should be provided of the sampling plans, the release specifications, and the analytical methods that will be implemented to assure the identify, strength, quality, purity, and bioavailability of the drug product. The accuracy, sensitivity, specificity, and reproducibility of the proposed test methods should be established and documented.

7. *Container closure systems.* Full information should be submitted regarding the physical, chemical, and biological characteristics of the container closer or other component parts of the drug product package to assure its suitability for the intended use. Test methods employed should be specified and the manufacturing process described. A description of the entire packaging operation and relevant in-process controls should also be included.

8. *Stability.* A complete and detailed description of, and data derived from, studies of the stability of the drug product should be submitted. Included would be information showing the suitability of the sampling plans, the analytical methods employed, and the stability protocol. Any additional stability studies under way or contemplated should be indicated. Stability data should be submitted for the finished dosage form in the container closure systems in which it is to be marketed. If the drug product is to be reconstituted at the time of dispensing, stability data should also be included for the solution prepared as directed. The expiration dating period should be clearly specified. If the stability protocol in the NDA submission will not be used to extend the expiration dating period via subsequent annual reports, this intention should be indicated.

Environmental Impact Analysis Report

An environmental impact analysis report must also be filed in accordance with the Code of Federal Regulations (21 CFR 25.1). The environmental impact (if any) of the manufacturing process and of the ultimate use of the drug product should be described.

Only after CDB has approved an NDA for safety and effectiveness, and has approved the labeling, may the drug go on the market. However, the manufacturer must continue to send periodic reports on adverse reactions and other aspects of drug experience. Because of dangers that are revealed, CDB may require changes of labeling or take other actions.

Each IND and NDA is reviewed by a team of FDA scientists: a physician, a pharmacologist, a chemist, a pharmacokineticist, a biometrician (usually), and in the case of antibiotics a biologist or a microbiologist. The center may also present important NDAs to advisory committees, whose recommendations are valued by FDA but are not binding on the agency.

If a manufacturer wants to change a drug with an approved NDA— for example, to claim a new use for it—a supplemental NDA may have to be filed and approved. Some useful new drugs have a potential for abuse. For these, CDB alerts the Drug Enforcement Administration before issuing approval so that the drugs can be placed in the appropriate schedule under the Controlled Substances Act, thus restricting access to them.

B. Premarket Approval Application

As indicated previously, the Center for Devices and Radiological Health (CDRH) is the FDA element responsible for ensuring that medical devices are safe, effective, and properly labeled for their intended use. Headquarters for CDRH are at 5600 Fishers Lane, Rockville, Maryland 20857, and 8757 Georgia Avenue, Silver Spring, Maryland 20910. CDRH is responsible for reviewing premarket approval applications.

Review of a premarket approval application is a four-step review process consisting of:

Administrative and limited scientific review by FDA staff to determine completeness ("filing review")

In-depth scientific and regulatory review by appropriate FDA scientific and compliance personnel ("in-depth review")

Review and recommendation by the appropriate advisory committee ("panel review")

Final deliberations, documentation, and notification of the decision by FDA

During the administrative and limited scientific review, FDA determines whether a PMA includes the type of information required by the FD&C Act and is suitable for filing. The filing of a PMA application not an approval. It merely means that FDA has made a threshold determination that the application is sufficiently complete to permit a substantive review. If the information is presented unclearly or incompletely, or is not capable of withstanding rigorous scientific review, FDA may consider the PMA incomplete and not file it. The filing date, therefore, is the date that FDA receives a PMA it considers to be suitable for filing. The 180-day review period provided by the FD&C Act begins on this filing date.

A PMA accepted for filing undergoes an in-depth scientific review by CDRH personnel and the advisory committee. CDRH then notifies the PMA applicant of any deficiencies. Within the 180-day review period, unless FDA and the applicant have agreed to a longer period, FDA will either approve or disapprove the PMA.

FDA will notify the applicant by letter of its decision, and a *Federal Register* notice will announce the decision and availability of a summary of the safety and effectiveness data on which the decision is based. The applicant and other interested persons are also given an opportunity for administrative review of the FDA approval or denial.

A PMA must be signed by the applicant or an authorized representative. If the applicant does not reside or have a place of business in the United States, the PMA must be countersigned by an authorized representative who does. In this case, the applicant must also submit the representative's name and address.

Contents of the Premarket Approval Application

Unless an omission is justified by the applicant [21 CFR 814.20(d)], a PMA must include all the following.

1. The name and address of the applicant.
2. A table of contents that specifies the volume and page number for each item referred to in the table.

    (a) The PMA must include separate sections on nonclinical laboratory studies and on clinical investigations involving human subjects. Six copies of the PMA are required, each bound in one or more numbered volumes of reasonable size. To facilitate review by the advisory committee(s), additional copies may be requested by FDA.

    (b) Trade secret or confidential commercial or financial information must be included in all copies of the PMA. The applicant must identify in at least one copy any information that it believes to be trade secret or confidential commercial or financial information.

3. A summary section in sufficient detail to provide a general understanding of the data and information in the application. The summary section must contain the following information.

(a) *Indications for use.* Give a general description of the disease or condition that the device will diagnose, treat, prevent, cure, or mitigate. Include a description of the patient population for which the device is intended.

(b) *Device description.* Explain how the device functions, the basic scientific concepts that form the basis for the device, and the significant physical and performance characteristics of the device. A brief description of the manufacturing process should be included if it will significantly enhance the reader's understanding of the device. The generic name of the device as well as any proprietary name or trade name should be included.

(c) *Alternative practices and procedures.* Describe any alternative practices or procedures for diagnosing, treating, preventing, curing, or mitigating the disease or condition for which the device is intended.

(d) *Marketing history.* Give a brief description of the foreign and United States marketing history, if any, of the device. Include a list of all countries in which the device has been marketed and a list of all countries in which the device had been withdrawn from marketing for any reason related to the safety or effectiveness of the device. The description must include the history of the marketing of the device by the applicant and, if known, the history of the marketing of the device by any other person.

(e) *Summary of studies.* Provide in this section (i) an *abstract* of any other data, information, or report described in the PMA under Section 814.20(b)(8)(ii) of 21 CFR 814 and (ii) a *summary* of the results of the clinical investigations and nonclinical laboratory studies conducted by or for the applicant.

The summary must describe the objective of each study or hypothesis tested, a brief discussion of how the data were collected and analyzed, and a brief description of the findings and conclusions, whether positive, negative, or inconclusive. This section must include (i) a summary of the nonclinical laboratory studies submitted in the application, and (ii) a summary of the clinical investigations involving human subjects, including a discussion of subject selection and exclusion criteria, study population, study period, safety and effectiveness data, adverse reactions and complications, patient discontinuation, device failures and replacements, results of statistical analyses of the clinical investigations, contraindications, precautions for use of the device, and other information from the clinical investigations as appropriate (any investigation conducted under an IDE must be identified).

(f) *Conclusions drawn from the studies.* Discuss how the data and information in the application constitute valid scientific evidence within the meaning of 21 CFR 860.7 (Determination of Safety and Effectiveness) and provide reasonable assurance that the device is safe and effective for its intended use. A concluding discussion must present benefit and risk considerations related to the device and must discuss any adverse effects of the device on health and any proposed additional studies or surveillance that the applicant intends to conduct following approval of the PMA.

The applicant's summary section should objectively link the medical claim(s) for the device to the hypotheses tested and conclusions drawn from the findings of all studies and investigations. Biased presentation of the study data and inclusion of promotional claims are to be avoided. When preparing the summary section, the applicant should be able to detect accountability discrepancies, as well as incomplete reporting and study design deficiencies that would be discovered in an in-depth scientific review. A properly developed summary section by the applicant can be the basis for FDA's summary of safety and effectiveness data and will facilitate the FDA and panel review process.

A full and explicit account of the clinical investigations and supporting data are needed to meet the legal requirements imposed by the FD&C Act.

4. A complete description of all the following:

(a) The device, including pictorial representations

(b) Each of the functional components or ingredients of the device if the device consists of more than one physical component or ingredient

(c) The properties of the device relevant to the diagnosis, treatment, prevention, cure, or mitigation of a disease or condition

(d) The principles of operation of the device

(e) The methods, facilities, and controls used in the manufacture, processing, packing, storage, and, where appropriate, installation of the device in sufficient detail to permit a person generally familiar with current good manufacturing practices to make a knowledgeable judgment about the quality control used in the manufacture of the device

5. Reference to any performance standard promulgated under Section 514 of the FD&C Act or the Radiation Control for Health and Safety Act of 1968 (42 USC 263b et seq.) in effect or proposed at the time of the PMA submission, and to any voluntary standard that is relevant to any aspect of the safety or effectiveness of the device.

    The applicant must provide adequate information to demonstrate how the device meets, or justify any deviation from, any of the above types of mandatory performance standards. The applicant must also explain any deviation from a voluntary standard.

6. Technical sections containing data and information in sufficient detail to permit FDA to determine whether to approve or disapprove the application. These sections and their contents are as follows.

    (a) A section containing results of the nonclinical laboratory studies with the device. This section must include information on microbiology, toxicology, immunology, biocompatibility, stress, wear, shelf life, and other laboratory or animal tests as appropriate. Information on nonclinical laboratory studies must include a statement that each such study was conducted in compliance with 21 CFR 58 (Good Laboratory Practices for Nonclinical Laboratory Studies) or, if not conducted in compliance with such regulations, a brief statement of the reason.

    (b) A section containing results of the clinical investigations involving human subjects. This section must include protocols; number of investigators and subjects per investigator; subject selection and exclusion criteria; study population; study period, safety, and effectiveness data; adverse reactions and complications; patient discontinuation; patient complaints; device failures and replacements; tabulations of data from all individual subject report forms; and copies of such forms for each subject who died during a clinical investigation or did not complete the investigation; results of statistical analyses of the clinical investigations, device failures, and replacements; contraindications and precautions for use of the device; and any other appropriate information from the clinical investigations. *Any investigation conducted under an IDE must be identified as such.* Information on clinical investigations involving human subjects must include the following.

        (i) A statement that each study either was conducted in compliance with institutional review board (IRB) regulations in 21 CFR 56 or was not subject to the

regulations (21 CFR 56.104 or 56.105), and that
it was conducted in compliance with the informed
consent regulations in 21 CFR 50. If not conducted
in compliance with these regulations, a brief statement of the reason is needed.

(ii) A statement that each study was conducted in compliance with the Code of Federal Regulations: Part
812 (Investigational Device Exemptions) or Part 813
(Investigational Exemptions for Intraocular Lenses).
If not conducted in compliance with those regulations, a brief statement of the reason is needed.

7. A justification showing why data and other information from
a single investigator are sufficient to demonstrate the safety
and effectiveness of the device and to ensure reproducibility
of test results if the PMA is based solely on data from one
investigator.

8. A bibliography of all published reports not already submitted,
whether adverse or supportive, that concern the safety or
effectiveness of the device. Also required are identification,
discussion, and analysis of any other data, information, or
report (foreign or domestic) relevant to an evaluation of the
safety and effectiveness of the device. This includes information from investigations other than those proposed in the application and from commercial marketing experience. Copies of
such published reports or unpublished information in the
possession of (or reasonably obtainable by) the applicant,
must be made available if requested by an FDA advisory committee or FDA.

9. One or more samples of the device and its components, if requested by FDA. If it is impractical to submit a requested
sample of the device, the applicant should name the location
at which FDA may examine and test one or more devices.

10. Copies of all proposed labeling for the device; such labeling
may include instructions for installation and any information,
literature, or advertising that constitutes labeling under Section 201(m) of the FD&C Act.

11. An environmental assessment under Part 25.22(a)(18) unless
the action qualifies for an exclusion. If the applicant believes
that the action qualifies for exclusion, the PMA must provide
information that establishes to FDA's satisfaction that the requested action is within the excluded category and meets the
criteria for the applicable exclusion.

12. Such other information as FDA may request.

If necessary, FDA will obtain the concurrence of the appropriate FDA
advisory committee with respect to the following.

Other information. Pertinent information already in FDA files and specifically referred to by an applicant may be incorporated into a PMA by reference. Information in a master file or other information submitted to FDA by a person other than the applicant cannot be part of a PMA unless such reference is authorized in writing by the person who submitted the information or the master file. If not referenced within 5 years after its submission to FDA, the master file is returned to the person who submitted it.

Omissions. If an applicant believes that certain required information under Section 814.20(b) is not applicable to the device and omits any such information from its PMA, the applicant must submit a statement that identifies the omitted information and justifies the omission. This statement is submitted as a separate section in the PMA and is identified in the table of contents. FDA will notify the applicant if it does not accept the justification for the omission.

Updates. An applicant must periodically update a pending application. He must supply any new safety and effectiveness information about the device acquired from ongoing or completed studies that may affect an evaluation of the safety and effectiveness of the device or the statement of contraindications, warnings, precautions, and adverse reactions in the draft labeling. The update report must be consistent with data reporting provisions of the protocol. The applicant must submit *three copies* of any update report and include in the report the PMA number assigned by FDA. These updates are considered as *amendments* to the pending PMA. The time frame for review of a PMA will not be extended due to the submission of an update report unless the update is a major amendment. An applicant must submit these reports 3 months after the filing date, following receipt of an approvable letter, and at any other time as requested by FDA.

Color additive. If a color additive is used in or on the device and has not previously been listed for such use, an applicant (in lieu of submitting a color additive petition under Part 71) may submit the information as part of the PMA. When submitted as part of the PMA, the information must be submitted separately in three copies, each bound in one or more numbered volumes of reasonable size. A PMA for a device with a color additive that is subject to Section 706 of the FD&C Act will not be approved until the color additive has been listed for use in or on the device.

VIII. GOOD MANUFACTURING PRACTICE FOR MEDICAL DEVICES

A. Introduction

In addition to the various premarketing requirements previously described, manufacturers must all comply with the Good Manufacturing Practice (GMP) for Medical Devices regulation during the production of most medical devices. Since the focus of our discussion is the regulation of drug delivery devices, our discussion will be limited to the GMP for medical devices regulation (21 CFR 820). The reader who is producing a new drug should conform to the Current Good Manufacturing Practice for Finished Pharmaceuticals regulation (21 CFR 211).

The GMP is a mandated quality assurance (QA) program for manufacturers of medical devices. If firms perform the activities required by the GMP regulation, there is a high probability that their devices would meet their quality claims and that these firms would be prepared for a GMP inspection of their manufacturing operations by an FDA investigator. The GMP encompasses environmental control, equipment maintenance, device master records, production control, quality audits, labeling, packaging, and complaints.

B. Flexibility of the Good Manufacturing Practice

The Code of Federal Regulations (21 CFR 820.5) outlines the requirement for medical device manufacturers to prepare and implement an appropriate QA program:

> Every finished device manufacturer shall prepare and implement a quality assurance program that is appropriate to the specific device manufactured and meets the requirements of this part.

Thus, the GMP rule is a flexible regulation. FDA has identified in the GMP the essential elements that a QA system must embody, without prescribing specific ways in which to establish them. Because the GMP regulation must embrace a broad spectrum of devices and manufacturing processes, it allows a certain leeway in the details of QA programs. It is left to manufacturers to determine the pertinence of, or necessity for, certain QA elements and to develop and implement specific procedures tailored to their particular manufacturing processes and devices.

Manufacturers must use good judgment when developing their GMP program and must apply the device GMP as appropriate for their specific products and operations (21 CFR 820.5). For complex devices and complex manufacturing processes, compliance with all requirements

of the GMP is usually necessary. For less complex products and manufacturing processes, however, strict adherence to the GMP becomes
less necessary and some requirements may not be necessary to assure
that the finished device will conform to specifications.

All manufacturers of medical devices must establish and implement
a QA program under the general umbrella of the medical device GMP
regulation that is specific to the nature of the device and the manufacturing processes used. How well the program meets GMP requirements
is monitored by audits. During the GMP self-audit, the auditor must
first identify the elements of the company's QA program, determine
how well each element is functioning, and determine its adequacy in
light of the intent of the device GMP regulation (i.e., to assure con-
formity to master record specifications) and adequacy with respect
to meeting the company's quality claims.

C. Good Manufacturing Practice Applications and Exemptions

Following is a summary of GMP applications and exemptions.

1. The GMP applies to the manufacture of finished devices com-
    mercially distributed for human use unless (a) there is an
    approved exemption in effect or (b) the device is manufac-
    tured exclusively for export and meets all the necessary con-
    ditions for export.
2. In some cases, components may be finished devices or acces-
    sories (e.g., blood tubing). Manufacturers of accessories
    are subject to the GMP when the devices are labeled and sold
    separately for health-related purposes.
3. The designation of a device as a "custom" device does not
    confer a GMP exemption.
4. Contract manufacturers and specification developers must com-
    ply with the sections of the GMP that apply to the functions
    they perform. Contract test laboratories are not routinely
    scheduled for GMP inspections. They are considered exten-
    sions of the manufacturer's QA program.

FDA has determined that certain types of establishments are exempt
from the GMP; and FDA has defined GMP responsibilities for others.
Exemption from the GMP regulation does not exempt manufacturers of
finished devices from keeping complaint files (21 CFR 820.198) or from
general requirements concerning records (820.180). Sterile devices
are never exempted from the GMP regulation.

Section 820.1 states that the GMP does not apply to component
manufacturers. Currently, FDA policy is to rely on the finished device manufacturer to assure that components are acceptable for use.

Devices such as tubing sets that are packaged, labeled, and distributed separately for health-related purposes are sometimes referred to
as components. However, FDA considers them to be finished devices
in that they are "suitable for use," and the manufacturer must comply
with the GMP. A device sold to supplement the performance of a
finished medical device is an accessory. Accessories are finished devices subject to Section 820.3(j) of the GMP.

A repacker or relabeler is a manufacturer, as stated in Section
820.3(k), and is subject to the applicable requirements of the GMP
regulation if the firm does one or more of the following:

1. Packages and/or labels previously manufactured finished
   devices
2. Receives finished devices in bulk (e.g., surgical tubing, syringes, media, etc.) and repacks them into individual packages
   and labels them
3. Receives previously manufactured devices, which have been
   packaged and labeled by another manufacturer, and combines
   them into a kit with other unpackaged devices, which are received in bulk

A firm is not a repacker or relabeler for purposes of the GMP if it
packs only previously packaged and labeled individual devices into
convenience packages.

A specification developer is a manufacturer and thus is subject
to the GMP requirements that apply to the activities conducted, such
as correct transfer of the design information to a contract manufacturer (820.100). This activity requires an adequate device master
record (820.181) and adequate change control. Furthermore, if the
product carries the specification developer's label, the developer is
responsible for maintaining a complaint file and processing complaints,
plus maintaining appropriate master records.

D. Quality Assurance Program

A quality assurance system consists of an organization that performs
a QA program according to documented policy and specifications to
achieve stated objectives. All activities and product quality data are
monitored and any deviations from policy and specifications are fed
back into the system, where the deviations may be corrected. "The
organization" is everyone in the company. The written policies and
objectives are set by management and are influenced by outside factors such as customer requirements, standards, and regulations. The
objectives are to produce safe and effective devices at a profit. The
documentation is the device master record, composed of product-specific
technical documentation, such as engineering drawings, and general
documentation, such as standard operating procedures.

If the required activities including the feedback are performed, the system is self-correcting and, thus, it is operating in a state of control. FDA requires manufacturers of medical devices to operate in a state of control.

E. Good Manufacturing Practice Versus Total Quality Assurance

An effective QA program is far more likely to prevent manufacture and shipping of defective products than a quality control (QC) program alone. Quality controls such as inspection and testing are important in feeding information back into the QA program. Here, action can be started to correct the root causes of problems. This is far better than superficial corrections by pass/fail quality control inspection of finished product or in-process assemblies.

Intrinsic, or desired quality is established by the design specifications for the product, its components, and the manufacturing process. Complying with the GMP assures that the manufacturing process can consistently achieve desired levels of quality and that the finished device meets its design or master record specifications. This is a significant quality step. However, the GMPs have a limitation. If the device as designed is of poor quality, the GMPs will only assure that the poor-quality device is consistently produced. To overcome this, many firms use an overall QA program embracing evaluation of customer needs, product design, development and evaluation, labeling development and control, all manufacturing and control activities, and customer feedback. The GMP actually covers all these areas except customer needs and initial product design. The GMP has a significant impact on the control of product design after production starts because of GMP requirements on changes to master records, data feedback, complaint processing, and corrective actions.

Because the intrinsic quality level is established during the design or preproduction phase, the QA program must include this phase to assure overall quality and to meet company quality claims. Quality assurance personnel should participate in the review, evaluation, and documentation of the product and process design. It is from data established during this phase that all other activities (i.e., processes, purchasing, and testing) derive. Development and evaluation data are also useful in cases of regulatory or product liability actions. They show that the design and manufacturing processes were well conceived and properly qualified, reviewed, and documented.

Component and raw material specifications developed during the design phase must be well conceived and adequate for their intended purpose. Manufacturing methods and processes to be used must be developed, equipment selected, and processes and methods qualified. Production specifications and methods employed in manufacturing must result in standard in-process and finished products without excessive sorting or reprocessing. Inspection and test methods must be developed that will adequately monitor product characteristics to ensure they are within the acceptable specifications. These methods should be developed, verified, and documented during the product and process development phase. They should be implemented at the beginning of routine production. Adverse effects that manufacturing processes, manufacturing materials, or equipment may have on product safety and function must be identified. Acceptance methods must be developed for accurate measurement of outgoing product quality.

The GMP requires that each manufacturer prepare and implement QA procedures adequate to assure that a formally established and documented QA program is performed. "Formally established" means not only formal documentation, but an obvious commitment to quality from top management. In many firms, this is accomplished through such means as a management policy, assignment of responsibilities and authorities, and general statements and actions that define and support the goals of the QA program. This policy is supported by a number of QA documents, such as qualification methods, sampling procedures, inspection/test procedures, product audits, and records indicating that measurement and monitoring of quality has occurred. The number of documents needed depends on the size and complexity of the operation and the characteristics of the product.

F. Organization of a Quality Assurance Program

FDA is more concerned with the adequacy and appropriateness of QA activities than it is with organizational structure. The regulations state that where possible, one or more designated individuals not having direct responsibility for the performance of a manufacturing operation shall be responsible for the QA program. The GMPs identify some of the objectives a QA system must embody but do not prescribe a specific organizational structure or specific ways to fulfill them.

One of the most important responsibilities of the QA unit is to identify QA problems, to recommend and provide solutions, and to verify implementation of the solutions [21 CFR 820.20(a)(3)].

The QA unit is also responsible for assuring that all components, packaging, labeling, and manufacturing materials have been approved for use and that contracted items and services are suitable. Additionally, the QA unit should assure that production records are reviewed before the product is distributed. These are the records required by the GMP for the device history record. They should be reviewed to verify that the operations they represent have been conducted and that the records are complete.

Typically, QA identifies problems with device quality through review of inspection/test data, trend analysis of history and repair records, failure analysis, analysis of complaints, and review of other objective data. In this regard, reduction in productivity is often an indicator of quality problems. Also, measurement of scrap and rework can highlight quality problems and reduce costs. These are examples of sources of feedback to the QA organization. Feedback is necessary to verify the adequacy of the manufacturing process and the controls used. It also helps trigger corrective action to solve root causes of quality problems, rather than just performing rework.

The QA unit must determine that all tests and inspections are performed correctly [21 CFR 820.20(a)(4)]. Some of the methods used to accomplish this are training, QA system audits, review of QA records, and product audits. However, simply instituting a QA control program and checking that it is conducted correctly is not enough to satisfy the GMP regulation. The GMP regulation also requires that QA controls be qualified to ensure they are appropriate and adequate for their purpose. The qualification should be done during final product development, pilot production, and, of course, whenever product and/or processes are modified.

G. Personnel Training and Responsibility

No matter how effective QA and production systems are as concepts, people still play the major role in producing a quality product. Personnel involved in QA activities must be properly trained, both by education and by experience. The GMP regulation requires QA training for manufacturing and QA personnel [21 CFR 820.25(a)]. Lack of training can lead to defective products and, sometimes, to regulatory or liability problems.

A QA system should maintain an ongoing formal program for training and motivating all personnel. All personnel should be made aware that product quality is not solely the responsibility of management. Quality is the responsibility of every employee—any employee can potentially generate a quality problem through negligence. It is extremely important to understand the following points with respect to typical quality-related functions.

1. Research and development has primary responsibility for designing quality into the device.
2. Technical services has primary responsibility for documenting the design.
3. Manufacturing, process, or "scaleup" engineering has primary responsibility for designing quality into the manufacturing processes.
4. Manufacturing personnel have primary responsibility for producing devices that have the maximum level of quality that can be achieved based on the product and process designs.

5. Quality assurance has primary responsibility for QA program management, status reports, audits, problem identification, data analysis, and so on.

A medical device manufacturer must never try to operate on the basis that the QA unit has primary and direct responsibility for the quality of the products. In reality, it is part of the responsibility of the QA unit to direct attention toward the correct department where the quality problem arises.

Where necessary, employees should be certified to perform certain manufacturing or QA procedures. Records of training and/or certification should be maintained. Personnel performing QA functions must:

Have sufficient, well-defined responsibilities and authority
Be afforded freedom to identify and evaluate quality problems
Be able to formulate, obtain, and recommend possible solutions
    for QA problems
Verify implementation of solutions to quality problems

When the QA program is operational, QA must continue to look for problem areas or factors that can have an impact on product quality. Many factors can have an impact on the quality program, such as:

Changes in, or absence of, personnel
Uncomfortable working conditions (e.g., breakdowns in air con-
    ditioning or heating equipment)
Increases in workload or production rates
Introduction of new production or inspection equipment
Changes in company incentive techniques (e.g., placing hourly
    employees on piecework can cause deterioration of product
    quality)
Changes in sources for purchased components and materials, as
    well as changes in components, products, or process tech-
    niques

H. Summary

Quality assurance must be an integrated effort. It is a total systems approach that satisfies the particular needs of a specific manufacturer, product, and user market. It must not consist merely of inspection and testing, or spot solutions. In all cases, quality must be considered at the earliest stages in every significant area that has an effect on the quality, safety, and effectiveness of the device. These areas include product development, design evaluation, component and/or vendor selection, documentation, development of labeling, design transfer, process development and validation, pilot production, routine manufacturing, testing/inspection, history record evaluation, distribution, service, and complaints. After the QA program has been put in place and checked, it must not be allowed to stagnate—it must continue to be dynamic. A QA program remains dynamic through continuous feedback, "big-picture" monitoring by system audits, and corrective action. Most important, management and employees must have the correct attitude if their QA program is to be effective. Quality consciousness must be developed in every employee. Each person must be made aware of the importance of his or her individual contributions in the effort to achieve an acceptable level of quality.

REFERENCES

1. U.S. Congress, House Committee on Interstate and Foreign Commerce, Medical Devices, Hearings before the Subcommittee on Public Health and the Environment, Oct. 23-24, 1973, Serial No. 93-61. Government Printing Office, Washington, DC, 1973.
2. Federal Food, Drug, and Cosmetic Act, as Amended Section 201(g). Government Printing Office, Washington, DC, 1985, p. 1.
3. Federal Food, Drug, and Cosmetic Act, as Amended, Section 201(h). Government Printing Office, Washington, DC, 1985, p. 2.
4. J. F. Stigi and A. C. Kohler, *Regulatory Requirements for Medical Devices—A Workshop Manual.* Government Printing Office, Washington, DC, 1985, p. III-5.
5. J. F. Stigi and A. C. Kohler, *Everything You Always Wanted to Know About the Medical Device Amendments . . . And Weren't Afraid to Ask.* Government Printing Office, Washington, DC, 1984, p. 9.
6. K. Mohan, Office of Device Evaluation, Food and Drug Administration, Silver Spring, MD. Personal Communication, June 30, 1986.
7. J. F. Stigi and A. C. Kohler, *Regulatory Requirements for Medical Devices—A Workshop Manual.* Government Printing Office, Washington, DC, 1985, p. VI-3.

Part Two
PUMPS AND IMPLANTABLE/ INFUSION SYSTEMS

4
Osmotic Pumps

JOHN W. FARA and NIGEL RAY / ALZA Corporation, Palo Alto,
California

I. INTRODUCTION

Drug delivery systems for routine use in preclinical and clinical research now provide the means for rate- and duration-controlled delivery of most drugs, locally or systemically, at rates chosen by the investigator. In preclinical studies, the use of implantable osmotic pumps for rate-controlled delivery of a wide variety of bioactive agents virtually has replaced the clumsy alternative of connecting small animals to heavy infusion pumps. Previously, the only implantable, long-duration, rate-controlled delivery devices were drug-containing Silastic tubes. These devices are restricted to their application to steroids and similar drugs because of the permeability characteristic of Silastic tubing. As their operation required the drug to diffuse across the wall of the tube, rate control was imprecise and the system required adjustment of membrane thickness and area for every specific compound studied. In contrast, osmotically powered delivery devices provide rate-controlled, unattended administration of a wide range of solutions or suspensions of drugs and other bioactive agents for days or weeks. Rates of administration from these devices are independent of the physical-chemical characteristics of the drug, allowing ionized drugs, peptides, and other macromolecules to be administered at a variety of rates.

Several pump designs utilizing osmotic energy for drug delivery have been described in the literature: the ALZET mini-osmotic pump [1,2] developed by the ALZA Corporation and widely used since it commercial introduction in 1977, and a device described by Shrock et al. and Baker in 1986 [3,4], which has yet to be proven in widespread experimental use. Both are variants of the Rose-Nelson pump [5], first described in 1955. Because of the extensive number of scientific studies published on the design and use of the Alzet pump, this chapter will focus on the two types of miniature, self-powered, osmotic pumps developed by ALZA.

ALZET pumps are designed to deliver solutions or suspensions continuously at controlled rates for prolonged periods. They have been used as subcutaneous or intraperitoneal delivery platforms in laboratory animals and have been used for site-specific administration by means of a catheter attached to the delivery port of the pump. Based

on similar technology, the OSMET drug delivery module developed by
ALZA is available for use for oral, vaginal, or rectal rate-controlled
administration of drugs in clinical research.
The impact of the use of these devices on basic pharmacological
research, on drug development, and on the future of therapeutics
will be discussed.

II. BACKGROUND AND DESIGN OF ALZET/OSMET DELIVERY SYSTEMS

A. Background

The osmotic delivery devices developed by ALZA became available for
investigational use in the mid-1970s, and researchers are now using
them routinely in very early stages of drug research, such as drug
screening, animal toxicology and pharmacology, and initial clinical testing. Additionally, applications in these areas are creating new therapeutic opportunities. For example, studies to define drug dosage
regimens—to minimize side effects, maximize therapeutic effect, and
optimize dosing frequency—can now be done early in the development
of a new drug. At both the experimental and clinical levels, use of
the osmotic pumps provides the logic for selecting the appropriate
drug dosage pattern for treatment and in the process eliminates the
need for painstaking empirical investigations. The same types of
investigation are also appropriate for the restudy of older drugs with
unfavorable therapeutic effects or inconvenient dosing schedules.

B. Design and Operation of the Miniature Osmotic Pump

ALZET osmotic pumps are capsular in shape and are manufactured in a
variety of sizes (Fig. 1). In cross section, they are composed of
three concentric layers (Fig. 2): the drug reservoir, the osmotic
sleeve, and the rate-controlling, semipermeable membrane. An
additional component, called the flow moderator, is inserted into the
body of the osmotic pump after filling.
At the core of the pump is the drug reservoir, a cylindrical cavity formed from a synthetic elastomer, which is open to the exterior
via a single portal. The compound the pump is to dispense is placed
in solution or suspension in this compartment. The wall of the drug
reservoir is chemically inert to most drug-vehicle combinations, including aqueous formulations, dilute acids, bases, and alcohols (Table 1).
It is also impermeable, blocking any passage of material between the
drug reservoir and the surrounding osmotic sleeve.
Outside the reservoir wall is the osmotic sleeve, a thin cylindrical
casing containing a high concentration of sodium chloride. The difference in osmotic pressure between this compartment and the aqueous

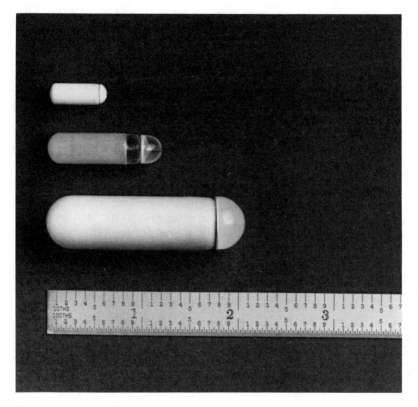

Fig. 1 The three sizes of ALZET osmotic pumps.

environment in which the pump is placed drives the delivery of the
test solution. After implantation of the filled pump, water from the
surrounding tissue enters the pump along the osmotic gradient and
is taken up by the osmotic sleeve, causing it to expand. Due to the
rigidity of the outer membrane, incoming water generates hydrostatic
pressure, resulting in compression of the flexible drug reservoir wall,
and a constant flow of the drug formulation up the flow moderator tube
and out through the delivery portal in the plastic end cap.

The rate at which water enters the osmotic sleeve, hence the pumping rate of the osmotic pump, is regulated by the porosity of the semipermeable membrane, its dimensions, and the osmotic pressure difference across the membrane. As a result, the delivery profile of the
pump is independent of the drug formulation dispensed. Agents of
various types, including ionized drugs, macromolecules, steroids, and
peptides, can be delivered at zero-order release rates. At manufac-

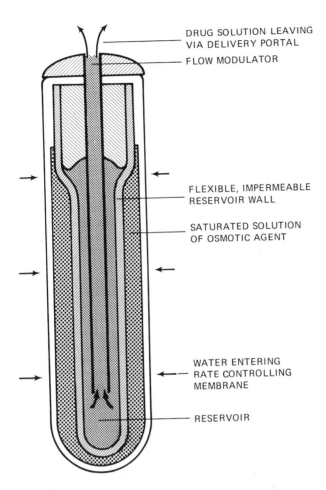

DRUG SOLUTION LEAVING
VIA DELIVERY PORTAL

FLOW MODULATOR

FLEXIBLE, IMPERMEABLE
RESERVOIR WALL

SATURATED SOLUTION
OF OSMOTIC AGENT

WATER ENTERING
RATE CONTROLLING
MEMBRANE

RESERVOIR

Fig. 2 Cross section of a functioning osmotic pump showing cylindrical reservoir for test solution, layer of osmotic driving agent, and semipermeable outer covering of pump.

ture, the rate at which water enters the osmotic sleeve and discharges the reservoir's contents is fixed. Pumps are available with a variety of delivery rates between 0.5 and 10 µl per hour and delivery durations between 3 days and 4 weeks (Fig. 3). Different mass delivery rates of test agents are achieved by varying the concentration of agent in the solution that is used to fill the pump.

The researcher fills the reservoir of the osmotic pump with the desired solution or suspension through the delivery portal, using a special filling tube attached to a syringe. For the pump to function

TABLE 1 Common Solvents Compatible with the
Reservoir Material of ALZET Osmotic Pumps

Distilled water or any aqueous solution

Isotonic NaCl or other salt solution

5% Dextrose in water or NaCl

Ethanol, up to 10% in water

Polyethylene glycol 300, neat or in water

2% Tween in water

DMSO to 50% in water

DMSO 50% + 10% ethanol

Propylene glycol, neat or in water

Glycerol

Dilute acids with pH greater than 1.8

Dilute bases with pH less than 14

Rat serum

Bacteriostatic culture media (1% benzyl alcohol
as bacteriostatic)

Artificial cerebrospinal fluid

---

correctly, all air must be displaced from the reservoir by the test solution. After filling, a flow moderator is inserted through the portal
into the body of the pump. The flow moderator functions to minimize
diffusion of the test agent out of the reservoir, ensuring that the osmotic process will control delivery, and provides a convenient attachment point for a catheter. The absence of air bubbles in the reservoir
can be determined by calculating the weight difference between the
unfilled pump and the filled pump with the flow moderator in place.

Delivery Rate in Vivo and in Vitro

Osmotic pumps are designed to deliver at a constant rate by incorporating into the sleeve compartment a mass of osmotic driving agent
that maintains a constant osmotic pressure difference across the semipermeable membrane throughout the life of the pump. Steady state
delivery is reached after an initial transient period arising from (a)
a time lag for water to enter the osmotic sleeve, (b) equilibration of
the temperature and hydrostatic pressure in the system, and (c)

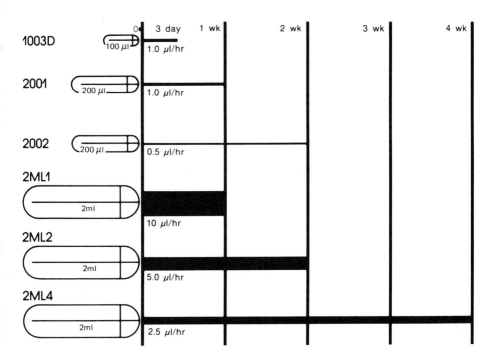

Fig. 3   Comparison of delivery rates and reservoir capacities of ALZET osmotic pumps.

relaxation of the semipermeable membrane to temperature and hydrated equilibria.

After equilibrium has been reached, the constant or zero-order mass delivery rate from the system is given by the equation:

$$Z = \frac{dV}{dt} C_d$$

Where C_d represents the concentration of drug formulated by the researcher and dV/dt the volume imbibition rate of water into the osmotic sleeve compartment.

With π_o the osmotic pressure of the osmotic agent, and the π_e the osmotic pressure of the pump environment, the volume delivery rate from the system can be written as follows:

$$\frac{dV}{dt} = K \frac{A}{h} (\pi_o - \pi_e)$$

In this equation A and h are the membrane area and thickness, respectively, and K is the osmotic permeability coefficient of the membrane.

Figure 4, an example of the volume delivery profile for the model 2002, is typical of the series as a whole. These data indicate that the in vivo and in vitro volume delivery rates of this ALZET pump are within 5% of the labeled rate (0.5 µl/hr). The in vivo delivery rate is obtained with the pump as an implant.

The in vivo and in vitro pumping rates of osmotic pumps are specified for 37°C operating conditions. As permeability and osmotic pressure are a function of the ambient temperature, the rate at which water crosses the semipermeable membrane and enters the osmotic sleeve, hence the release rate of the pump as a whole, is a function of temperature (Fig. 5). The actual pumping rates at temperature T for two models of Alzet pump are given by the following equations:

Model 2001: $Q_T = Q_0 (0.135 \exp(0.054T) - 0.004\pi + 0.03)$

Model 2ML1: $Q_T = Q_0 (0.141 \exp(0.051T) - 0.007\pi + 0.12)$

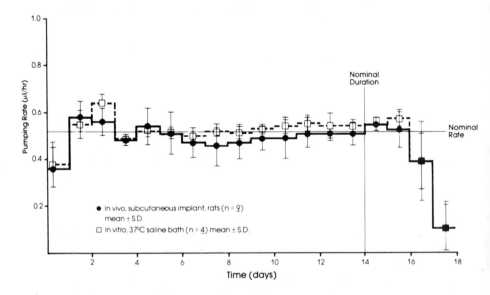

Fig. 4 Example of delivery rates (µl/hr) for model 2002 ALZET osmotic pump in vivo and in vitro. In vivo data were derived from subcutaneous implants in nine rats. In vitro data were obtained from four mini-osmotic pumps immersed in a 37°C bath of 0.9% saline. The in vivo and in vitro rates are shown to be within 5% of each other. The nominal delivery rate is 0.5 µl/hr.

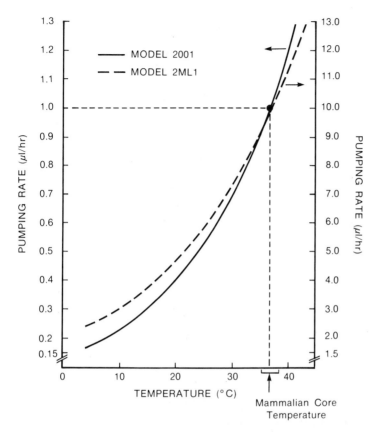

Fig. 5 Temperature dependence of the delivery rate (μl/hr) for models 2001 and 2ML1 from 4°C to over 40°C in 0.9% saline.

Where Q_0 is the specified pumping rate of the pump at 37°C (μl/hr), T is the ambient temperature (°C), and π is the osmotic pressure of the pump environment (atm). Alzet pumps have been used to infuse agents at a variety of body temperatures from fish at 21°C [6] to chickens at 41°C [7].

III. MINIATURE OSMOTIC PUMPS IN BASIC RESEARCH

A. Introduction

Since the introduction of the Alzet pumps nearly 10 years ago, more than 1700 publications have appeared in the scientific literature. Within this broad publication list, more than 500 agents have been delivered

TABLE 2 Classification of Agents Delivered by ALZET Osmotic Pump

Amino acids	Growth factors
Anesthetics	Heavy metals
Antibiotics	Lymphokines
Antibodies	Metabolites
Anticancer agents	Neurotransmitters
Anticoagulants	Nerve growth factors
Antiepileptics	Nucleosides
Antigens	Nucleotides
Antihypertensives	Peptides and peptide hormones
Antiparasitic agents	Prostaglandins
Anti-Parkinson agents	Radioisotopes
Ascitic fluid	Renin-angiotensin system
Catecholamines	hormones/inhibitors
Chelators	Steroids
Cholinergics	Thyroid-related hormones
CNS-acting agents	Toxins
Enzyme inhibitors	Vitamins
Gastrointestinal motility modulators	

using the pumps (Table 2 and chapter appendix) in various animals, including mice, rabbits, rats, dogs, baboons, and sheep (Table 3). Indeed, several novel approaches have been used in cold-blooded animals, including fish, hermit crabs, snakes [8], and iguanas [9]. Review of these publications reveals several general areas of application of rate-controlled delivery at the preclinical level utilizing these osmotic delivery systems.

B. Rate-Controlled Modulation of Hormone Levels

One experimental method employed in endocrinology is to remove an organ or part of an organ by surgery or other means and then observe the resulting effect on the remaining organ systems. Replacement of substances normally produced by the removed organ or tissue can be used to explore the mechanisms of hormone release and hormone

TABLE 3 Major Animal Species in Which ALZET
Pumps Have Been Used

Baboon	Iguana
Cat	Leopard
Cattle	Mouse
Cheetah	Monkey
Chicken	Marmoset
Dog	Pig
Fish (cichlids and trout)	Pigeon
Frog	Rabbit
Gerbil	Rat
Guinea pig	Sheep
Hamster	Squirrel
Horse	Toad

action. This approach has been applied to the adrenals, pancreas,
pituitary, and many other endocrine structures.

As an artificial pancreas, delivery systems have been implanted
to infuse insulin to rats with experimentally (streptozotocin) induced
diabetes [11]. Large pulses of insulin release—typical of meal-eaters—
do not ordinarily occur in this species because the rat does not eat
meals, but instead nibbles day and night. Thus, continuous infusion
provides a means for assaying the total daily need for insulin.

In one study, miniature osmotic pumps were filled with different
concentrations of unmodified crystalline bovine insulin in isotonic saline and implanted subcutaneously to infuse doses of 2, 4, and 10 units
per 200 g rat per day. Isotonic saline-filled pumps were implanted
subcutaneously in other (control) rats with induced diabetes. The
temporal dose-response curve (Fig. 6) showed that a dose of 2 U/day
was sufficient to return the streptozotocin-diabetic rat to normogly-
cemic levels of 90 to 120 mg% [11].

In another study, Patel [12] utilized the osmotic pumps for insulin
replacement in diabetic rats to maintain normoglycemia and normogluca-
gonemia in studies that spanned 60 to 80 days. Prolonged administration was accomplished by repeated serial replacement of osmotic pumps
of 2 weeks' duration. This author's careful attention to detail is illustrated by contrasting the design of Patel's study with that of another
investigation [13], which virtually catalogues the technical problems

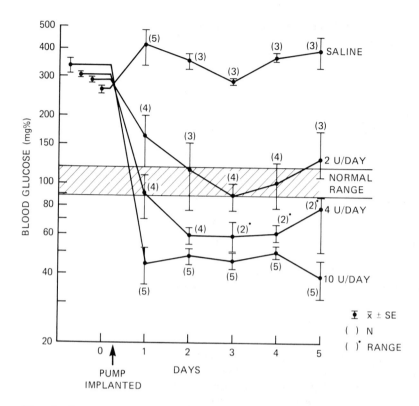

Fig. 6 Dose-response curves of insulin in the streptozotocin-diabetic rat. (From Ref. 11.)

that can confuse the assessment of continuous delivery of a peptide hormone.

In other studies the osmotic pump has been utilized to supply re-placement therapy in animals that have undergone surgical removal of single or multiple endocrine glands such as the thyroid [14,15], pineal [16,17], adrenal [18,19], parathyroid [20,21], hypophysis [22, 23], kidney(s) [24,25], gonads [26-28], or nervous system structures (ganglionectomy, laminectomy, denervation) [29-31]. It has also been utilized for replacement therapy in vitamin-deficient animals.

C. Schedule Dependency of Drug Actions

The literature provides a growing number of examples [20,32-39] of the way that regimen or rate of drug administration can influence the expression of drug actions. Not only anticancer drugs but those used in a variety of therapeutic situations demonstrate a changing range of actions depending on the dosing schedule. Basically, regimen dependence or schedule dependence signifies a shift of the dose-response curve to the right or left according to the time pattern of drug administration. That is, the same total dose of the drug given over the same time period produces different actions when the schedule of its administration changes.

Scaling

Understanding the pharmacokinetics that most drugs have in small laboratory animals is basic to understanding regimen-dependent expressions of drug action. In general, small animals metabolize and/or excrete drugs much more rapidly than humans. Thus, the problem in early drug and toxicity screening and testing is one of scaling, that is, designing the study to permit extrapolating its results from animal to man.

Although experimental designs generally take body weight differences fully into account, they tend to ignore the consequences of time differences in drug metabolism and excretion. Yet differences in plasma half-lives produce very different patterns of drug concentration in species that differ as markedly as mouse and man. The most important consequence of a short drug half-life in small animals is that with a regimen of daily injections, a rapidly absorbable drug quickly reaches high peak concentrations in blood and tissues, then within a short period of time declines to very low levels. In fact, drug will be absent for some time in each dosage interval when a rapidly absorbed and excreted drug is administered to small animals according to the usual (48 times daily) regimen.

According to several investigators [39], scaling in terms of the plasma half-life is on the order of the body weight to the one-quarter power. Thus, in rats and mice plasma half-lives would be one-tenth or less of those in humans. For example, in a recent study by Nau and his colleagues, the plasma half-life of valproate in the mouse is only 0.8 hr, compared to 8 to 16 hr in humans [32].

Extrapolating the results of a mouse toxicity data to humans can therefore give rise to two types of error. The higher peak levels in mice may lead to overestimating human toxicity of a drug; or conversely, the long periods of no detectable drug in mice may lead to underestimating its human toxicity.

Efficacy studies are subject to the same sources of error. Does the test drug's therapeutic action (as has been suggested with some antibiotics) depend on sharp peaking concentrations [40]? If so, then the relatively higher peaks obtained in small animals may lead to false expectations of efficacy in humans. However, if a drug's effectiveness depends on its maintenance in plasma at certain critical levels that dosage three or four times a day could maintain in humans, then the drug's recurrent absence in plasma in preclinical testing on a similar regimen can lead to underestimating its therapeutic potential.

Recent studies by Nau, Sikic, and others show that by comparing two types of drug regimen (e.g., pulsed vs. continuous drug delivery), it is possible to identify the effects associated with peak and trough levels and those associated with constant plasma concentrations. Such protocols illustrate an interesting technique for achieving a more valid basis for extrapolation of animal data to the human.

The Injection-Infusion Comparison (IIC) Protocol

Nau et al. [32] administered valproic acid (VPA) by two different regimens in the same total dose to pregnant mice from days 7 to 15 of gestation: by injection once daily and by continuous, constant-rate infusion from implanted pumps. The injections caused drug concentrations in plasma to peak and decline quickly (Fig. 7); in fact, for long periods between injections, the drug was undetectable. In humans the peaks

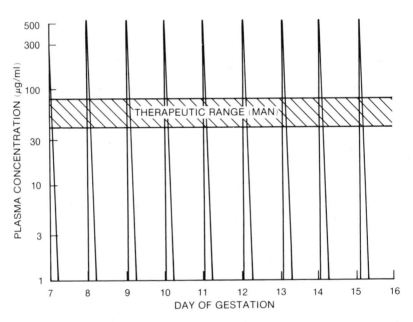

Fig. 7 Concentrations of valproic acid in mice following once daily subcutaneous administration of the drug (400 mg/kg) between days 7 and 15 of gestation. The shaded area represents the range of human plasma concentrations during pregnancy, and the curves show experimental data. (From Ref. 32.)

with the usual therapeutic regimen are only one-tenth as high, but the trough concentrations are many times higher. These differences arise because the half-life of this widely used antiepileptic drug is only 0.8 hr in the mouse but 8 to 16 hr in humans.

The continuous infusion in mice maintained drug and metabolite levels within a narrow range (Fig. 8). Moreover, Nau found that with the infusion mode, higher total dose was required to produce embryotoxicity (resorptions and exencephaly) than with daily injections (Figs. 9 and 10). Thus, the infusion regimen shifted the dose-response curve for embryotoxicity to the right (Fig. 11), such that a 10-fold higher dose was required with the infusion regimen to yield the same resorption rate observed with the injection regimen.

Sikic et al. [33] had previously observed regimen dependence for both the toxic and therapeutic actions of the anticancer drug bleomycin. These workers administered doses of the drug in three different 5 day regiments: injections twice daily, alternate-day injections, and continuous infusions by implanted osmotic pumps. Results associated with drug infusion differed in two ways from results obtained with either injection regimen: at equal total doses, the infusion reduced

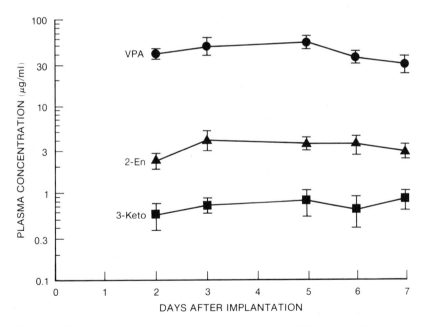

Fig. 8 Plasma concentrations of valproic acid (VPA) and its metabolites (2-En and 3-Keto) in mice after subcutaneous implantation on day 7 of gestation of two osmotic pumps containing 400 mg/ml sodium valproate and deliverying 1 μl/hr of drug. (From Ref. 32.)

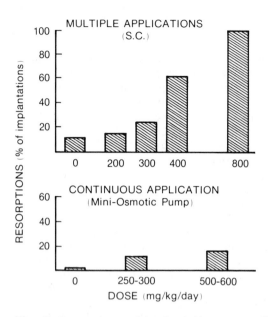

Fig. 9 Percentage of implantation resorptions in mice after administration of valproic acid between days 7 and 15 of gestation. (From Ref. 32.)

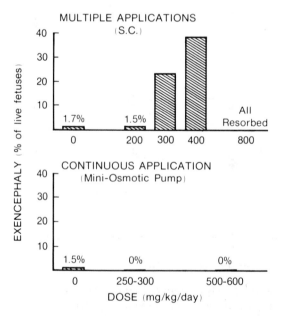

Fig. 10 Incidence of exencephaly in mice following administration of valproic acid between gestational days 7 and 15. (From Ref. 32.)

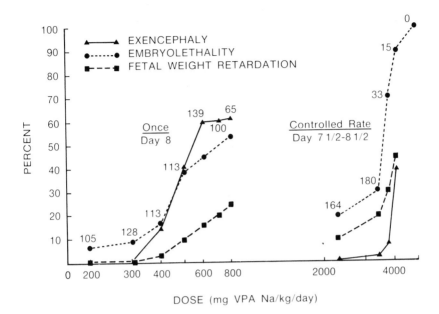

Fig. 11 Dose-response curves for the embryotoxicity (lethality and fetal weight retardation) and teratogenicity (exencephaly) following single subcutaneous injections of VPA on day 8 or controlled-rate administration via subcutaneously implanted mini-osmotic pumps between days 7 and 8 of gestation. The exencephaly rates are given as percentage of live fetuses (controls: water-injected, 0%; water-filled mini-osmotic pumps, 1%). The embryolethality was calculated as percentage resorptions per total implantations (controls: water-injected, 8.3%; water-filled mini-osmotic pumps, 12%). The fetal weight retardation is given as the weight reduction in percent of the weights of the control group (1.18 ± 0.09 g). The numbers of live fetuses examined in each group are given as numerals.

the drug's toxicity (Fig. 12) but increased its antitumor efficacy (Fig. 13). This enhanced efficacy observed with continuous infusion of bleomycin was confirmed by Peng and colleagues [35]. Thus, continuous infusion shifted the dose-response curve for bleomycin toxicity to the right, while shifting the dose-response curve for efficacy to the left. These two observations lead to the conclusion that bleomycin's therapeutic index is widened by use of the infusion regimen and narrowed by the injection regimen. Subsequent clinical studies also appear to confirm the prediction that the human use of bleomycin may be made both safer and more efficacious by use of a constant-rate infusion regiment [40,41].

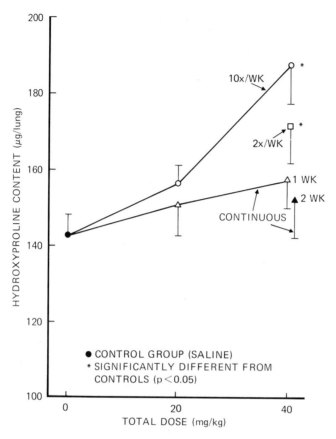

FIG. 12 Effect of various doses and regimens of bleomycin on pulmonary toxicity in nontumored mice, as measured by the hydroxyproline content of lung after 10 weeks of treatment. (From Ref. 33.)

Other experimental studies of regimen dependence using continuous infusion have involved exogenous administrations of hormones, whose effects have long been recognized as rate dependent rather than dose dependent. For example, the action of parathyroid hormone [20], human growth hormone [36], and triiodothyronine [37] have now been studied in comparative injection-infusion protocols.

Several studies using the IIC protocol indicated that the net effect of parathyroid hormone on bone formation and resorption depended on the regimen used. These investigations are described briefly.

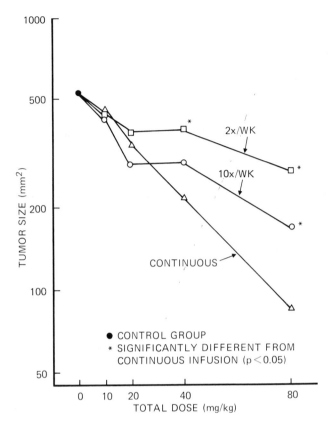

Fig. 13 Dose-response curve of bleomycin administered by three regimens against Lewis lung carcinoma. Measurements shown were made on day 15 of treatment but are representative of differences that existed throughout the course of treatment. (From Ref. 33.)

Tam et al. [20] compared the effects of bovine parathyroid hormone when administered by either daily subcutaneous injections or by continuous infusion in thyroparathyroidectomized rats. The infusion resulted in increased bone apposition and an increase in both bone formation and resorption surfaces, with a net decrease in trabecular bone. Equal doses given as a subcutaneous injection increased bone apposition rate and bone formation surface but did not increase resorption surfaces; in this case bone volume increased. The authors conclude that the subcutaneous injection regimen provides a way of separating the resorptive effects of parathyroid hormone from its effects on apposition rate and that intermittent doses of the hormone would be more effective than continuous infusion in promoting anabolic skeletal effects.

Podbesek et al. [42], using the IIC protocol in intact greyhounds to explore the effects of administering parathyroid hormone (hPTH 1-34) by subcutaneous injections or by continuous infusion, also found that the injection regimen increased trabecular bone volume while the infusion regimen decreased it. Results with injections were in agreement with those in patients similarly treated. The authors concluded that an intermittent dosage regimen, despite providing only transiently elevated PTH levels, appears more promising for the treatment of osteoporosis than the infusion regimen, which they suggest may inhibit the full expression of osteoblastic new bond formation by the "persistently supraphysiologic levels of the peptide" that it maintains.

Connors and Hedge [37] explored quantitative relationships in the control of thyroid hormone secretion in unanesthetized, thyroidectomized rats (Fig. 14). Physiological amounts of triiodothyronine (T_3) administered by continuous infusion maintained near normal T_3 plasma levels, while thyroid stimulating hormone (TSH) levels rose steadily over 144 hr; at higher levels in the physiological range, T_3 was elevated and TSH was in the normal range. Equivalent amounts of T_3 given twice daily by subcutaneous injection produced a twice-daily

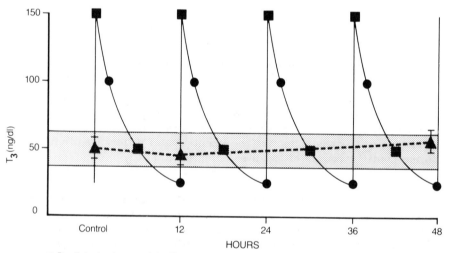

■ Predicted values, sc injections
• Measured values, sc injections
▲ Measured values, continuous infusion
Shaded area: ━ ━ ━ ━ ━

Fig. 14 Plasma concentrations of T_3 following subcutaneous injections of 161 mg of T_3 per 100 g every 12 hr and with continuous infusion in thyroidectomized rats. The shaded area is the range of plasma concentrations of T_3 in intact rats. (From Ref. 37.)

nonphysiological peak-and-trough pattern of T_3 concentrations and suppressed TSH to below prethyroidectomy levels. The injection regimen also reduced responsiveness to TRH to a greater degree than the infusion. In a second study, the authors administered thyroxine (T_4), 5 g or 1 g per 100 g of body weight per day, in drinking water or by subcutaneous injection (0.5-2.0 g per 100 g of body weight per day.) At the lower dose, the drinking water regimen produced a rise in plasma T_4 and TSH and a decrease in T_3; the higher dose produced a greater elevation in T_4, only a transient decrease in T_3, and no change in TSH. Continuous replacement of T_4 caused dose-dependent elevation of T_4, little plasma T_3 generation, and inhibition of the post-thyroidectomy use in plasma TSH. The authors concluded that T_4 in plasma exerts a negative-feedback effect on TSH secretion in addition to that due to plasma T_3. In the control of pituitary TSH secretion, T_4 acts as both a hormone—conveying feedback information to the pituitary—and as a prohormone, giving rise to a large fraction of plasma T_3. In addition, small amounts of T_4 replacement enhance the TSH responsiveness to exogenous TRH in short-term hypothyroid rats.

To determine the most efficient way to administer the limited amounts of human growth hormone (hGH) available, Cotes et al. [36] examined the effects in hypophysectomized rats of various dose regimens and vehicles for administering hGH. Human growth hormone administered by continuous subcutaneous infusion induced a greater growth response than hGH administered in higher doses by intermittent daily injection. Though it is known that in the rat (and normal child) GH secretion is episodic, the potency of the hormone administered by infusion was 169% of that administered in intermittent injections of hGH solution.

Obie and Cooper [43] demonstrated that constant exogenous subcutaneous input of calcitonin (CT) or parathyroid hormone (PTH) for one week in rats produced consistently elevated levels of these agents, but the hypocalcemia produced by CT was transitory, as was the hypercalcemia caused by PTH. Rather than illustrating receptor "downregulation," this phenomenon was attributed to counterregulatory action of the other hormone—that is, the experiment illustrated a double-feedback system.

These are only a few examples of the growing number of studies under way to test the advantages or disadvantages of constant-rate infusion (versus intermittent injections in the administration of endogenous and exogenous substances. As the reports above indicate, no general or predictable result emerges, emphasizing the importance of running the IIC protocol for each agent.

D. Time-Varying Drug Administration Regimens

Although osmotic pumps are designed to provide constant-rate delivery, they can be adapted to deliver drugs or hormones at rates that vary over time. Various investigators have devised techniques utilizing differentially loaded catheters attached to the exit port of osmotic pumps to achieve these patterns of infusion. Since it is not yet clear which drugs or bioactive agents are best given by a constant rate regimen and which require a pattern of differential administration rates to obtain an optimal regimen, this adaptation is an exciting development in drug delivery research. It facilitates investigation of the regimen dependence of drug effects and permits reproductive enhancement of free-running exotic animals. Work with this technique has shown that the true physiological effect of some hormones may be observable only when the agent is given by an on/off or phasic/tonic administration.

For example, a common temporal pattern of endogenous signals is the circadian rhythm. An adaptation of the osmotic pump [16,17] has recently permitted mimicking this pattern for melatonin. Lynch and colleagues connected an osmotic pump to a coil of fine-gage polyethylene tubing loaded with a sequence of melatonin-containing solutions alternating with drug-free spacer solutions (see Fig. 15). In the lumen of the catheter, these two solutions do not mix because the vehicle solution is not miscible in the drug solution or is separated from it by a small bubble of air. The pump and attached coil are then subcutaneously implanted in rats, and the constant inflow of fluid from the pump into the coil displaces the alternating sequence of vehicle/ melatonin solutions, resulting in the delivery of melatonin in an on/off time pattern over 6 days. To verify the functioning of the pump-coil assembly, the agent was recovered from urine in a pattern equivalent to its subcutaneous delivery (Fig. 16). This early use of osmotic pumps to achieve a time-varying pattern of delivery has stimulated other experiments to mimic or uncover the effects of temporal administration patterns.

Pulse administration of luteinizing hormone releasing hormone (LHRH) by this technique has successfully superovulated otherwise infertile exotic animals [9,10,44[. Thus animals, infertile due to seasonal anestrous or captivity-associated stress, may be successfully bred. In addition, this technique has permiteed investigation of the behavioral and hormonal components of seasonal mating. Phillips et al. [44] treated adult female green iguanas with repetitive pulses of gonadotropin releasing hormone (GnRH) for 6 days. Not only did prolong pulsatile administration induce estrous, these investigators observed an increase in mating behaviors in untreated male lizards caged with treated females. Estrogen levels in female iguanas were supressed by pulsatile GnRh administration.

Kobil's work [38] provides another example of a dynamic mode of rate-controlled administration. Using an on/off pattern of delivery, he demonstrated that the physiological actions of GnRH—and attempts to mimic those actions in therapy--depend on frequency and amplitude

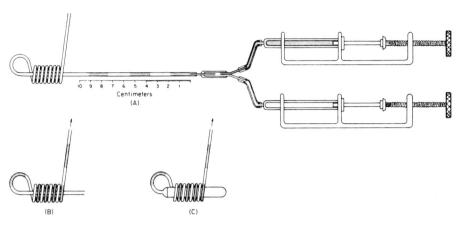

Fig. 15 Programmed microinfusion apparatus. (A) Individual components of the infusate program are forced from microsyringes, via a manifold, into the straight feeder portion of a thermoformed capillary tubing forming the linearly arrayed program. (B) The program is driven, with additional vehicle, into the coiled portion of the tubing. (C) The feeder portion of the tubing is cut off, a saline-filled mini-osmotic pump is attached, and the assembly is ready for implantation.

of its administration. Neither dose nor fixed rate provides a rational basis for understanding this hormone's actions. Such results should stimulate the explorations of time-varied patterns in the administration of many other biological substances to determine the extent to which their actions depend on frequency or amplitude of administration.

E. Organ- or Tissue-Specific Targeted Drug Delivery

Osmotically powered delivery systems eliminate important experimental difficulties that have hampered studies of agents with site- or tissue-specific effects. For example, by introducing agents directly into cerebrospinal fluid, these pumps circumvent the blood-brain barrier, facilitating the study of agents with central system effects. Osmotic pumps can permit localized delivery not only to specific organs over prolonged periods, but also microperfusion of discrete tissue areas of those organs. The osmotic pump has now been used for chronic delivery of drugs to the surface of the eye, into the uterus and vagina, into the cerebral ventricles and brain tissue, into the kidney via the renal artery, into bone, into spinal cord, into the stomach, into the testes, and to microperfuse selected areas of the visual cortex and peripheral nerves.

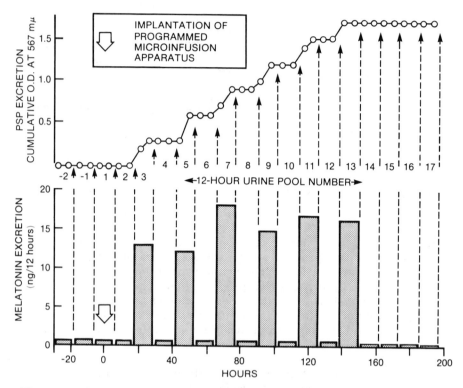

Fig. 16 Rhythmic infusion of melatonin. A programmed infusate, consisting of 10 µg of melatonin in phenolsulfonephthalein (PSP) solution alternating with melatonin-free mineral oil, was implanted in a pinealectomized rat. After 6 hr urine samples had been collected and pooled according to the cyclic appearance of PSP, the melatonin content of the urine samples was measured.

Infusion of drugs via these routes allows the buildup of a relatively high concentration in one organ—or in one area of an organ—with low systemic levels, and low levels in areas of an organ not being perfused. For example, after 6 days of continuous intracerebroventricular (ICV) or subcutaneous infusion of propanol, the ratio of concentrations by the two routes respectively were close to 1 in plasma, heart, lungs, and liver, compared with 50 to 600 in different regions of the brain [45]. On pharmacokinetic grounds, it can be shown that the gain obtained by long-term perfusion into tissues in terms of selectivity of tissue concentration depends primarily on tissue blood flow, the blood/tissue partition coefficient of the drug, and the clearance of the drug [46].

Constant-rate targeted infusions—by eliminating time-dependent, regimen-induced fluctuations in drug levels and actions—provide a high degree of ability to discriminate between a drug's central and peripheral modes of action. Smits et al. [47], using intracerebroventricular and subcutaneous influsion of tritium-labeled propanolol, demonstrated unambiguously in hypertensive rats that the antihypertensive actions of the drug depends on its peripheral action rather than its CNS actions. A similar infusion technique [48] also demonstrated the CNS locus of clonidine's antihypertensive effect in the spontaneously hypertensive rat. With continuous subcutaneous injections of the drug, a 10-fold shift of dose-response curve to the right occurred versus its continuous intracerebroventricular infusion.

Struyker-Boudier [49] also devised a technique for single-organ infusion via the cardiovascular system by implanting a catheter attached to an osmotic pump into the right suprarenal artery of a conscious, unrestrained, uninephrectomized rat to selectively infuse the right kidney (Fig. 17). Investigation of various indicators of kidney function showed no changes induced by the catheter itself. The technique was subsequently employed for the intrarenal administration of vasoactive drugs and represents a means of achieving in vivo pharmacological manipulation of intrarenal processes [50]. It was also successfully used for administration of the immunosuppressive drug prednisolone in local treatment of renal allograft rejection [80,81].

Kasamatsu et al. [51] used continuous microperfusion to demonstrate the effect of neocortical catecholamines (CAs), specifically norepinephrine, on cortical plasticity, as indicated by the marked visual cortical changes in ocular dominance that follow monocular deprivation in kittens. The investigators utilized two separate osmotic pump/cannula systems to deliver norepinephrine and control solutions, respectively, corresponding sites in the left and right visual cortices. They found that—in kittens that had lost their susceptibility to the effects of monocular lid suture because of prior treatment of the visual cortex with 6-hydroxydopamine (6-OHDA)—norepinephrine restored plasticity as shown by a shift in ocular dominance. Older animals that had outgrown susceptibility to the effects of monocular deprivation also showed a decrease in binocularity with norepinephrine treatment. The authors cited the following advantages for the microperfusion technique over the intraventricular infusion approach used previously:

Ability to localize drug effects to a specific brain region and thus to pinpoint more precisely the anatomical locus of drug effect
Ability to utilize a corresponding site in the opposite hemisphere or a distant site of the same hemisphere as a control in the same animal
Elimination of side effects that often occur with repeated intraventricular injections (reported by a number of authors)

OSMOTIC PUMP

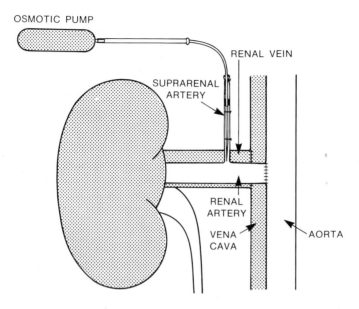

Fig. 17 Schematic outline of the experimental model used for drug infusion into the renal artery of a transplanted kidney. A catheter is introduced into the suprarenal (or testicular) artery of the transplanted kidney and connected to an osmotic pump implanted in the abdominal cavity. The osmotic pump delivers the drug in a continuous fashion from day 0 until day 13. (From Ref. 80.)

F. New Animal Models for Drug Screening

One difficulty in preclinical early drug screening and pharmacotherapeutic studies is that of creating a suitable animal model of the disease for which the test drug is indicated. Chronic duodenal ulcers, for example, do not naturally occur in species traditionally used for the testing of antiulcer drugs. Histamine injected subcutaneously in bolus doses has long been used to produce hypersecretion of gastric acid, but it has not been highly effective in ulcerogenesis. Use of continuous infusion of histamine however—at doses up to 15 mg per kilogram of body weight per day in adult rats—produced multiple ulcers [52]. Responses were dose related: at higher delivery rates some perforations occurred. In contrast, 50 mg/kg/day given as a single subcutaneous injection was not ulcerogenic. The animal models for both acute and chronic ulcerogenesis permitted comparisons of agents that stimulate gastric acid secretion and evaluation of drug antagonists. Infusion of water in control animals demonstrated that neither the pump implantation procedure or the pump's presence changed gastric or duodenal mucosa.

G. Minimization of Animal Stress

In experimental situations, a variety of factors—handling of animals, subjecting them to frequent injections, or confining them during infusions—can all introduce stress into experimental animals. The biochemical or physiological changes that result can alter drug metabolism or action, or change drug-related physiological parameters, skewing test results. For example, Riley [53] has shown that the appearance of mammary tumors in female mice of the C3H He strain carrying an oncogenic virus can be dramatically increased or accelerated by stressful factors, including handling. Less obvious manifestations of the stress response to environmental stimuli, the hypersecretion of adrenal steroids, may interact with the test agent in undesired and undetected ways.

The usual means of differentiating the effects of stress from the effects of the agent under study is to administer only vehicle to a control group of animals, according to the same regimen and procedures used to administer drug to treated animals. Rather than eliminating stress, this procedure compares the effects of drug in stressed animals to the effects of no drug in stressed animals. Therefore, stress is probably an unintended, unmeasurable variable in a large proportion of the endocrine or pharmacological studies.

Implantable delivery systems, by administering drug over prolonged time periods (up to 4 weeks) can eliminate virtually all stress due to repeated animal handling during dosage. A number of investigators have commented in their publications that neither implantation of the pump nor any other procedure for its use is stressful [29,54-61]. In general, data on the action of the agent being inferred in the unstressed physiological state can be obtained after the first day of the experiment. That change can presumably lead to very different results from those seen when stress is present.

H. Use of Osmotic Pumps in Isotope Labeling Studies

Tritium-labeled thymidine is incorporated into the DNA of proliferating cells and so can be used to measure cell turnover. In vivo, [^{3}H]thymidine has a very short plasma half-life. Studies to determine the length of various portions of the cell cycle (S, G$_2$, G$_1$, M, C) exploit the kinetics of [^{3}H]thymidine to label cells at a discrete point in their cell cycle. Cell cycle length is calculated from measurements on the rate at which labeled mitoses, as a proportion of total mitoses, appear over time following a single exposure to a pulse of [^{3}H]thymidine.

To study cell cycle dynamics over an extended period of time, prolonged administration of [^{3}H]thymidine is necessary. This can be achieved by repeated injections, but the short half-life of [^{3}H]thymidine necessitates the giving of injections every 4 hr or less if exposure is to be maintained [62]. This is costly both in time and effort needed to maintain this injection schedule around the clock. In addition, the repeated handling of animals during complex injection schedules can elicit hormonal changes that alter the biochemistry of the tissues under study [63]. Moreover, if handling occurs at different times during the diurnal cycle, hormonal fluctuations may alter cell cycle kinetics [63].

Osmotic pumps offer an alternative method of prolonged exposure to [^{3}H]thymidine with several advantages. In addition to obviating the need for nighttime and weekend dosing, continuous infusion minimizes the handling of animals, reducing experimental artifacts. Because the animal is exposed to a continuous low dose, more reliable lableing is achieved with a less prominent background gradient [64]. As [^{3}H]thymidine clearance is minimized, better autoradiographs result from the use of less isotope [64]. Also, prolonged infusions of [^{3}H]thymidine are an excellent method of labeling slowly proliferating cells, which are difficult to label with pulse techniques [63,64]. ALZET osmotic pumps have been used in a wide variety of applications in research on cell proliferation.

IV. OSMET OSMOTIC PUMPS IN CLINICAL RESEARCH

The same osmotic technology described for use in preclinical studies has been adapted to provide for oral or rectal administration of drug solution or suspensions. Although somewhat bulkier than conventional tablets, the capsule shaped modules transit the gastrointestinal tract in the same manner. The smaller 0.2 ml capacity modules deliver continuously to the gastrointestinal tract at a near-constant rate for 8, 12, or 24 hr. The 2 ml capacity modules for rectal or vaginal administration deliver for 15 or 30 hr.

A. Oral Drug Administration

Several studies have been done in which OSMET modules were radiolabeled and their transit through the gastrointestinal tract of man monitored by gamma scintigraphy. Additionally, the pump can be filled with a second radiolabel and its release and distribution both visualized and calculated [65,66]. In these studies, it was found that the release rate of the marker in vivo approximates a zero-order release rate profile and is almost equal to that obtained in vitro. Furthermore, the position of the device in the gastrointestinal tract did not affect the release profile, nor did the presence of food, indicating that drug delivery from the osmotic system is independent of pH and motility in the gastrointestinal tract. While the release rate was independent of the presence of food, the gastric residence time of the pump was greatly influenced by food intake. For instance, when the Osmet modules were taken after a heavy breakfast, they were retained in the stomach for at least 9 hr, during which time the breakfast and the release radiolabel emptied from the stomach. Indeed, the release and distribution of the radiolabel could be monitored throughout its transit into the colon.

In other studies, it was demonstrated that these OSMET modules move through the small intestine in about 200 min, similar in time to that of pellets, tablets, and solutions, independent of food intake [67-69].

An important application of the OSMET module is to define whether and to what extent a drug-specific window of absorption exists along the gastrointestinal tract. With the assurance that the rate of drug release in vivo equals that in vitro for the OSMET module, one can deduce the absorption characteristics of a compound from the plasma concentration versus time profile by using deconvolution techniques without the need for radiolabeled compounds or gamma scintigraphy (ALZA data).

B. Rectal Drug Delivery

Breimer and colleagues in Leiden have used the 2 ml OSMET modules for zero-order rectal drug administration in several studies in healthy subjects [70,71]. Initial studies focused on the in vivo performance of the osmotic devices when introduced and kept in the human rectum for several days, and subsequent clinical trials explored the pharmacokinetics and pharmacodynamics of vairous drugs.

With the model drugs antipyrine and theophylline (as its choline salt), almost perfect zero-order infusion-type plasma concentration curves were obtained, with very constant steady state levels reached after about four times the elimination half-life of the parent drugs [72, 73] (Figs. 18 and 19). Just after defecation a new system was inserted, and neither this procedure nor renewal of the system after a 24 hr interval caused irregularities in the plasma concentration profile. The volunteers had no difficulties in keeping systems in the rectum over a several-day period of periodic insertion/defecation cycles, and no topical irritation or disruption in bowel habits was observed. In all studies, the in vivo pumping rate appeared to be nearly identical to the in vitro pumping rate.

The results of these studies clearly indicate that the 2 ml OSMET module can be used as a tool in clinical pharmacology. It is easy to use, is well-tolerated, and can provide near-steady-state plasma concentrations. Indeed, the use of this device with some compounds may be regarded as an alternative to zero-order intravenous infusion.

Beyond studies of pump performance and tolerability, several significant reports have appeared describing clinical pharmacological studies using the OSMET modules, including:

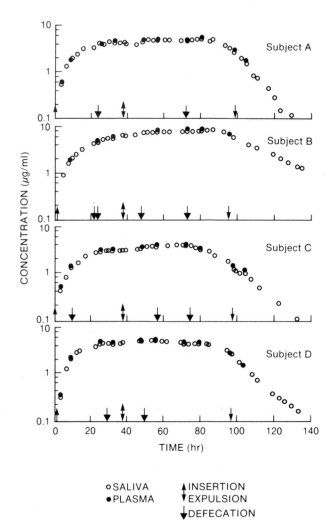

o SALIVA   ▲ INSERTION
● PLASMA   ▼ EXPULSION
               ↓ DEFECATION

Fig. 18 Concentrations of antipyrine in plasma and saliva following administration of an osmotic rectal delivery system (delivering 43 µl/hr antipyrine) in four subjects. (From Ref. 72.)

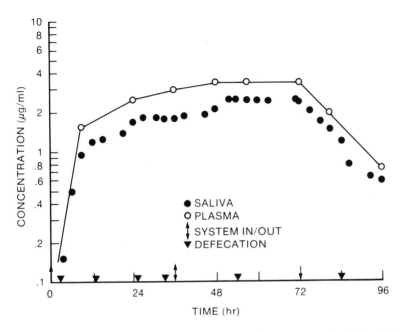

Fig. 19 Concentrations of theophylline in plasma and saliva after administration of an osmotic rectal delivery system (delivering 11 mg/hr theophylline) in one subject. (From Ref. 73.)

Steady state pharmacokinetics and β-adrenergic receptor blockade by propranolol [74]

Possible development of tolerance during assessment of performance and sleep with continuous rectal infusion of triazolam [75]

Pharmacokinetic interaction between cimetidine and antipyrine during steady state [76]

Site-specific rectal administration of lidocaine in relation to the extent of first-pass elimination [77]

In a broader consideration of dosage form design, rate-controleld rectal drug delivery with the OSMET modules can be regarded as an excellent tool to help set design specifications for oral, transdermal, and intravenous drug delivery systems. One specific and dramatic example of this is illustrated in the work of Kleinbloesem et al. [78] in which the pharmacodynamics of nifedipine was compared between a constant drug input from an OSMET module with that of a conventional dosing regimen. In this study, the investigators clearly show that by giving this calcium channel blocker at relatively slow rates of input, the desired antihypertensive effect of nifedipine could be dissociated from the undesired tachycardia observed with immediate release dosing.

Studies such as this dramatically illustrate the usefulness of such pharmacological tools, and in a practical sense they represent the opportunity to build, at an early stage, the rationale or therapeutic basis for the development of rate-controlled dosage forms.

V. CONCLUSIONS

Until rate-controlled osmotic delivery systems became available, drug assessment was severely hampered at both the preclinical and clinical levels by the difficulties of exploring the pharmacodynamics of drug actions. Single-dose pharmacokinetic studies have yielded only limited information in comparison with that now obtainable by studying the agent in a wide array of temporally varied delivery modes. Moreover, the advent of these implantable osmotic pumps has greatly facilitated rate-controlled drug admistration in preclinical studies by dispensing with the need for animal restraint and special equipment.

For these reasons—and because of the availability of therapeutic rate-controlled dosage forms—researchers are beginning to view the study of drug actions at steady state or in programmed, time-varying patterns of delivery as matters of practical importance and not merely of academic interest. Specifically, they are beginning to explore the effects of regimen variation in both pharmacological and pharmacotherapeutic research. In the next decade such studies should bring about several developments:

Testing, registration, and marketing of a growing number of products in which innovation is based on rate-controlled release of established agents rather than on synthesis of new chemical entities

Use in routine outpatient therapy of agents with half-lives too short or therapeutic indices too narrow to permit their administration in conventional bolus dosage forms

Optimization of regimens early in the development phase of new drugs and revision of the regimens of many older drugs in the light of data now obtainable from rate-controlled preclinical and clinical studies

APPENDIX

COMPOUNDS ADMINISTERED BY ALZET OSMOTIC
PUMP LISTED BY COMPOUND CATEGORY

Neurotransmitters and Nerve Growth Factors

Acetylcholine
Dopamine
Endorphine
Enkephalins
Epinephrine
Histamine
Hydroxydopamine
Melatonin
Nerve growth factors
Neuroregenerative agents
Norepinephrine
Serotonin

Peptides and Peptide Hormones

ACTH
Atrial natriuretic factor
AVP (arginine vasopressin)
Bombesin
Buserelin
Calcitonin
Cerulein
Cholecystokinin
Dermorphin
DDAVP (1-Desamino-8-Arginine Vasopressin)
Dynorphin
Endorphins
Enkephalins
Follicle stimulating hormone (FSH)
Glucagon
Gonadotropin releasing hormone (GnRH)
Growth hormones
Insulin
Insulinlike growth factor (IGF)
Luteinizing hormone (LH)
Luteinizing hormone releasing hormone (LHRH)
Luteinizing hormone releasing hormone analogues, antagonists
α-Melanocyte stimulating hormone
Neurotensin
Oxytocin

Parathyroid hormone (PTH)
Pituitary extract
Prolactin
Somatostatin
Thyroid releasing hormone (TRH)
Thyroid stimulating hormone (TSH)
Vasopressin
Wy-40972 (GnRH antagonist)

Prostaglandins

PGA_2
PGE_1
PGE_2
PGF_2a
TPT (analogue)

Agents Acting on the Central Nervous System

Amitriptyline
Amphetamines
Apomorphine
Clorgyline
Desipramine
Endorphins
Enkephalins
Enkephalin analogues, antagonists
Fentanyl
Haloperidol
LSD
Morphine
Naloxone
Naltrexone
Phenobarbital
Scopolamine
Serotonin
Sufentanyl
Tetrahydrocannabinol (THC)

Cholinergics

Carbachol
Physostigmine
Pyridostigmine

Gastrointestinal Motility Modulators

Metoclopramide
Scopolamine

Metabolites

Fructose
Glucose
Glycerol
Vitamin D_3 metabolites

Radioisotopes

^{14}C labeled
[^{109}Cd]Cl
^{51}Cr labeled
^{59}Fe labeled
^{3}H labeled (usually tritiated thymidine)
^{125}I labeled
^{35}S labeled

Renin-Angiotensin System and Inhibitors

Angiotensin II
Angiotensin II antagonists
Captopril

Steroids

Alderosterone
Catecholestrogens
Corticosterone
Dexamethasone
DOCA
Estradiol
Estriol
Estrone
Progesterone
Progestin
Testosterone

Thyroid and Thyroid-related Hormones

Melatonin
T_3

T_4
Thyrotropin
Thyroid releasing hormone (TRH)
Thyroid stimulating hormone (TSH)
Thyroxine

Toxins

Endotoxin
Picrotoxin
Tetrodotoxin

REFERENCES

1. F. Theeuwes and S. I. Yum, *Ann. Biomed. Eng.*, 4:343 (1976).
2. F. Theeuwes and B. Eckenhoff, *Controlled Release of Bioactive Materials* (R. Baker, ed.). Academic Press, New York, 1980, p. 61.
3. P. Shrock, V. Helm, and R. W. Baker, *Proceedings of Controlled Release Society Meeting*, Norfolk, VA, 1986, p. 7.
4. R. W. Baker and L. M. Sanders, in *Controlled Release Delivery Systems* (P. M. Bungay et al., eds.). Reidel, Dordrecht, 1985, p. 581.
5. S. Rose and J. F. Nelson, *Aust. J. Exp. Biol.*, 33:415 (1955).
6. K. T. Rodrigues and J. P. Sumpter, *J. Endocrinol.*, 101:277 (1984).
7. T. F. Davison, B. M. Freeman, and J. Rea, *Gen. Comp. Endocrinol.*, 59:416 (1985).
8. J. Urquhart, J. Fara, and K. L. Willis, *Annu. Rev. Pharmacol. Toxicol.*, 24:199 (1984).
9. B. L. Lasley and A. Wing, *Proceedings of the American Association of Zoo Veterinarians*, Tampa, FL, 1983, p. 14.
10. D. Lindburg, S. Millard, and B. Lasley, *Annu. Proc. AAZPA*, 2:560 (1985).
11. B. Eckenhoff, F. Theeuwes, and J. Urquhart, *Pharm. Technol.*, 5(1):35 (1981).
12. D. G. Patel, *Proc. Soc. Exp. Biol. Med.*, 172:74 (1983).
13. G. D. Lopaschuk, A. G. Tahiliani, and J. H. McNeill, *J. Pharmacol. Methods*, 9:71 (1983).
14. D. P. Rose and K. G. Mountjoy, *Cancer Res.*, 43:2588 (1983).
15. J. G. Brown and D. J. Millward, *Biochim. Biophys. Acta*, 757:182 (1983).
16. H. J. Lynch, R. W. Rivest, and R. J. Wurtman, *Neuroendocrinology*, 31:106 (1980).
17. H. J. Lynch and R. J. Wurtman, in *Biological Rhythms and Their*

Central Mechanism (M. Suda, O. Hayaishi, and H. Nakagawa, eds.). Elsevier/North Holland, Amsterdam, 1979, p. 117.

18. P. C. Will, R. N. Cortright, and U. Hopfer, *J. Pharm. Sci.*, 69:747 (1980).

19. D. J. Morris and C. J. Kenyon, *Clin. Exp. Hyper. Theory Pract.*, A4:1613 (1982).

20. C. S. Tam, J. N. M. Heersche, T. M. Murray, and J. A. Parsons, *Endocrinology*, 110:506 (1982).

21. E. Hefti, U. Trechsel, H. Fleisch, and J. P. Bonjour, *Am. J. Physiol.*, 244:E313 (1983).

22. L. L. Ewing, T. Y. Wing, R. C. Cochran, N. Kromann, and B. R. Zirkin, *Endocrinology*, 112:1763 (1983).

23. E. Schoenle, J. Zapf, and E. R. Froesch, *Endocrinology*, 112:384 (1983).

24. W. Fried, J. Barone-Varelas, T. Barone, and A. Anagnostou, *J. Lab. Clin. Med.*, 99:520 (1982).

25. J. C. S. Kelinjans, J. F. M. Smits, C. M. Kasbergen, H. T. M. Vervoort-Peters, and H. A. J. Struyker-Boudier, *Clin. Sci.*, 65:111 (1983).

26. M. Cervantes, R. Ruelas, and C. Beyer, *Psychoneuroendocrinology*, 4:245 (1979).

27. R. Bochskanl and C. Kirchner, *Wilhelm Roue Arch. Entwicklungsmech. Org.*, 190:127 (1981).

28. R. N. Clayton, *Endocrinology*, 111:152 (1982).

29. J. C. de la Torre, and M. Gonzalez-Carvajal, *Lab. Animal Sci.*, 31:701 (1981).

30. M. F. Bear, M. A. Paradiso, M. Schwartz, S. B. Nelson, K. M. Carnes, and J. D. Daniels, *Nature*, 302:245 (1983).

31. D. I. Diz, P. G. Baer, and A. Nasjletti, *Am. J. Physiol.*, 241:F477 (1981).

32. H. Nau, R. Zierer, H. Spielmann, D. Neubert, and C. Gansau, *Life Sci.*, 29:2803 (1981).

33. B. I. Sikic, J. M. Collins, E. G. Mimnaugh, and T. E. Gram, *Cancer Treat. Rep.*, 62:2011 (1978).

34. H. S. Brown, G. Meltzer, R. C. Merrill, M. Fisher, C. Ferre, and V. A. Place, *Arch. Ophthalmol.*, 94:1716 (1976).

35. Y. M. Peng, D. S. Alberts, H. S. Chen, N. Mason, and T. E. Moon, *Br. J. Cancer*, 41:644 (1980).

36. P. M. Cotes, W. A. Bartlett, R. E. G. Das, P. Flecknell, and R. Termeer, *J. Endocrinol.*, 87:303 (1980).

37. J. M. Connors and G. A. Hedge, *Endocrinology*, 106:911 (1980).

38. E. Knobil, *Recent Prog. Hormone Res.*, 36:53 (1980).

39. G. Levy, M. Rowland, and H. Nau, personal communications.

40. G. Coonely, D. Vugrin, C. LaMonte, and M. J. Lacher, *Proc. Am. Assoc. Cancer Res.*, 22:369 (1981).

41. K. R. Cooper and W. K. Hong, *Cancer Treat. Rep.*, 65:419 (1981).

42. R. Podbesek, C. Edouard, P. J. Meunier, J. A. Parsons, J. Reeve, R. W. Stevenson, and J. M. Zanelli, *Endocrinology*, 112:1000 (1983).
43. J. F. Obie and C. W. Cooper, *J. Pharmacol. Exp. Ther.*, 209: 422 (1979).
44. J. A. Phillips, N. Alexander, W. B. Karesh, R. Miller, and B. L. Lasley, *J. Exp. Zool.*, 234:481 (1985).
45. H. A. J. Struyker-Boudier, *Labo-Pharma Probl. Tech.*, 298:373 (1980).
46. H. A. J. Struyker-Boudier, *Trends Pharmacol. Sci.*, 3:162 (1982).
47. J. F. M. Smits, H. van Essen, and H. A. J. Struyker-Boudier, *J. Pharmacol. Exp. Ther.*, 215:221 (1980).
48. H. A. J. Struyker-Boudier and H. van Essen, *Naunyn-Schmiedebergs Arch. Pharmakol.*, 311 (Suppl.):R49 (1980).
49. J. F. M. Smits, C. M. Kasbergen, H. van Essen, J. C. Kleinjans, and H. A. J. Struyker-Boudier, *Am. J. Physiol.*, 244:H304 (1983).
50. J. C. Kleinjans, J. F. Smits, H. van Essen, and H. A. Struyker-Boudier, *Fed. Proc. Am. Soc. Exp. Biol.*, 41:1660 (1982).
51. T. Kasamatsu, J. D. Pettigrew, and M. Ary, *J. Comp. Neurol.*, 185:163 (1979).
52. S. Hosada, I. Hachiro, and T. Saito, *Gastroenterology*, 80:16 (1981).
53. V. Riley, *Science*, 189:465 (1975).
54. K. Jarnagin, R. Brommage, H. F. DeLuca, S. Yamada, and H. Takayama, *Am. J. Physiol.*, 244:E290 (1983).
55. S. W. T. Cheng, W. G. North, and M. Gellai, *Ann. N.Y. Acad. Sci.*, 394:473 (1982).
56. S. A. Beyler, L. J. D. Zaneveld, *Contraception*, 26:137 (1982).
57. J. S. Kroin and R. D. Penn, *Neurosurgery*, 10:349 (1982).
58. J. E. Krause, J. P. Advis, and J. F. McKelvey, *Endocrinology*, 111:344 (1982).
59. T. R. L. Gould, D. M. Brunette, and J. Dorey, *J. Peridontal Res.*, 17:662 (1982).
60. F. B. Akhtar, G. R. Marshall, E. J. Wickings, and E. Nieschlag, *J. Clin. Endocrinol. Metab.*, 56:534 (1983).
61. H. A. J. Struyker-Boudier, J. F. M. Smits, and C. Kasbergen, *Naunyn-Schmiedebergs Arch. Pharmakol.*, 319 (Suppl.):R50 (1982).
62. M. Tatematsu, R. H. Ho, T. Kaku, J. K. Ekem, and E. Farber, *Am. J. Pathol.*, 114(3):418 (1984).
63. T. R. L. Gould, D. M. Brunette, and J. Dorey, *J. Periodontal Res.*, 17:662 (1982).
64. A. N. Hirshfield, *Biol. Reprod.*, 30:485 (1984).
65. S. S. Davis, J. G. Hardy, M. J. Taylor, A. Stockwell, D. R. Whalley, and C. G. Wilson, *J. Pharm. Pharmacol.*, 36:740 (1984).

66. S. S. Davis, in *Topics in Pharmaceutical Sciences 1983* (D. D. Breimer and P. Speiser, eds.). Elsevier Biomedical Press, Amsterdam, 1983, p. 205.

67. S. S. Davis, J. G. Hardy, M. J. Taylor, D. R. Whalley, and C. G. Wilson, *Int. J. Pharm.*, 21:331 (1984).

68. S. S. Davis, J. G. Hardy, M. J. Taylor, D. R. Whalley, and C. G. Wilson, *Int. J. Pharm.*, 21:167 (1984).

69. S. S. Davis, J. G. Hardy, and J. W. Fara, *Gut*, 27(8):886 (1986).

70. D. D. Breimer, L. G. J. De Leede, and A. G. De Boer, *Proceedings of the Second World Conference on Clinical Pharmacology and Therapeutics*, Bethesda, MD, 1984, pp. 431-443.

71. D. D. Breimer, L. G. J. De Leede, and A. G. De Boer, in *Rate Control in Drug Therapy* (L. F. Prescott and W. S. Nimmo, eds.). Churchill & Livingstone, Edinburgh, 1985, p. 54.

72. L. G. J. De Leede, A. G. De Boer, and D. D. Breimer, *Biopharm. Drug Disp.*, 2:131 (1981).

73. L. G. J. De Leede, A. G. De Boer, S. L. Van Velzen, and D. D. Breimer, *J. Pharmacokinet. Biopharm.*, 10:525 (1982).

74. L. G. J. De Leede, C. C. Hug, Jr., S. De Lange, A. G. De Boer, and D. D. Breimer, *Clin. Pharmacol. Ther.*, 35:148 (1984).

75. D. D. Breimer, R. Jochemsen, H. A. C. Kamphuizen, A. N. Nicholson, M. B. Spencer, and B. M. Stone, *Br. J. Clin. Pharmacol.*, 19:807 (1985).

76. M. W. E. Teunissen, C. H. Kleinbloesem, L. G. J. De Leede, and D. D. Breimer, *Eur. J. Clin. Pharmacol.*, 28:681 (1985).

77. L. G. J. De Leede, A. G. De Boer, C. D. Feijen, and D. D. Breimer, *Pharm. Res.*, 3:129 (1984).

78. C. H. Kleinbloesem, J. Van Harten, L. G. J. De Leede, P. Van Brummelen, and D. D. Breimer, *Clin. Pharmacol. Ther.*, 36:396 (1984).

79. P. Tran Ba Huy, P. Bernard, and J. Schacht, *J. Clin. Invest.*, 77:1492 (1986).

80. T. J. M. Ruers, W. A. Buurman, J. F. M. Smits, C. J. van der Linden, J. J. van Dongen, H. A. J. Struyker-Boudier, and G. Kootstra, *Transplantation*, 41(2):156 (1986).

81. T. J. M. Ruers, W. A. Buurman, J. F. M. Smits, C. J. van der Linden, J. J. van Dongen, E. E. M. Spronken, and G. Kootstra, *Transplant. Proc.* XVIII(5):1106 (1986).

5

Ambulatory Infusion Devices

PETER LUKACSKO and GRAHAM S. MAY / Pharmacia Deltec, Inc.,
St. Paul, Minnesota

I. INTRODUCTION

Parenteral therapy got off to an inauspicious start when, in 1492, physicians attempted to treat the dying pope by transfusing blood from three healthy men. The pontiff and all the donors died, presumably as the result of blood incompatibility and air emboli. Subsequently, such procedures were banned in Europe for more than a century.

With the description of the circulation by Sir William Harvey in the early 1600s, physicians once again entertained the idea of intravenous therapy. At approximately the same time, Johann Taylor and Christopher Wren described their techniques by which a device composed of a goose quill and an animal bladder could be used to inject fluids directly into the veins of men and animals. The plunger type of syringe was introduced in the mid-1800s, but it was not until late in the same century that sterilization of the syringe and solution was stressed. Techniques of parenteral drug therapy have advanced steadily but slowly over the past 200 years [1,2], in contrast with current innovations in drug delivery, which are often obsolete before they have been fully evaluated.

The gravity feed intravenous administration set is one of the most common and simplest techniques used currently. Typically, the solution is contained in a glass bottle or polymeric bag that is hung at a height of about 1 m to provide the necessary pressure to cause flow. The rate at which the fluid is delivered to the patient is regulated by a clamp that is preset manually on the administration set tubing. However, since the flow rate of a simple gravity feed system is variable, this arrangement is not ideal when the amount of drug to be delivered is critical.

Infusion controllers were developed to improve the accuracy of gravity feed systems. Although controllers basically count drops and are still gravity dependent, the rate of flow is regulated automatically rather than by a manual clamp. In addition to more precise flow control, electronic controllers incorporate in-built safety features; they may shut off or alarm when air is in the line, when the reservoir is empty, when flow is inadequate, or when tissue infiltration occurs. However, since controllers rely on gravity for their driving pressure, their use in parenteral drug delivery is also limited.

Infusion pumps rely on an electric or mechanical power source and, for the most part, eliminate the restrictions of gravity feed systems. Since infusion pumps can maintain a constant pressure over time, they can deliver a precise flow rate even against a resistance such as arterial pressure. As most infusion pumps are programmed to deliver milliliters rather than drops, they are generally referred to as volumetric pumps.

II. RATIONALE FOR OUTPATIENT INFUSION THERAPY

The health care system in the United States has recently been presented with a formidable challenge, namely to maintain or improve the standard of medical care without exceeding the economic boundaries imposed by the diagnostic related grouping (DRGs). One way to meet this challenge is to reduce hospital overhead by providing treatment, when possible, in an ambulatory outpatient setting.

There are also less obvious benefits of outpatient treatment. It has been estimated that nosocomial infections affect 1 of every 20 patients hospitalized in the United States [3]. These alone may increase health care costs by as much as $10 billion. Under the DRG program, an institution is not entitled to reimbursement for extra costs incurred, either for additional medication or for per diem charges.

At present, there is little information regarding the actual cost savings of outpatient ambulatory therapy. However, the annual cost to the hospital of using a volumetric pump (one device plus 240 intravenous administration sets) has been estimated at $1700 [4]. Potentially, ambulatory infusion therapy could in one year save an average hospital more than $100,000 as the result of fewer dressing changes and about $200,000 in reduced nursing costs [4]. Another report [5] has shown that a regimen of antibiotic therapy given in an outpatient setting costs only one-third as much as the same regimen given in hospital. Considering that health care costs for the nation in 1984 were estimated to be #387 billion [6], even a small percentage reduction would have a significant impact.

Finally, the ambulatory patient is spared the overwhelming financial and emotional burden of prolonged hospitalization. The individual has the possibility of returning to work and the potential to enjoy a more normal lifestyle. Moreover, several ambulatory pumps allow a degree of patient interaction in controlling the dosing regimen, which gives the patient some sense of autonomy over the treatment. In some institutions receiving therapy in the outpatient setting is no longer considered an option but is expected by both physician and patient.

III. CAUTIONS AND CONCERNS

Despite the obvious incentives for outpatient treatment, caution must be exercised with the use of ambulatory pumps [7]. It is important to remember that treatment with these devices is still in a relatively early stage. As with any new treatment modality, a readily available and comprehensive data bank of information for easy reference has yet to be developed. Anyone authorizing the use of an ambulatory pump must assume the responsibility for ensuring its reliability and performance characteristics, the stability of the drug to be infused, the selection of the appropriate patient, and the ability of the patient to manage a pump malfunction or adverse drug reaction.

Since 1976, when the Medical Devices Amendments to the Food, Drug, and Cosmetics Act were passed, it has been necessary to obtain the evaluation and approval of the Food and Drug Administration before any such device can be distributed commercially in the United States (see Chapter 4). Unlike the extensive review process to which drugs are subjected, evaluation of many medical devices is concerned primarily with mechanical and electronic performance criteria rather than the effectiveness of the treatment modality involved. Many new devices are presented to the FDA as being "substantially equivalent" to similar devices available prior to 1976. The agency's review of such products does not necessarily involve an extensive evaluation of either safety of efficacy data. It remains incumbent on the physician and user of the pump to assess whether the device will perform according to the specifications claimed. This judgment may be heavily influenced by the reputation of the manufacturer.

Ambulatory pumps may use a syringe, PVC bag, or a cassette-type cartridge as the drug reservoir. Since the drug may remain in contact with the reservoir for several days, it is important for the reservoir to be constructed of material that is compatible with the drug under the conditions encountered in the outpatient setting. Since many ambulatory infusion pumps can accurately delivery small volumes over extended periods, the drug may be in prolonged contact not only with the complex materials of the reservoir but also with those of the extension tubing and vascular access catheter. Moreover, any single drug molecule may be in transit for a long time before reaching the patient's circulation. Each molecule of drug may be exposed to changes in temperature (ambient to body) and light (indoor or outdoor), as well as to oxygen that may have diffused through the various components of the administration set. Clearly, the issues of drug compatibility, stability, and solubility require special consideration when recommending ambulatory therapy.

Selection of appropriate patients is also important. The patient and at least one other member of the family must fully understand how to use the pump and must be aware of any complications that may occur, such as extravasation, needle dislodgement, kinking of extension sets, leaking Luer fittings, air in line, catheter occlusions, and any adverse effects of the drug. It is essential for the patient to understand the meaning of the various pump alarms and what action to take should one go off. It may also be necessary for the patient to know how to reload the drug reservoir and prime the extension tubing and how to maintain the power source for the pump. Both the medical staff and the manufacturer share the obligation to ensure that the patient is fully informed of all these issues when using an ambulatory pump.

IV. TYPES OF AMBULATORY INFUSION PUMP

One of the earliest ambulatory infusion pumps was developed by the University of Minnesota and patented in 1972 [8]. The university awarded the Metal Bellows Corporation the right to manufacture and market the device that is presently referred to as the Infusaid Implantable Pump.

The objective in developing the pump was to provide a system that could be totally implanted subcutaneously and would deliver a constant intravenous infusion. The pump is roughly the size of a hockey puck (8.7 cm diameter, 2.8 cm thick) and weighs about 208 g empty. The pump is filled with drug through a septum accessed by hypodermic needle puncture and holds about 50 ml. Usually the reservoir empties slowly over a 7 to 14 day period through a catheter that has been introduced into a central vein. The drug is delivered at a constant rate that is predetermined by internal flow restrictors. This rate cannot be changed.

The source of power for delivering the solution is derived from a fluorocarbon that, at body temperature, is in equilibrium between the liquid and gaseous phase. The expandable chamber containing the drug solution is surrounded by a second inflexible chamber containing the fluorocarbon, so that when the drug chamber is filled, the fluorocarbon gas is compressed into the liquid state. This gradually reverts to the gaseous phase, and the resulting pressure expels the solution at a slow and constant rate. Recharging of the power source can theoretically continue indefinitely.

The advantages of an implantable system are obvious. Maintenance requirements are minimal, so little patient involvement is necessary. Since both pump and catheter are subcutaneous, the system may be more cosmetically acceptable to the patient and the risk of infection is minimized. A drawback is that the pump does not allow for changes in the rate of drug delivery. The rate at which the fluorocarbon changes from the liquid to the gaseous phase depends on temperature and atmospheric pressure, so significant changes in the delivery rate may occur should the patient become febrile or travel by airplane. Another disadvantage is that the pump cannot be turned off unless the drug solution is removed or the device explanted. As the level of drug cannot be checked visually, the reservoir may empty inadvertently. Cost is an additional factor. The model 400 is priced at about $3750, excluding implantation fees, and it is intended for single patient use only.

As an alternative to implantable systems, a number of externally worn ambulatory pumps are now available. These pumps may be generally classified further as either the syringe or peristaltic variety, although others such as the Travenol Infusor are elastomerically driven. Syringe pumps are relatively simple mechanically in that the plunger of the syringe is depressed by a battery-powered electric motor. The syringe may be filled manually by a health professional, but for some pumps proprietary prefilled syringes are provided by the manufacturer. These may cost more initially, but there is no charge for filling.

Ambulatory syringe pumps range in simplicity from, for example, the Provider 3000 (Pancretec), which delivers only at a fixed incremental volume of 0.06 ml at 90 min intervals, to the more adaptable Graseby MS 16A or MS 26 (Intermedics Infusaid Inc.), to programmable computerized microinfusion pumps, such as the CADD-LD (Pharmacia Deltec). The CADD-LD pump delivers incremental volumes of 0.005 ml at programmable time intervals with a maximum delivery rate of 0.5 ml/min.

Peristaltic pumps propel fluid by applying an external force against tubing originating from the drug reservoir. As the external force moves along the tubing, the contained solution is propelled in the same direction. Peristaltic pumps are either of rotary or linear design. In rotary pumps, the pumping action is produced by an eccentrically placed roller on a rotating cam. The tubing is squeezed between the roller and a stationary wall. Perhaps one of the most popular rotary ambulatory pumps marketed in the United States is supplied by Cormed, Inc. Several Cormed pumps are available, depending on the flow rate required and the intended use. All are self-contained units in which a polymeric reservoir is back-filled with the drug solution. The power source for all models is a rechargable nickel-cadmium (NiCad) battery.

Linear peristaltic pumps propel fluids by means of a series of contact points that compress the tubing in a sequential manner against a stationary back plate. Popular examples of this type of pump are the Infumed 200 (MedFusion System Inc.) and the CADD-1 and CADD-PCA pumps (Pharmacia Deltec). Each model is a self-contained unit to which a collapsible drug reservoir is attached. The drug reservoir is not attached directly to the Infumed 200 but instead is worn on a remote site on the body. The reservoir or the CADD pump is contained within a hard plastic cassette attached directly to the pump. These pumps are all powered by disposable alkaline batteries.

V. SELECTING A PUMP

It is not surprising that there is often uncertainty with regard to the sort of pump to be selected for a specific therapeutic application and to the manufacturer from which to purchase it. The choice of pump is often determined by little more than the physician's or nurse's personal preference and the claims of the manufacturer's representative.

Considering the cost of current technology, it would be wise for any hospital or clinic contemplating the purchase of an ambulatory infusion pump to first define carefully its present and future applications. A committee comprised of members from the medical staff, IV nursing team, pharmacy, engineering, and purchasing should evaluate whether the features of a proposed pump are appropriate for its intended use. They should also assess the overall cost effectiveness of patient care, taking into account the cost of disposable items.

It should not be forgotten that an expensive pump can soon become obsolete, especially if it was originally purchased for a limited indication. Once a pump has been accepted for one indication, the medical staff may wish to expand its use. A state-of-the-art device should not be self-limiting in its clinical application. Purchasing a pump with somewhat greater programming capacity than that needed initially may permit the necessary flexibility to enable later use of the pump in new indications. A device that can accommodate upgrading of microprocessor function without replacement of the entire pump is obviously desirable.

The pump should be relatively tamper resistant. It should be designed to preclude accidental or intentional altering of the delivery parameters. The drug reservoir should withstand normal wear and tear and should be designed to discourage unauthorized access. These features are especially important when dealing with narcotic delivery for pain management.

Any ambulatory infusion pump used in an outpatient setting should be equipped with alarms and automatic shutoff in case of potential or actual malfunction. Audible and/or visual alarms may warn of the following circumstances: microprocessor or motor fault, improper delivery, low and empty drug reservoir, line occlusion, low battery, and air in line. The pump should have the capacity to be preset for total volume to be infused and to turn itself off when the infusion is completed. The pump should have a continuous and cumulative readout to inform the user of the amount of drug already infused and the volume remaining in the present delivery cycle. Pumps that allow for visual review of the programmed delivery parameters are preferable. Since the pumps will be used outside the hospital, additional issues such as static protection and water resistance should also be considered.

Ambulatory infusion pumps should be accurate. Unfortunately, many pump manufacturers do not provide ratings with their promotional literature. Even when the accuracy is given, this may be of limited use since the same reported value for two pumps may not indicate equivalence. Manufacturers do not necessarily test their pumps under the same range of operating conditions, because no standard criteria presently exist within the industry.

It has been suggested [9] that the delivery rate should not deviate by more than 10% from the programmed setting. The same article suggested that deviations of as much as 25% might be acceptable for some drugs. A more recent report [10] states that a "flow rate accu-

racy of ±10% is generally acceptable" but qualifies this statement by
saying that flow rate deviations of ±5% are more appropriate in certain
circumstances (e.g., in infants, for drugs with a narrow therapeutic
range, etc.).
   Although patients should use an accurate pump especially when
in the outpatient setting, it should be remembered that the flow rate
is only one of many factors that determine the plasma concentration
of a drug, thereby influencing both its therapeutic efficacy and the
adverse effects profile. Drug bioavailability, distribution, metabolism,
and excretion will vary between formulations and individuals so, although accuracy is a consideration when choosing a pump, its importance should be kept in perspective.
   Although programmable infusion pumps may simplify a therapeutic
regimen, they introduce still another level of complexity for the medical profession. For the most part, difficulties with pumps arise not
out of malfunction of the device but because its operation and performance characteristics are poorly understood. As the complexity
of the pump increases, it becomes paramount for the equipment manufacturer to provide educational literature and personal support for
both medical staff and patient. When selecting a pump, the commitment
of the manufacturer to providing this documentation, as well as ongoing in-servicing for medical staff, should be considered. Prospective buyers should also ask the manufacturer about the procedures
for repairing pumps, should the need arise, and whether the pumps
can be recertified on a routine basis.

VI. PARADE OF AMBULATORY INFUSION PUMPS

Dozens of infusion pumps are manufactured and sold in the United
States. To qualify for ambulatory status, the pump and drug reservoir combined should not weigh much over a pound and preferably
less. Overall weight and size are probably the most important criteria for the patient.
   The review of ambulatory pumps that follows is representative
rather than exhaustive. Every effort has been made to accurately
and fairly portray some of the major ambulatory pumps presently marketed in the United States. Some specific features of representative
pumps are shown in Tables 1 to 10 and Figs. 1 to 10.

VII. CLINICAL APPLICATIONS

The preferred route of administration of most drugs is by mouth. It
is convenient, noninvasive, and acceptable to the patient. However,
drugs given orally must resist digestion in the gut; they must be

TABLE 1 Cormed Models 6-4 and 6-6

Manufacturer	Cormed Inc. 591 Markar Street Medina, New York 14103
Cost	$1325
Pumping mechanism	Rotary peristaltic
Dimensions	8.3 cm wide × 12.7 cm high × 3.8 cm thick
Weight	540 g
Power source	2.5 V rechargeable NiCad battery
Battery life	7 days
Program modes	Continuous infusion only, adjustable rates
Security level	None
Flow rates	Model 6-4: 4-20 ml/24 hr Model 6-6: 10-50 ml/24 hr
Accuracy	Not available
Automatic KVO rate[a]	No
Prime function	No
Digital readout	No
Memory	Not applicable; set by adjustable flow rate meter
Alarms	No
Automatic shutdown	No
Drug reservoir type	Dedicated polymeric reservoir bag, disposable
Volume	50 ml

[a]KVO = keep vein open.

TABLE 2 The Cormed II

Manufacturer	Cormed Inc. 591 Mahar Street Medina, New York 14103
Cost	$1595
Pump mechanism	Rotary peristaltic
Dimensions	10.7 cm wide × 12 cm high × 3.8 cm thick
Weight	482 g
Power source	5 V rechargeable NiCad battery
Battery life	5 days
Program modes	Continuous infusion only, adjustable rates
Security level	None
Flow rates	6-50 ml/24 hr
Accuracy	Not available
Automatic KVO rate	No
Prime function	No
Digital readout	Yes (LCD)
Memory	Not applicable; set by adjustable dial
Alarms	Yes: audible and visual for low battery low flow high flow[a] electronic malfunction[a]
Automatic shutdown[a]	Yes
Drug reservoir type	Dedicated polymeric reservoir bag, disposable
Volume	60 ml

[a]Automatic shutdown when flow exceeds 49% of set flow or during pump malfunction.

TABLE 3 Graseby MS 16A or MS 26

Manufacturer	Intermedics Infusaid Corp. 1400 Providence Highway Norwood, Massachusetts 02062
Cost	$1150 each
Pumping mechanism	Syringe
Dimensions	16.5 cm long × 2.3 cm wide × 5.3 cm high
Weight	175 g
Power source	9 V alkaline battery
Battery life	About 1-1/2 months
Program modes	Intermittent pulses only
Security level	None
Flow rates	MS 16A: 1-99 mm/hr[a] MS 26: 1-99 mm/24 hr
Accuracy	±5%
Automatic KVO rate	No
Prime function	Yes
Digital readout	No
Memory	No

Alarms	Yes: audible and visual
	  empty syringe
	  occlusion
	  overperfusion
	  low battery
	  system malfunction

Automatic shutdown	Yes
Drug reservoir type	Hypodermic syringes
Volume	5-35 ml

[a]Depending on volume of syringe, flow rates range from 0.2 to 33 ml/hr for MS 16A or 0.12 to 44 ml/24 hr for MS 26.

TABLE 4 The Provider Plus Series 2000 and 4000

Manufacturer	Pancretec Inc. 3878 Ruffin Road San Diego, California 92123
Cost	$2398 (2000+) or $2498 (4000+)
Pumping mechanism	Rotary peristaltic
Dimensions	8.6 cm wide × 15 cm high × 4 cm thick
Weight	660 g
Power source	8.5 V rechargeable NiCad battery
Battery life	24 hr (2000+) or 10 hr (4000+) at maximum flow
Program modes	Continuous or intermittent
Security level	Patient lockout
Flow rates	2000+: 0.2-83.0 ml/hr 4000+: 0.4-200.0 ml/hr
Accuracy	± 5%
Automatic KVO rate	Yes: 0.1 ml/hr (2000+), 0.2 ml/hr (4000+)
Prime function	Yes
Digital readout	Yes
Memory	Yes (30 sec without battery support)
Alarms	Yes: audible and visual infusion complete air-in-line occlusion improper cartridge insertion low battery low reservoir program error memory loss prime overuse system malfunction
Automatic shutdown	Information not provided
Drug reservoir type	Any external collapsible reservoir
Volume	Dependent on reservoir

TABLE 5 The Pharmacia Deltec CADD-1 5100HF

Manufacturer	Pharmacia Deltec 1265 Gray Fox Road St. Paul, Minnesota 55112
Cost	$2395
Pumping mechanism	Linear peristaltic
Dimensions	16 cm high × 8.9 cm wide × 2.8 cm thick (includes 50 ml reservoir cassette)
Weight	465 g
Power source	9 V alkaline battery
Battery life	10 days
Program modes	Continuous or extended bolus[a]
Security level	Yes (three patient lockout levels)
Flow rates	1-200 ml/24 hr or 90 ml/hr[a]
Accuracy	±10%
Automatic KVO rate	No
Prime function	Yes
Digital readout	Yes (LCD)
Memory	Yes (20 year with battery out)

Alarms	Yes: visual and audible
	  low battery
	  pump stopped
	  pump malfunction
	  low volume
	  occlusion

Automatic shutdown	Yes
Drug reservoir type	Dedicated cassette
Volume	50 or 100 ml or remote reservoir adapter for use with any collapsible reservoir

[a]Extended bolus mode pumps at a fixed rate of 90 ml/hr.

TABLE 6 The Pharmacia Deltec CADD-PCA 5200P

Manufacturer	Pharmacia Deltec, Inc. 1265 Gray Fox Road St. Paul, Minnesota 55112
Cost	$2995
Pumping mechanism	Linear peristaltic
Dimensions	16 cm high × 8.9 cm wide × 2.8 cm thick (includes 50 ml reservoir cassette)
Weight	465 g
Power source	9 V alkaline battery
Battery life	10 days
Program modes	Continuous, bolus, or continuous plus bolus
Security level	Yes (three patient lockout levels)
Flow rates	0.05-10.0 ml/hr
Accuracy	±10%
Automatic KVO rate	No
Digital readout	Yes (LCD)
Memory	Yes (20 years with battery out)

Alarms	Yes: audible and visual
	  low battery
	  pump stopped
	  pump malfunction
	  low volume
	  occlusion

Automatic shutdown	Yes
Drug reservoir type	Dedicated cassette
Volume	50 or 100 ml cassette

TABLE 7 The Travenol Infusor Models: 2C1070, 2C1080, and 2C1073

Manufacturer	Travenol Laboratories, Inc. Hospital Division Deerfield, Illinois 60015
Cost	$30
Pumping mechanism	Constant pressure
Dimensions	16 cm long × 3 cm diameter
Weight	90 g (full)
Power source	Balloon, elastomeric energy
Battery life	Not applicable
Program modes	Continuous infusion only, not adjustable
Security level	None
Flow rates	2 ml/hr (2C1070), 0.5 ml/hr (2C1080), 5 ml/hr (2C1073)
Accuracy	Not available
Prime function	No
Digital readout	No
Memory	No
Alarms	No
Automatic shutdown	No
Drug reservoir type	Balloon reservoir back-filled through a filling port[a]
Volume	60 ml

[a]The unit is intended for single use only. The Infusor must not be refilled or resterilized.

TABLE 8 The Infumed 200

Manufacturer	Medfusion Systems, Inc. 3070 Business Park Drive Norcross, Georgia 30071
Cost	$1595
Pumping mechanism	Linear peristaltic
Dimensions	11.2 cm wide × 10.2 cm high × 4.6 cm thick
Weight	320 g
Power source	9 V alkaline battery
Battery life	3.5 days at maximal flow
Program modes	Continuous infusions only, adjustable
Security level	None
Flow rates	0.1-9.9 ml/hr
Accuracy	±5%
Automatic KVO rate	No
Prime function	No
Digital readout	Yes, flow rate dial set on number
Memory	Not applicable; set by adjustable dial
Alarms	Yes low flow high flow low battery system malfunction
Automatic shutdown	Yes
Drug reservoir type	Any external collapsible polymeric container
Volume	Depends on reservoir; MedFusion supplies 70 ml reservoir

TABLE 9 The Infusaid Model 400

Manufacturer	Intermedics Infusaid Inc. 1400 Providence Highway Norwood, Massachusetts 02062
Cost	$3750
Pumping mechanism	Constant-pressure bellows
Dimensions	8.7 cm diameter × 2.8 cm thick
Weight	208 g
Power source	Freon gas vapor pressure
Battery life	Not applicable
Program modes	Continuous infusion only, not adjustable
Security level	None, but implanted subcutaneously
Flow rates	1-6 ml/24 hr, depending on outlet flow restrictors
Accuracy	Not available
Automatic KVO rate	No
Prime function	No
Digital readout	No
Memory	No
Alarms	No
Automatic shutdown	No
Drug reservoir type	Drug chamber built into pump
Volume	50 ml

TABLE 10 Betatron II

Manufacturer	Cardiac Pacemakers, Inc. 4100 North Hamline Avenue St. Paul, Minnesota 55164
Cost	$2850
Pumping mechanism	Positive displacement
Dimensions	6.6 cm wide × 9.9 cm high × 2.0 cm thick
Weight	163 g
Power source	Rechargeable NiCad battery with 3 V backup battery
Battery line	30 hr main battery, 6 months backup battery
Program modes	Multiple basal rates, meal bolus
Security level	Patient lockout
Flow rates	1-150 U/24 hr basal rate; 0.1-20.0 U meal bolus
Accuracy	±3%
Automatic KVO rate	Not applicable
Prime function	Yes
Digital readout	Yes
Memory	Yes, battery dependent
Alarms	Yes low battery catheter block motor fault microcomputer fault reservoir empty memory fault
Automatic shutdown	No
Drug reservoir type	Syringe
Volume	1.5 ml

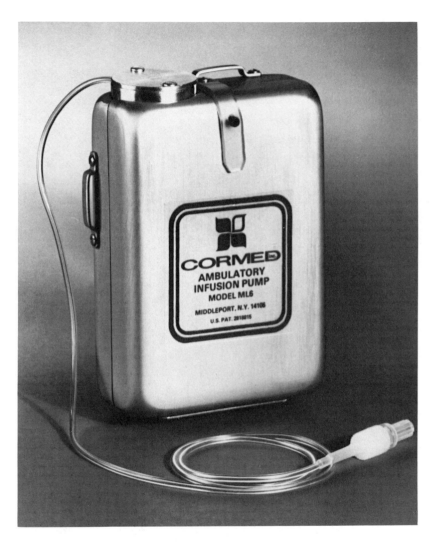

Fig. 1 The Cormed model ML6.

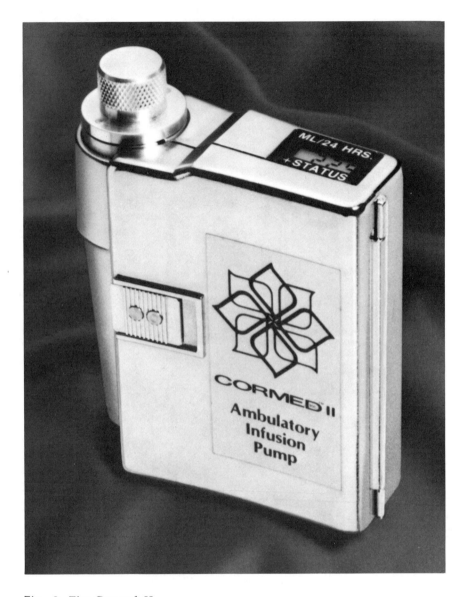

Fig. 2 The Cormed II.

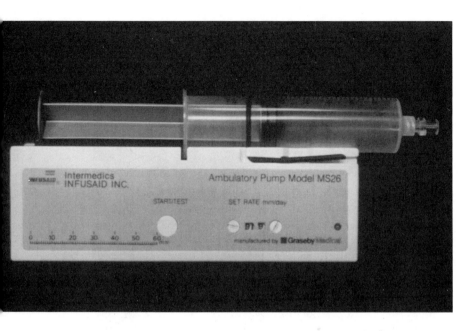

Fig. 3 The Graseby MS 26.

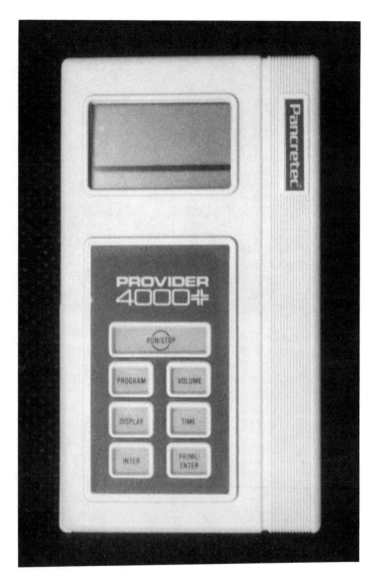

Fig. 4 The Provider Plus 4000+.

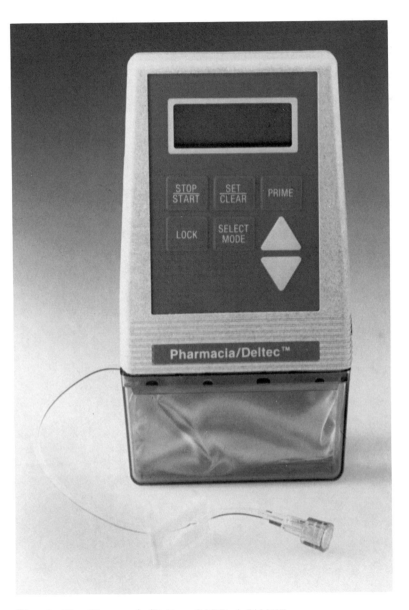

Fig. 5 The Pharmacia/Deltec CADD-1 5100HF.

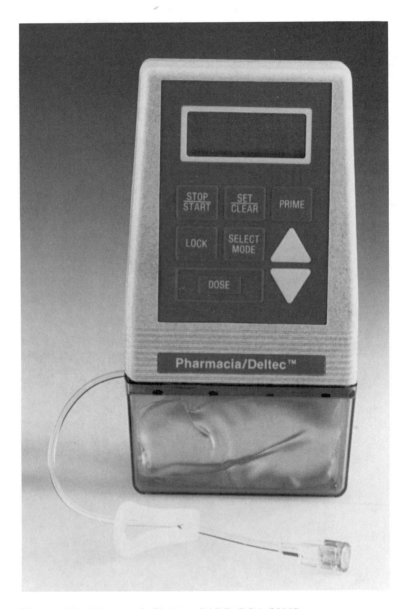

Fig. 6 The Pharmacia/Deltec CADD-PCA 5200P.

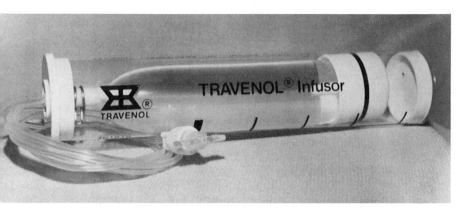

Fig. 7 The Travenol Infusor.

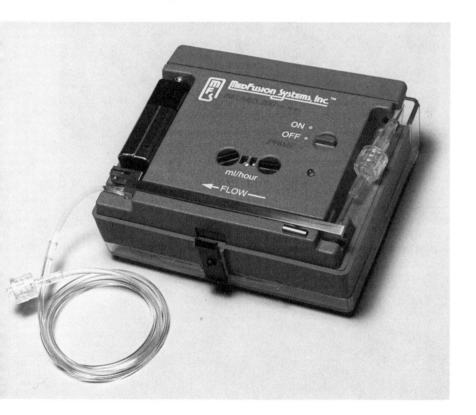

Fig. 8 The Infumed 200.

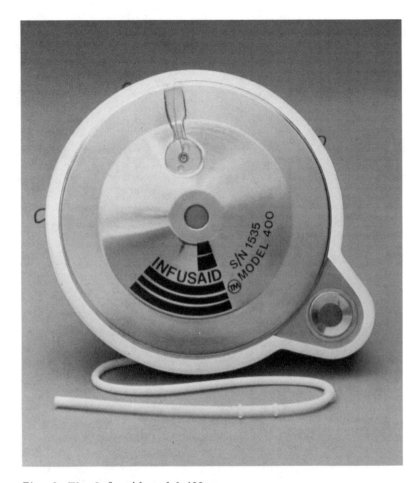

Fig. 9 The Infusaid model 400.

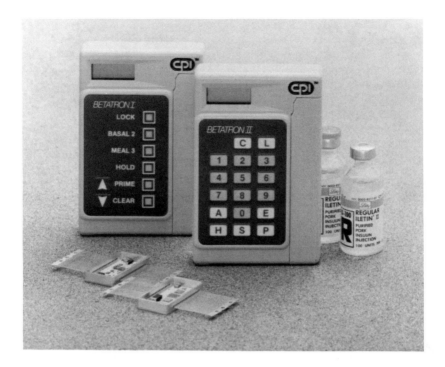

Fig. 10 The Betatron I and II.

transported across the bowel in their active form, and they must reach the systemic circulation in quantities sufficient for therapeutic efficacy. The digestive tract must be relatively resistant to any adverse effects of the agent, since the highest concentration of the drug occurs in the bowel. Many pharmacological agents either cannot be given by mouth or, when given by this route, have an effect that is unpredictable. Such drugs must be given by parenteral injection.

For optimal efficacy, a drug should be present in the plasma within a specific therapeutic range. Despite this, most drugs are given by intermittent bolus injection, a method of administration that often results in plasma concentrations oscillating between therapeutic failure and toxic levels. Continuous infusion pumps should be considered when wide variations in plasma concentrations are to be avoided.

A. Insulin

Insulin was isolated from pancreatic β cells in 1922 [11]. In 1974 a division of Miles Laboratories developed an improved version of a closed-loop system for the administration of insulin. The system, named the Biostator Controller, consisted of a biosensor for the frequent determination of plasma glucose, a computer-controlled motor for processing the data, and a pumping mechanism for delivering the appropriate dose of insulin [12]. These bulky, extracorporeal systems required constant attention by a trained professional and obligated the patient to remain in bed.

In 1978 a portable infusion device (the Mill Hill Pump) was described [13] that was much reduced in size and complexity but lacked feedback control, a so-called open-loop system. Subsequently, others also reported [14,15] that open-loop portable infusion pumps could be used successfully for the subcutaneous or intravenous infusion of insulin in many insulin-dependent diabetic patients.

However, the development of ambulatory infusion pumps for the delivery of insulin was not the breakthrough for the diabetic that might have been expected. Even though these early studies showed that good control of blood glucose could be achieved with portable open-loop pumps, the maintenance of normoglycemia was not always significantly better than that achieved using multiple bolus injections of insulin. In fact, it could be argued that without definitive evidence of additional benefit, the need to wear a continuous infusion pump may actually be an added inconvenience and expense for the patient.

The use of portable pumps also resulted in a number of complications [16] that were not encountered with subcutaneous injections of insulin. Insulin tends to self-associate to form macromolecular aggregates, and the resulting insulin fibrils may obstruct the pump tubing. Insulin fibrillization, which is enhanced by an increase in temperature and by motion, results in the progressive inactivation of the insulin in the pump reservoir. Obstruction of the tubing is a concern, as any interruption in the insulin supply may have serious consequences.

Only very small volumes (0.05-0.2 ml/hr) of insulin are necessary when given as a continuous infusion. Delivery accuracy and functional integrity are important, since the administration of inappropriate doses of insulin to the diabetic may result in clinically significant hypo- or hyperglycemia. Ambulatory insulin pumps are usually of the syringe rather than the peristaltic type, since these are usually more accurate for administering small volumes. Moreover, syringe pumps unlike peristaltic pumps do not cause excessive motion of the insulin, so fibrilization is less likely to occur.

It is estimated that the normal pancreas, on average, releases between 50 and 80 units of insulin per 24 hr period and that half the total daily production is associated with meals. It follows that any open-loop insulin pump should allow the user to select multiple infusion rates and should automatically revert to the basal mode of delivery after the completion of a meal bolus.

B. Antineoplastics

Most antineoplastic agents express their anticancer activity by inter-
fering with DNA replication during cell division. Since all tumor cells
do not reproduce simultaneously, a constant therapeutic plasma level
of the drug should be more effective in inhibiting tumor growth than
the wide fluctuations between high and low concentrations that typically
accompany sequential bolus dosing [17]. However, the relative efficacy of a drug when given by continuous infusion or bolus injection
is still unresolved. It is not within the context of this chapter to de-
bate the effectiveness of various dosing regimens, but some improvement in the therapeutic index has been reported for certain antineoplastic agents when given by continuous infusion.

A variety of ambulatory infusion pumps have been evaluated for
the continuous infusion of chemotherapy. One study [18] reports that
the Travenol Infusor was successfully used for the long-term infusion
of 5-fluorouracil. A new Infusor was filled each day by the patient
and delivered 48 ml/day, with the length of infusion ranging from 54
to 324 days. These systems are simple to use but since they pump
a fixed volume, the concentration of the drug solution must be calculated and adjusted so as to deliver the desired amount of medication.
With the development of programmable microprocessor-based pumps,
it should be possible to enter only the amount of drug to be delivered
and the concentration of the drug solution. The pump could then calculate the appropriate volume to be infused. This would greatly facilitate tailoring of a prescribed dosing regimen to an individual patient.

The amount of antineoplastic drug that can be administered by
intravenous bolus and, therefore, its efficacy, may be limited by the
production of adverse systemic effects. To overcome this, some investigators have advocated delivering of the drug intra-arterially just
upstream from the target organ. Intra-arterial delivery should produce a continuously high drug concentration at the tumor site with a
reduced circulating level and, hence, less adverse effects.

Intra-arterial organ-specific chemotherapy was initially evaluated
in the 1950s [19]. However, the numerous mechanical, vascular, and
septic complications that resulted from the use of percutaneous arterial
infusion lines and the limited clinical benefit seen discouraged widespread acceptance. The development of a safe, long-term vascular
access infusion system in the early 1970s revived interest in the therapeutic application of continuous regional chemotherapy. In 1980 Buchwald et al. [20] reported that in 1977 they had implanted infusion
pumps in four patients with metastatic disease of the liver. The catheters were placed in the hepatic artery for delivery of chemotherapy.
This small study clearly demonstrated the feasibility of regional chemotherapy by means of an implantable pump. A number of investigators
have since used various portable infusion pumps for the continuous

intra-arterial delivery of antineoplastic drugs, both into the hepatic artery for the treatment of colorectal hepatic metastases [21-23], and into the carotid artery for head and neck cancer [24].

C. Pain Management

Acute pain following surgery is typically managed by repeated intramuscular bolus injections of narcotic analgesics. The inadequacies of this regimen for pain management have been discussed [25,26]. Usually, after first complaining of pain the patient must wait for the nurse to respond, then wait for the nurse to prepare the medicaiton, wait for the dose to be given, and finally wait for the medication to take effect. Frequently, the dose administered is either too large or too small, resulting in either sedation or inadequate pain relief.

In contrast, when an analgesic is administered intravenously, the drug is distributed rapidly resulting in a faster onset of action. The immediate biological effect of a narcotic when given intravenously allows more precise adjustment of the dose to achieve safe analgesia.

More recently, the concept of administering an analgesic by continuous infusion coupled with the ability to give intermittent bolus injections on patient demand has been recognized. This method, which has been termed patient-controlled analgesia (PCA), allows the patient to trigger, within preset dose and time limitations, a bolus injection usually in addition to a background maintenance infusion. In this way, the patient has some ability to titrate analgesic administration to the level of pain experienced [27,28].

A PCA pump provides some combination of analgesic infusion coupled to patient-triggered bolus injections. Most in-hospital PCA devices cannot reasonably be classified as ambulatory. The two most popular devices are the Bard PCA (10 lb) and Abbott Lifecare PCA (14 lb) pumps. Because of their weight and size, these pumps are obligated to a pole mount. Only three ambulatory PCA devices are currently available, the Pharmacia CADD-PCA, the Travenol Infusor, and the Minimed (Pacesetter Systems Inc.) pump.

Ambulatory PCA devices for postoperative pain management may encourage earlier ambulation, enhance speed of recovery, and allow for greater social interaction. They may be especially useful after caesarean section, since the mother remains mobile, allowing a closer relationship with the infant. These potential benefits, however, remain to be substantiated by controlled clinical trials.

Ambulatory pumps have found a special niche in the management of chronic pain due to cancer. It is claimed that well over half of all patients with cancer eventually develop pain that will require some therapy [29]. Oral narcotics are usually the first choice for palliative pain relief, but in many instances the pain persists, or oral narcotics are not well tolerated. In such cases, parenteral management of the pain is indicated. However, the traditional large doses of narcotics, given by intermittent intramuscular or intravenous injection, result in widely fluctuating plasma levels that are often associated with adverse effects or analgesic failure. Alternatively, the analgesic can be given by continuous intravenous infusion but, until lately, this has meant confining the patient to bed. Today, ambulatory pumps are being used by physicians for the intravenous [30], subcutaneous [31], and epidural/intrathecal [32] administration of narcotic analgesics. With few exceptions, pain appears to be adequately controlled, and neither respiratory depression nor opiate tolerance is a limiting factor in the cancer patient.

D. Antibiotics

There are few treatments with respect to which the economic pressures (e.g., DRGs) can be as easily addressed without compromising the quality of care. Antibiotic therapy is one such area. The number of antimicrobials available to the clinic has doubled in the past decade. Many of the newer generation antimicrobials are more stable, have extended half-lives, and are less toxic. With the recent development of ambulatory pumps, outpatient treatment is becoming more feasible. Intravenous antibiotic therapy for the ambulatory outpatient should, however, be limited to infections for which there is a need to achieve high tissue levels of a drug, or when oral medication is inappropriate or not possible. Outpatient intravenous antibiotic therapy may be considered for infections such as osteomyelitis, deep wound sepsis, infected prosthetic devices, endo- and pericarditis, nephritis, meningitis, and possibly as prophylaxis in patients with cystic fibrosis or neutropenia secondary to bone marrow transplantation.

One recent publication [33] has convincingly demonstrated both the improved efficacy and cost-saving advantages of an outpatient antibiotic regimen using an ambulatory pump. These authors reported on 14 patients with active osteomyelitis who had failed treatment with conventional antibiotic regimens and surgical debridement. Each of these patients received an ambulatory pump (Infusaid model 400) with the distal end of the catheter placed near the infected sinus. The pumps were filled with the appropriate concentration of an antibiotic as determined by blood cultures and serum levels of the drug. In this way, high concentraitons of the drug were achieved at or near the site of infection but were associated with low systemic levels. This resulted in a high cure rate and a low incidence of side effects. Eleven of the 14 patients showed no recurrence of infection after a follow-up of one year.

Furthermore, this study and others [34,35] provide clear evidence of the significant cost savings that may be achieved with outpatient antibiotic therapy. The mean time on the pump was 63 days, but the

mean length of the hospitalization was only 24 days. Obviously, a
reduction in hospitalization of about one month represents a substantial cost savings with no compromise in therapeutic efficacy. Other
less tangible benefits such as permitting a more normal lifestyle, reduction in the emotional trauma and anxiety of hospitalization, and a return
to work must also be considered as beneficial to the patient and to
the community.

Although antibiotic outpatient therapy using portable infusion
pumps has definite advantages, it is not appropriate for all patients
nor for all types of infection. The importance of patient selection has
been stressed [36]. Patients should have no medical problems other
than the need for intravenous antibiotics. Only after patients have
been stabilized on antibiotic therapy in hospital should they be considered for outpatient treatment. The patient or a member of the family
must be taught how to adequately care for the intravenous system.

E. Other

Patients with Parkinson's disease have been treated successfully in
the home with dopaminergic agonists infused parenterally with ambulatory pumps [37]. In one small study, the investigators reported that
three patients with difficult-to-treat, long-standing Parkinsonism were
placed on a continuous subcutaneous infusion of Lisuride (agent not
approved in the United States). All patients were discharged with
good control of motor function. Patient selection and follow-up are
again essential, since severe vomiting, confusion, hallucinations, and
blood pressure and inotropic effects have been reported to occur as
the result of dopaminergic drug administration.

Some patients with severe congestive heart failure may not toler-
ate or may remain refractory to conventional therapy such as diuretics,
nitrates, or angiotensin-converting enzyme inhibitors. Intravenous
infusion of dobutamine, however, has been shown to produce marked
symptomatic improvement in these patients. One report [38] describes
the use of an ambulatory pump for the administration of dobutamine
in a patient with congestive heart failure. Dobutamine was administered intermittently for 48 hr at weekly intervals. The patient died
after 8 months on ambulatory therapy. During the course of treatment,
marked improvement in exercise tolerance and a reduction in fatigue
were noted.

VIII. FUTURE TRENDS

It is expected that cost containment measures will result in an exponential growth of the ambulatory infusion pump market in the next
10 years. To speculate on the technology of tomorrow in this dynamic

setting is beset with pitfalls. Nevertheless, some future trends are already evident.

For ambulatory pumps to realize their full potential, the parenteral administration of drugs in the outpatient must become more widely accepted among health professionals. Once this has been realized, infusion pumps will be developed to encompass an even wider therapeutic spectrum.

Drug administration in the home and at work is certain to raise concern not only about the efficacy and safety of the treatment regimen, but also regarding the reliability of infusion pumps. Sensitive, reliable alarms to warn of existing or imminent problems with an ongoing infusion will be mandatory. Automatic shutdown features to preclude inappropriate drug delivery in the event of pump malfunction will be an essential safeguard. It is probable that more reliance will be placed on basing drug delivery on pharmacokinetic and pharmacodynamic considerations.

With the evolving interest in biosensors, closed-loop systems will be developed for indications other than insulin administration. Infusion pumps will automatically adjust drug delivery depending on plasma levels of the agent or the resulting physiological response. Pumps are currently available that permit an infusion in two stages. These mimic the current practice of giving an initial bolus as a loading dose followed by a prolonged lower rate of infusion. In this way the plasma level of the drug is rapidly elevated and then maintained within the effective therapeutic range with less chance of toxic adverse effects.

Real-time programming has already arrived and will be given a further boost if the claims of chronotherapy are verified. It is reported that the effect and toxicity of some therapeutic agents may be influenced by the actual time of day they are administered. Pulsatile hormone delivery is an indication that also lends itself to real-time capabilities [39].

It is obvious that a new level of sophistication will be developed for ambulatory pumps. However, this must not be at the expense of apparent simplicity and user friendliness. More extensive programming capacity may enable an infusion pump to be used in a variety of therapeutic situations. Although it is difficult to predict the precise path of future innovation, new infusion systems will enable the medical profession to provide treatment to the patient at reduced cost while not comprising the standard of care. The future development of ambulatory infusion pumps is an exciting area, which holds much promise both for the medical profession and for the patient.

REFERENCES

1. R. K. Ausman, *Intravascular Infusion Systems.* MTP Press Limited, Lancaster, 1984, p. 9.

2. C. E. Bortecchi, *S. Med. J.*, 75:61 (1982).
3. R. P. Wenzel, *Am. J. Med.*, 78:3 (1985).
4. B. Bivins, R. Rapp, and H. McKean, *Arch. Surg.*, 115:70 (1980).
5. A. C. Kind, D. N. Williams, G. Persons, and J. A. Gibson, *Arch. Intern. Med.*, 139:413 (1979).
6. K. Levit, H. Lazenby, D. Walder, and L. Davidoff, *Health Care Finance Rev.*, 7:1 (1985).
7. I. H. Pitman, *Med. J. Aust.*, 144:78 (1986).
8. R. L. Hansen and G. A. Carlson, Implantable drug delivery pumps. In *Proceedings of Business Opportunities in Drug and I.V. Fluid Therapy*, New Orleans, 1985, pp. 4.1-4.11.
9. *Health Devices*, 4:193 (1975).
10. *Health Devices*, 8:103 (1979).
11. F. Banting, C. Best, J. Collip, and J. Macleod, *Trans. R. Soc. Can.*, 5 (1922).
12. W. Clarke and J. Santiago, *Artif. Organs*, 1:78 (1977).
13. J. Pickup, H. Keen, J. Parsons, and K. Alberti, *Br. Med. J.*, 1:204 (1978).
14. M. Champion, G. Shepherd, N. Rodger, and J. Dupre, *Diabetes*, 29:206 (1980).
15. P. Raskin, A. Pietri, and R. Unger, *Diabetes*, 28:1033 (1979).
16. D. S. Schade, J. V. Santiago, J. S. Skyler, and R. A. Rizza, *Intensive Insulin Therapy*. Excerpta Medica USA, New York, 1983, p. 302.
17. N. A. Vogelzang, *J. Clin. Oncol.*, 2:1289 (1984).
18. G. A. Caballero, R. K. Ausman, and E. J. Quebbeman, *Cancer Treat. Rep.*, 69:13 (1985).
19. C. T. Klopp, T. C. Alfordd, and J. Bateman, *Ann. Surg.*, 132:811 (1950).
20. H. Buchwald, T. B. Grage, P. P. Vassilopoulus, et al., *Cancer*, 45:866 (1980).
21. W. Ensminger, J. Niederhuber, S. Dakhil, et al., *Cancer Treat. Rep.*, 65:393 (1981).
22. R. von Roemeling, M. MacDonald, T. Langevin, et al., *Oncol. Nurs. Forum*, 13:17 (1986).
23. N. J. Vogelzang, M. Ruane, and T. R. DeMeestu, *J. Clin. Oncol.*, 3:407 (1985).
24. S. Frustaci, L. Barzan, S. Tumolo, et al., *Cancer*, 57:1118 (1986).
25. J. E. Utting and J. M. Smith, *Anesthesia*, 34:320 (1979).
26. R. M. Marks and E. J. Sachar, *Ann. Intern. Med.*, 78:173 (1973).
27. D. A. Graves, T. S. Foster, R. L. Batenhorst, et al., *Ann. Intern. Med.*, 99:360 (1983).
28. R. L. Bennett, R. L. Batenhorst, B. A. Bivins, et al., *Ann. Surg.*, 195:700 (1982).

29. M. L. Citron and A. Johnson-Early, *Arch. Intern. Med.*, 146: 734 (1986).
30. J. D. Adams, L. F. Diehl, and J. P. Wilson, *Drug Intell. Clin. Pharm.*, 18:138 (1984).
31. N. Coyle, A. Mauskop, J. Maggard, and K. M. Foley, *Oncol. Nurs. Forum*, 13:53 (1986).
32. D. W. Coombs, R. L. Saunders, M. S. Gaylor, et al., *JAMA*, 250:2336 (1983).
33. C. R. Perry, J. K. Ritterbusch, and S. H. Rice, *Am. J. Med.*, 80:222 (1986).
34. A. C. Kind, D. N. Williams, G. Persons, and J. A. Gibson, *Arch. Intern. Med.*, 139:413 (1979).
35. L. F. Harris, T. F. Buckle, and F. L. Coffey, *South. Med. J.*, 79:193 (1986).
36. M. B. Grizzard, *Postgrad. Med.*, 78:187 (1985).
37. J. A. Obeso, M. R. Luquin, and J. M. Martinez-Lage, *Lancet*, 1:467 (1986).
38. M. Bergen and C. K. McSherry, *Chest*, 88:295 (1985).
39. J. C. Marshall and R. P. Kelch, *New Engl. J. Med.*, 315:1459 (1986).

6

The Infusors: Complete Self-Powered Continuous Infusion Systems

DAVID A. WINCHELL and JOEL A. TUNE / Baxter Healthcare Corporation, Round Lake, Illinois

I. INTRODUCTION

Advances in infusion device technology have resulted in greater accuracy, flexibility, and ease of use, and in more infusion safeguards. Portable devices have facilitated in-hospital ambulation and have allowed outpatient and at-home treatment of patients for whom continuous infusion therapy has been prescribed.

This chapter describes the technology, preparation and use, and specific clinical applications of the Infusor. This innovation, from Baxter, has resulted in a complete, self-powered infusion system that is accurate, highly portable, disposable, and simple to use.

The initial application of the Infusor technology was in continuous infusion of chemotherapy for cancer. This has been expanded to include analgesia, notably patient-controlled analgesia (PCA), and other drug categories are being evaluated in the system.

The Infusor requires no batteries or external power source. A constant flow rate is maintained by the kinetic elastomer material of the balloon reservoir. The flow rate is preset in manufacturing. Varitions in drug dosage and infusion duration are managed by changes in concentration and fill volume, respectively.

II. INFUSOR TECHNOLOGY

A. Development Objectives

Several objectives were set for development of the Infusor technology, based on a recognized clinical need for a cost-effective, easily managed infusion system that could be used in the hospital, for outpatients, and at home.

Goals were to avoid bulkiness and weight associated with existing portable pumps, as well as the need for a power source, the sometimes complex settings or adjustments, the maintenance requirements, and the high cost.

The primary objectives, therefore, for Infusor development were for a unit that would be:

Accurate
Easy to operate and monitor
Lightweight
Disposable
Cost effective

B. Infusor Design

Four Infusor models are currently available. The basic design is the same for all. There are, however, differences in filling procedure,, location of the rate controller in the system, and flow rates; in addition, a control module can be added for patient-controlled analgesia.

Basic Infusor Design

The basic Infusor system comprises a balloon reservoir within a housing unit and 36 in. nonkinking tubing for attachment to the catheter (Fig. 1).

Balloon reservoir function is based on kinetic elastomer technology, in which memory is established by controlled cross-link density of carbon-carbon double bonds in polyisoprene. The bonds provide a low level of hysteresis in the material. These unique material properties, when combined with the cylindrical reservoir shape, provide a consistent pressure on the fluid regardless of the volume in the reservoir.

This constant-pressure reservoir is matched to a microbore glass capillary to provide the desired flow rate. The performance of this system is governed by Poiseuille's law of capillary flow, as shown in the following equation for intravenous infusion:

$$Q = \pi r^4 \frac{P}{8\mu l}$$

where
Q = infusion rate
r = inner radius of the glass flow restrictor
P = reservoir pressure minus venous pressure
μ = viscosity of drug/diluent
l = length of glass flow restrictor

The system can also be used for arterial, epidural, intrathecal, and subcutaneous infusions. In all cases except arterial infusions, the flow rate is the same because reservoir pressure is several times greater than the resisting pressure of the system. With arterial infusions, the flow rate will be about 12% slower.

Viscosity of the drug has an inversely proportional effect on flow rate. With typical drug concentrations, the diluent is the primary factor in determining fluid viscosity. The device flow rate is calibrated for the use of 5% dextrose as the diluent. Other diluents such as 0.9% saline, Ringer's lactate, or sterile water may also be used and will provide a flow rate 10% faster than the baseline with 5% dextrose.

The remaining factors, namely the glass flow restrictor dimensions, are stringently controlled in manufacturing through a series of tests and product release points.

The reservoir is filled through the injection site to a maximum of 65 ml. After filling and removal of the syringe, the injection site self-

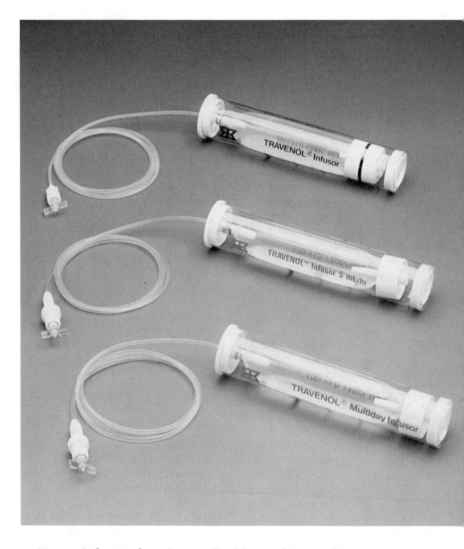

Fig. 1 Infusors from Baxter Healthcare Corporation.

seals. Filling forces the solution into the tubing which, after priming, is capped to form a closed system for delivery to the floor or to the patient.

The Infusor weighs 4 oz. when filled and has the following dimensions: length, 6 in.; diameter, 1-1/4 in.

Infusor Models

The four Infusor models are described below, and their application in patient-controlled analgesia is introduced.

Single-Day Infusor

The Single-Day Infusor (Fig. 2) was the first to be developed and is used for continuous infusions up to 24 hr, primarily for cancer chemotherapy. It is filled using a syringe with a needle, has the flow regulator at the distal end of the Infusor housing, and has a preset flow rate of 2 ml/hr. The Infusor housing should be worn close to the skin to provide optimal performance (Table 1).

Easy-Fill Infusors

The three Easy-Fill Infusor models (see, e.g., Fig. 3) can also be used in cancer chemotherapy or for any continuous infusion. They are designed for single-day, half-day, and multiple-day continuous infusions. All three Easy-Fill Infusors are filled directly from the syringe Luer connector to the fill site, without a needle. This decreases the number of filling steps, making the unit easier to fill and helping to decrease potential exposure to cytotoxic agents.

The flow regulator in the Easy-Fill Infusors is located at the distal end of the tubing, allowing more flexibility in wearing the device, because only the regulator must be worn next to the skin (rather than the unit itself).

The three Infusors differ only in preset flow rates, which permit continuous infusions of differing durations. Variations in drug dosage are made by changing concentration of the drug solution, and duration of the infusion is based on fluid volume. The three Easy-Fill models are summarized below and in Table 1.

Easy-Fill model	Flow rate (ml/hr)	Course of therapy
Single-day	2	to 24 hr
Half-day	5	to 12 hr
Multi-day	0.5	to 5 days

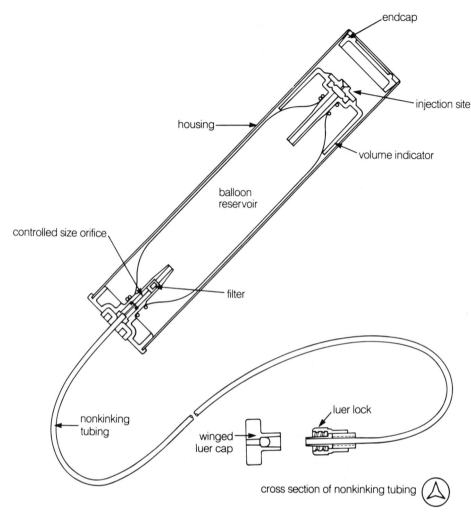

Fig. 2 A Single-Day Infusor.

Patient-Controlled Analgesia

For patient-controlled analgesia (PCA), which is described in more detail in Section IV, an Infusor is used with a wristband control module set in the tubing between the regulator and the Luer connector for the catheter tubing (Fig. 4). The control module includes a Velcro wristband, a 0.5 ml reservoir, a medication demand button, and tabs that indicate when the reservoir is filled and another analgesic dose may be administered (Fig. 5).

TABLE 1 Major Infusor Characteristics

All Infusors	
Maximum fill volume	65 ml
Tubing	36 in., nonkinking
Dimensions	6 in. × 1-1/4 in.
Filled weight	4 oz.
Dosage variation	by drug concentration
Infusion time variation	by fill volume

Individual Infusor models	Flow rate (ml/hr)	Duration of infusion (hr)	Filter size (μm)	Regulator site
Single-Day	2.0	to 24	10	Unit
Easy-Fill				
Single-Day	2.0[a]	to 24	5	Tubing
Half-Day	5.0[b]	to 12	5	Tubing
Multi-Day	0.5	to 120	5	Tubing

[a]For PCA, wristband reservoir is filled at 15 min intervals.
[b]For PCA, wristband reservoir is filled at 6 min intervals.

Any Infusor model can be used with the wristband control module. For PCA, the most commonly used model has a set flow rate of 5 ml/hr (e.g., the Easy-Fill Half-Day Infusor), which allows filling of the wristband reservoir every 6 min. A flow rate of 2 ml/hr (as in the Single-Day Infusors) allows filling of the reservoir at 15 min intervals.

III. INFUSOR PREPARATION AND USE

A. Dose Calculation

The flow rate is preset at a fixed rate for all Infusor models. Therefore, dosage alterations are made by changing *drug concentration*, and duration of the infusion is determined by the *fill volume*.

The Infusors were designed for use with 5% dextrose as the final diluent for flow at the specified rate for the Infusor. If 0.9% sodium chloride or Ringer's lactate is used, the viscosity will be lower and the flow rate will be 10% greater than the specified rate for the Infusor. Formulas for dosage calculation are given below.

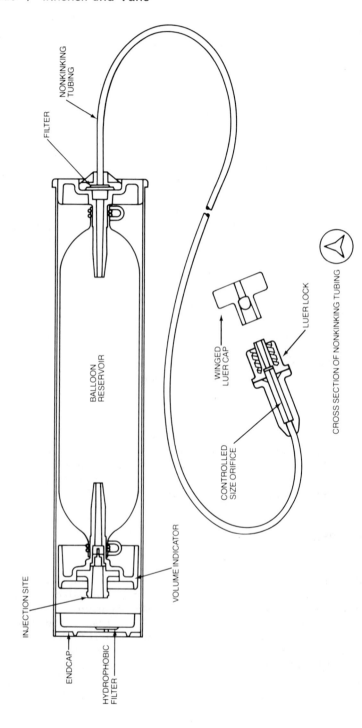

Fig. 3 An Easy-Fill Infusor.

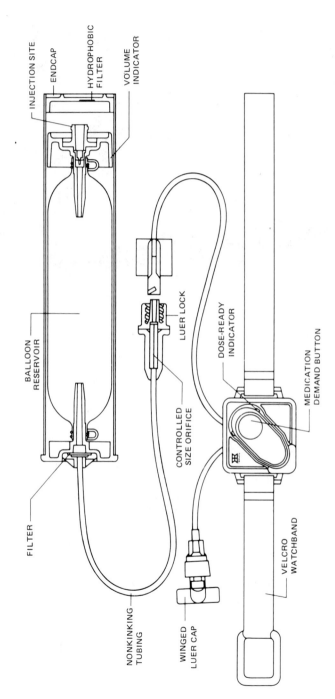

INJECTION SITE

ENDCAP

HYDROPHOBIC FILTER

VOLUME INDICATOR

BALLOON RESERVOIR

LUER LOCK

DOSE-READY INDICATOR

MEDICATION DEMAND BUTTON

CONTROLLED SIZE ORIFICE

FILTER

VELCRO WATCHBAND

NONKINKING TUBING

WINGED LUER CAP

Fig. 4 Infusor for patient-controlled analgesia.

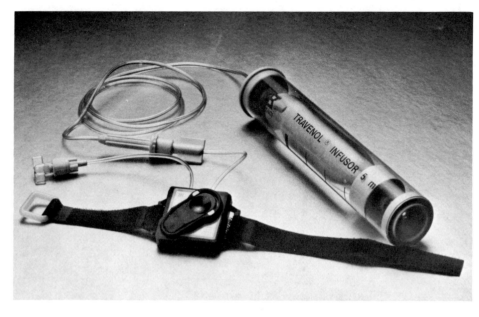

Fig. 5 Infusor for patient-controlled analgesia.

    The Single-Day Infusor has a residual volume of 2 ml and the Easy-Fill, 1 ml, after the reservoir is empty. If there is a need to compensate for the residual volume, dosage should be increased as shown below.

    The fill volume is first calculated, then the total medication. Equations shown below are appropriate for 5% dextrose. If sterile normal saline or Ringer's lactate is used, the fill volume should be 10% greater (to a maximum of 65 ml) because the flow rate will be 10% faster than with D5W. These equations can be used for infusion times less than those specified for a given Infusor model.

    Total medication (including compensation for the residual volume) will be 4% greater than the desired dose for the Single-Day Infusor, and 2% greater for the Easy-Fill Infusors.

Single-Day Infusor

fill volume = (flow rate × infusion time) + 2 ml residual

$$\text{total medication} = \text{desired dose} \times \left(\frac{\text{fill volume}}{\text{fill volume} - 2} \right)$$

Easy-Fill Infusors

fill volume = (flow rate × infusion time) + 1 ml residual

$$\text{total medication} = \text{desired dose} \left(\frac{\text{fill volume}}{\text{fill volume} - 1} \right)$$

B. Filling the Infusor

The filling procedure is the same for all Infusors, except that a syringe with a needle is used with the Single-Day Infusor and a direct Luer connection is used with the Easy-Fill models (Fig. 6). The list that follows is a convenient abridgement of the steps described in Fig. 6.

1. Mix drug solution.
2. Fill 60 ml syringe (use 20-22 gage needle with Single-Day Infusor).
3. Insert Luer connector (or needle) into fill site.
4. Keeping the Infusor unit vertical, place the head of the syringe plunger on a work surface.
5. Pull down on the syringe to force fluid into the reservoir. (More than 9 psi will be required.)
6. Remove Infusor from syringe. Filling site will automatically seal.
7. Insert endcap.
8. Prime tubing.
9. Secure Luer cap.
10. Label.
11. Place in storage bag.

C. Infusor Setup and Wearing

In the hospital, the housing of the Easy-Fill Infusors may be attached to an IV pole, to a bed, or to the patient's clothing. The unit may be vertical or horizontal. A primary consideration is that the flow regulator on the tubing be next to the patient's skin to ensure proper temperature. (The Single-Day Infusor, which has the flow regulator in the unit, does not lend itself to use with an IV pole.)

Ambulation in the hospital or at home is facilitated because the unit is small, lightweight, and can be concealed under clothing. With the Single-Day Infusor, the housing unit must be next to the skin in one of several recommended locations on the upper body (Fig. 7). The unit may be vertical or horizontal, but should not be worn on the arm, leg, or between the breasts, as body temperatures are too low or too high for optimal performance.

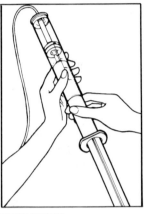

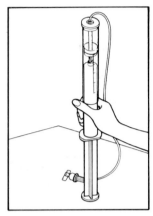

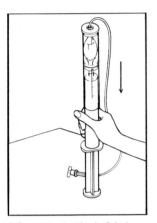

TO FILL INFUSOR:

1. Grasp volume indicator through housing and attach syringe Luer tip to filling port. DO NOT ATTACH NEEDLE TO SYRINGE. DO NOT REMOVE WINGED LUER CAP UNTIL UNIT IS FILLED.

2. Place head of syringe plunger on work surface keeping the unit vertical.

3. Grasp syringe barrel and pull slowly downward to gradually force fluid into balloon reservoir. DO NOT GRASP INFUSOR HOUSING, as this will interfere with normal filling and may cause damage to the balloon reservoir. A pressure in excess of 9 psi will be required to inflate the reservoir.

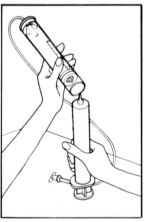

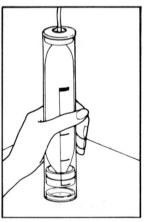

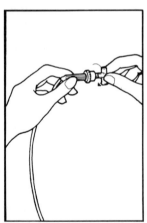

4. When the reservoir is filled, grasp the volume indicator through the housing and remove syringe. The filling port is designed to seal the contents of the reservoir against the pressure created by the inflated reservoir.

5. Place end cap on work surface. Grasp the housing and by using downward force on the work surface, push the end cap into the housing until flush.

6. Remove the winged Luer cap and allow fluid to fill set and expel air. The medication will automatically fill the delivery tubing. NOTE: If the set does not start to prime, attach an empty syringe to the Luer body using a male-to-female adapter. Pull syringe plunger until fluid appears in tip of syringe and disconnect adapter.

Fig. 6 Infusor filling procedure.

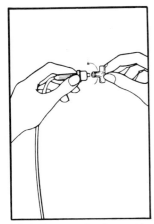

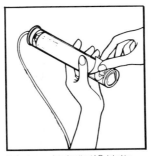

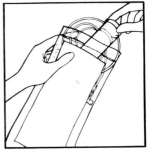

7. To stop flow, secure winged Luer cap into the Luer connector by turning Luer cap in a clockwise rotation. NOTE: Clamping the delivery tubing will not stop flow.

8. Apply completed patient I.D. label to Infusor in space provided.

9. Package filled Infusor in transparent dispenser bag for transport to patient.

Fig. 6 (*continued*)

The Easy-Fill Infusor units may be worn without regard to location. The flow regulator on the tubing, however, must be next to the skin. Infusors should not be exposed to sunlight when worn. This protects both the drug solution and the device.

D. Monitoring the Infusion

The infusion can be generally monitored by observing the level of the volume indicator line in relationship to the infusion scale (Fig. 5). The Infusor should be changed when the volume indicator line is level with the lowest scale line and the reservoir has returned to its empty shape.

IV. CLINICAL APPLICATIONS OF THE INFUSOR

Uses of the Infusor for cancer chemotherapy, analgesia, and other therapies are described in this section. In addition, in-hospital and at-home applications are discussed.

Central and peripheral venous infusions and subcutaneous, epidural, and arterial infusions have all been used with the Infusors. Solution flow in arterial infusions is decreased to 42 ml/24 hr, compared with 48 ml/24 hr, due to arterial resistance.

Many different types of catheter can be used with continuous infusion therapy. Tunneled subclavian, subclavian, jugular, and multi-

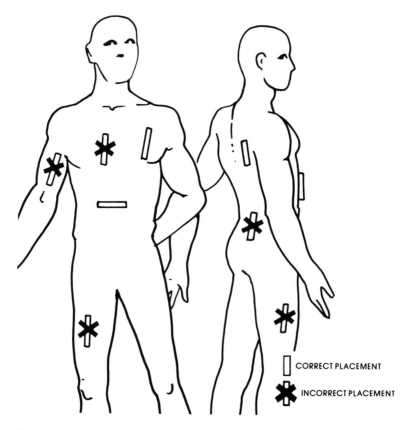

Fig. 7 Wearing the Single-Day Infusor.

lumen subclavian catheters, percutaneously inserted central venous catheters, and implanted ports have been used for central line administration. For peripheral administration, peripheral catheters, percutaneously inserted central line catheters, and scalp vein infusion sets have been used.

A. Drug Categories

Cancer Chemotherapy

Intravenous infusions of antineoplastic agents are common in cancer chemotherapy. Continuous infusions, made practical by advances in pump technology, are used increasingly because there is potential for retaining or increasing efficacy while decreasing systemic toxicity because of longer exposure, lower dose drug administration [1].

Vogelzang [2] cited three reasons for consideration of continuous infusion chemotherapy, noting that drug concentration in the body is of paramount importance for both efficacy and safety:

1. Because most chemotherapeutic agents are effective only against actively cycling tumor cells, continuous presence of the agent may be beneficial.
2. Drugs with short half-lives might be more effective with continuous infusion.
3. Length of exposure of tumor cells to cytotoxic agents may increase potential for transport into the cell.

Not all antineoplastic drugs or regimens are appropriate for continuous infusion chemotherapy. Most published clinical experience to date has been with 5-fluorouracil, methotrexate, cytosine arabinoside, doxorubicin, bleomycin, mitomycin C, vincristine, vinblastine, vindesine, hydroxyurea, and cisplatin. Controlled studies of these and other agents will further define appropriate applications of continuous infusion protocols [2].

In addition to safety and efficacy benefits, continuous infusion chemotherapy administered at home allows improved quality of life by facilitating normal activities and decreasing the need for repeated hospitalization for cancer chemotherapy.

Infusors were included in a study of ambulatory continuous infusion of 5-fluorouracil in 23 patients [3]. Many patients returned to work or resumed other normal activities while infusion therapy was in progress. The authors noted a conspicuous absence of toxicities commonly associated with 5-fluorouracil therapy. They suggested that because there was no bone marrow toxicity, it may be possible to use more aggressive concurrent therapy with other anticancer drugs or radiation.

Notable clinical responses were reported in a study of 29 patients with advanced, refractory multiple myeloma [4]. Infusors were used for continuous infusion of vincristine and doxorubicin in the VAD regimen (which also includes orally administered dexamethasone).

Table 2 is an overview of the use of typical protocols for continuous infusion chemotherapy using the Single- or Multi-Day Infusors. Stability parameters for some common antineoplastic agents are shown in Table 3.

Analgesia

When a patient has requested an analgesic because of severe pain, the drug may not be administered for 30 min or more due to the extensive record keeping required for narcotics and busy nursing schedules [5]. This time interval allows both pain and anxiety to increase, which

TABLE 2 Typical Protocols for Continuous Infusion Chemotherapy

Drug	Typical protocols	Infusor use	
		Single-Day	Multi-Day
Bleomycin	15-20 U/m^2/day for 5 days 15 U/m^2/day for 7 days 10-20 U/m^2/week or biweekly	Yes	Yes
Cisplatin	100 mg/m^2/day for 1 day 20 mg/m^2/day for 5 days for 3-4 weeks	Yes	No
Cyclophos- phamide	400-2000 mg/m^2/day for 3 weeks Initial: 40-50 mg/kg over 2-5 days Maintenance: 10-15 mg/kg every 7-10 days Maintenance: 3-5 mg/kg biweekly	Yes	Limited[a]
Dacarbazine	200-250 mg/m^2/day for 5 days every 3-4 weeks 375 mg/m^2/day for 15 days every 3-4 weeks 650-1450 mg/m^2/day weekly every 4-6 weeks 400 mg for 4 days	Yes	No
Doxorubicin	60-75 mg/m^2/day for 1 day every 3 weeks 20-30 mg/m^2/day for 3 days every 4 weeks 15 mg/m^2/day for 4 days 50-60 mg/m^2/day for 4 days 40 mg for 4 days 60-75 mg/m^2/day for 1 day every 3 weeks 20-30 mg/m^2/day for 3 days every 4 weeks	Yes	Limited[b]
Fluorouracil	400-600 mg/m^2/day for 5 days 20 mg/kg/day for 7 days 500 or 800 mg daily 12 mg/kg for 4 days, then 6 mg/kg on 6th, 8th, 10th, and 12th days	Yes	Limited[c]
Methotrexate	100-150 mg/m^2/day for 5 days 15 mg/m^2/day for 24 hr Initial: 15-30 mg/m^2/day IM over 5 days	Yes	Yes

TABLE 2 (*continued*)

Drug	Typical protocols	Infusor use	
		Single-Day	Multi-Day
Mitomycin	Maintenance: 30 mg/m^2 IM biweekly or 50 mg IM per week 10-20 mg/m^2 every 6-8 weeks Intrahepatic: 15 mg/m^2/day for 5 days	Yes	No
Vinblastine	4-6 mg/m^2 every week 1.5 mg/m^2 day for 5 days 3.7-18.5 mg/m^2 every week	Yes	Yes
Vincristine	2 mg every week 0.5 mg/m^2/day for 5 days 1.4-2.0 mg/m^2 every week	Yes	Yes

[a]Although the initial therapy protocol for cyclophosphamide recommended in *Physician's Desk Reference* cannot be placed in the Multi-Day Infusor, the maintenance protocol can.
[b]At the recommended (2 mg/ml) concentration of doxorubicin, the lower dosage (15-20 mg) 3 and 4 day protocols can be given in the Multi-Day Infusor but not higher dosage protocols. At the 5 mg/ml concentration Baxter Chemotherapy Service is using, the majority of doxorubicin protocols can be given in the Multi-Day Infusor; the only exception is the higher dosage protocols (60-70 mg) given for more than 2 days.
[c]The majority of typical 5-fluorouracil drug protocols cannot be given in the Multi-Day Infusor. The only exception is the protocol for colorectal cancer (1-300 mg/ml/day for 3-5 weeks), which can be given in the Multi-Day Infusor.

    may contribute to inadequate analgesia that has been reported following surgery [6].
    In efforts to improve analgesia, small, repeated bolus doses [7] and continuous infusion of low doses of narcotic analgesics [8-11] have been evaluated in comparison with intramuscular injections. While satisfactory analgesia was achieved with lower total doses of narcotics, duration of analgesia was shorter.
    Improved analgesia with lower total doses was reported when intravenous bolus injections were administered on patient demand [12]. While successful, it was considered to be impractical because of the requirement for a great deal of nursing time.

TABLE 3 Stability and Storage Characteristics of Common Chemotherapeutic Agents

Drug	Dosage preparation	Final drug concentration (mg/ml)	Storage temperature	Chemical stability
Cyclophosphamide	Reconstituted with sterile water for injection USP and then diluted to final concentration with 0.9% sodium chloride injection USP	2-20	2-8 °C Room temperature	48 days 2 days[a]
Doxorubicin hydrochloride	Reconstituted and diluted as required with 0.9% sodium chloride injection USP	0.2-1.0	2-8 °C Room temperature	30 days 2 days[a]
Fluorouracil	Liquid dosage form undiluted or diluted as required with 0.9% sodium chloride injection USP or 5% dextrose injection USP	5-50	Room temperature 33 °C	15 days 4 days[b]
Methotrexate sodium, preservative-free	Reconstituted and diluted as required with 0.9% sodium chloride injection USP	1.25-12.5	2-8 °C Room temperature	105 days 2 days[b]
Vinblastine sulfate	Reconstituted and diluted as required with 0.9% sodium chloride injection USP	0.015-0.5	2-8 °C 33 °C	21 days 5 days[c]
Vincristine sulfate	Reconstituted and diluted as required with 0.9% sodium chloride injection USP	0.2	2-8 °C Room temperature	51 days 2 days[a]
Vincristine sulfate	Reconstituted and diluted as required with 0.9% sodium chloride injection USP	0.04-<0.2	2-8 °C Room temperature	29 days 2 days[a]

[a]Room temperature stability applies for storage at room temperature immediately after compounding or after refrigerated storage not exceeding stated limits.

[b]Stability at 33°C applies for storage at 33°C immediately after compounding or after room temperature storage not exceeding stated limit.

[c]Stability at 33°C applies for storage at 33°C immediately after compounding or after refrigerated storage not exceeding stated limit.

Patient-controlled analgesia, first reported in the early 1970s [13-15], offers important benefits. Studies have shown that the total analgesic dose is lower and pain relief greater than with intramuscular injections. Analgesic blood levels are maintained within a narrow therapeutic range, which helps avoid both pain and sedation.

With PCA it has been reported that sedation is minimal, sleep disturbances are fewer, and respiratory depression is uncommon. It is thought that the patient's control over analgesic dosing contributes to decreased anxiety, an important factor in pain perception. Circadian patterns of pain are reflected in the way patients self-administer analgesics. And, finally, potentials for shorter hospitalization and for cost and time savings have been noted in published reports [16-22].

Efficacy of PCA with the Infusor was evaluated using morphine for postoperative analgesia in a clinical study conducted at the University of Kentucky at Lexington [23]. Fifty-three patients participated in the study. They were given Infusors upon recovery from general anesthesia following abdominal surgery. With PCA, a maximum of 1 mg of morphine (in 0.5 ml) could be self-administered every 6 min. Some patients received a loading dose of 1 or 2 mg of morphine. Patients were evaluated for narcotic usage, pain relief, sedation, and respiratory depression. In addition, patients filled out a self-assessment questionnaire at the end of the study.

Fifty patients completed the study. Three withdrew from the study because of severe nausea (two patients), thought to result from either general anesthesia or morphine, and one because of a rash attributed to morphine.

Patients received an average of 18 mg of morphine or its equivalent in other narcotic analgesics before, during, or immediately after surgery. With PCA, the average dose of morphine was 1.4 mg/hr.

Morphine doses were typically highest immediately after surgery and on the morning of the first postoperative day, which coincided with increased activity levels and ambulation. An increased analgesic requirement in the morning is similar to a circadian pattern reported by Graves et al. [19].

Dosage adjustments were made for 10 patients; for one, dosage was decreased due to sedation. Dosage increases in nine patients were attributed to more extensive surgery, recent multiple surgical procedures, or greater body surface area. (The protocol did not allow initiating analgesia with larger doses for patients with greater body surface area. In general clinical usage, this type of adjustment will be made, and it is anticipated that few dosage adjustments will be required.)

Seventy percent of patients reported that they felt comfortable or had only mild discomfort 4 hr after surgery. This increased to about 90% or more 8 hr later and remained at this level throughout hospitalization.

The level of sedation was evaluated by nurses. About 45% of patients were wide awake or slightly drowsy during the first 8 hr after surgery. By 16 hr, the same assessments had increased to 85%, and to about 90% at 24 hr. Respiratory depression was not observed in any patient.

An overall rating of mild to moderate pain was reported by 90% of patients in the poststudy questionnaire. Overall, 78% of patients reported that they were only mildly uncomfortable during the time after surgery. A preference for PCA over intramuscular injections was expressed by 92% of patients.

PCA was continued for an average of 68 hr after surgery, and each patient used two Infusors and one control module, on the average. Investigators reported that pain was well controlled in more than 90% of patients and that there was no evidence of oversedation or respiratory depression. Average morphine consumption (1.4 mg/hr) was similar to that in another report [18].

Other Drugs

Infusors were used for continuous intravenous infusion of metoclopramide for the treatment of chronic nausea that did not respond to oral metoclopramide [24]. Infusions were continued for an average of 10 days, with notable relief of nausea, decreases in vomiting episodes, and/or increased food intake. The authors suggested that ambulatory continuous infusion with the Infusor might be very useful in the treatment of nausea and vomiting associated with chemotherapy.

In a study of three patients who received at-home continuous infusion of heparin using the Infusor, it was reported that the patients were successfully anticoagulated and transferred to oral anticoagulants [25]. It was noted that shorter hospitalization provided an average of more than $5000 in cost savings for these patients and that quality of life was improved.

Other potential uses of the Infusor are suggested by reports of subcutaneous continuous infusion of chelating agents for the prevention of iron-related cardiac toxicity in patients with thalassemia major [26] and intrathecal infusions of baclofen to treat severe spasms resulting from spinal cord damage [27]. Diabetes, hormone imbalances, drug addiction, and alcoholism are among other disorders for which continuous infusion with the Infusor may be practical.

B. Infusor Usage: Hospital and Home

Hospital Infusor Usage

Continuous infusions of both chemotherapeutic and analgesic regimens are practical for use in the hospital. The Infusor is filled in the pharmacy. On the floor, setup and monitoring are convenient, and

ambulation is facilitated. Instructing patients on the use of PCA with
the Infusor is neither difficult nor time-consuming.

No capital expenditures, leasing agreements, maintenance, or equipment tracking is required with the Infusors.

Exposure of hospital personnel to cytotoxic agents may be decreased
with the use of the Infusor. In a study of exposure of nursing personnel to these agents during routine admixing and administration procedures, the Infusor was associated with the lowest percentage of skin
exposure [28].

At-Home Continuous Infusion with the Infusor

At-home use of the Infusor has been primarily for cancer chemotherapy
regimens. While PCA can be used in a home setting, clinical reports
to date are of postsurgical use with narcotic analgesics, which is limited
to several days and does not require posthospital administration. Another consideration is the increased potential for abuse outside the
hospital environment. For terminally ill patients, however, at-home
PCA with narcotics is not only outside these considerations but may
contribute significantly to the quality of life of the user.

Studies have shown that patients are easily taught to use Infusors
at home for cancer chemotherapy. They are provided with prefilled
Infusors from the pharmacy and given instructions on how and when
to change the Infusor.

The filled Infusors are generally stored under refrigeration and
allowed to warm to room temperature for 30 min prior to use. Changing
the Infusor involves clamping the catheter, removing the used Infusor,
attaching the new Infusor, and carefully disposing of the used Infusor.

REFERENCES

1. R. W. Carlson and B. I. Sikic, *Ann. Intern. Med.*, 99:823 (1983).
2. N. J. Vogelzang, *J. Clin. Oncol.*, 2:1289 (1984).
3. G. A. Caballero, R. K. Ausman, and E. J. Quebbeman, *Cancer Treat. Rep.*, 69:13 (1985).
4. B. Barlogie, L. Smith, and R. Alexanian, *New Engl. J. Med.*, 310:1353 (1984).
5. E. Vaché, *New Engl. J. Med.* (letter), 307:55 (1982).
6. R. M. Marks and E. J. Sachar, *Ann. Intern. Med.*, 78:173 (1973).
7. B. B. Roe, *Arch. Surg.*, 87:912 (1963).
8. K. L. Austin, J. V. Stapleton, and L. E. Mather, *Anesthesiology*, 53:460 (1980).
9. E. N. S. Fry, *Br. Med. J.* (letter), 2:817 (1976).
10. R. Schad, *Therapeutics*, 39:3 (1981).
11. J. V. Stapleton, K. L. Austin, and L. E. Mather, *Anesthesiol. Intensive Care*, 7:25 (1979).

12. P. H. Sechzer, *Anesthesiology*, 29:209 (1968).
13. W. H. Forrest, Jr., P. W. R. Smethurst, and M. E. Kienitz, *Anesthesiology*, 33:363 (1970).
14. M. Keeri-Szanto, *Can. Anesthesiol. Soc. J.*, 18:581 (1971).
15. P. H. Sechzer, *Anesth. Analg.*, 50:1 (1971).
16. P. F. White, *Semi. Anesth.*, IV:255 (1985).
17. D. A. Graves, T. S. Foster, R. L. Batenhorst, R. L. Bennett, and T. J. Baumann, *Ann. Intern. Med.*, 99:360 (1983).
18. R. Bennett, R. Batenhorst, D. A. Graves, T. S. Foster, W. O. Griffin, and B. D. Wright, *Pharmacotherapy*, 2:50 (1982).
19. D. A. Graves, R. L. Batenhorst, R. L. Bennett, J. G. Wettstein, W. O. Griffin, B. D. Wright, and T. S. Foster, *Clin. Pharm.*, 2:49 (1983).
20. J. Chrubasik and K. Wiemers, *Anesthesiology*, 62:263 (1985).
21. A. Tamsen, C. Hartvig, B. Fagerlund, B. Dahlstrom, and U. Bondesson, *Anaesthesiol. Scand.*, 74:157 (1982).
22. T. J. Baumann, R. L. Batenhorst, D. A. Graves, T. S. Foster, and R. L. Bennett, *DICP*, 20:297 (1986).
23. D. P. Wermeling, T. S. Foster, R. P. Rapp, D. E. Kenady, and E. F. Munson, *Clin. Pharm.*, 6:307 (1987).
24. E. Bruera, N. MacDonald, C. Brenneis, I. Simpson, and D. LeGatt, *Ann. Intern. Med.*, 104:896 (1986).
25. Data on file, Baxter Healthcare Corporation.
26. L. Wolfe, N. Olivieri, D. Sallan, S. Colan, V. Rose, R. Propper, M. H. Freedman, and D. G. Nathan, *New Engl. J. Med.*, 312:1600 (1985).
27. R. D. Penn and J. S. Kroin, *Lancet*, 2:125 (1985).
28. M. M. Cloak, T. H. Connor, K. R. Stevens, J. C. Theiss, J. M. Alt, T. F. Matney, and R. W. Anderson, *Oncol. Nurs. Forum*, 12:33 (1985).

7

Implantable Infusion Pumps

THOMAS D. ROHDE and HENRY BUCHWALD / University of
Minnesota, Minneapolis, Minnesota

PERRY J. BLACKSHEAR / Duke University Medical Center,
Durham, North Carolina

I. INTRODUCTION

New drugs are being developed and made available for clinical use at an amazing pace. Unfortunately, simply making available new compounds that have therapeutic potential does not provide benefit to patients unless an effective means of administration exists. When given orally, a drug must be protected against denaturation in the gastrointestinal tract, and it must be capable of absorption across the wall of the stomach or the intestine. Upon reaching the portal circulation, it must be resistant to a variety of hepatic enzymes. The turnover rate of the compound in the circulation must be slow enough to ensure that blood levels within the therapeutic range are maintained, at least between doses. Finally, the amount of intact drug that ultimately reaches the site of activity must be adequately large to achieve the desired therapeutic effect but insufficient to cause untoward side effects.

Many new protein or peptide drugs with great therapeutic potential now available from genetic engineering techniques are vulnerable to the adverse conditions described above and, thus, will be unsuitable for oral administration. Parenteral delivery has generally been an unsuitable alternative to oral delivery because of the requirement for long-term maintenance of percutaneous catheterization with its attendant hazards. Furthermore, in the past, parenteral drug administration generally meant hospitalization. With the advent of implantable infusion pumps, drug delivery rate can be precisely controlled and the substance can be provided to almost any location in the body on an indefinite basis. These capabilities enable outpatients to receive continuous parenteral drug therapy without interference in their daily lives.

In this chapter, we will use a rather narrow definition of implantable drug infusion pumps, including only devices with intrinsic power sources and means of replenishment of the reservoir contents while implanted. Excluded are passive devices such as Ommaya reservoirs and Levene shunts, implantable pellets and capsules, osmotic pumps, and other entities that might be classified broadly as implantable infusion devices. We will discuss pharmacokinetic principles as they apply to drug therapy by continuous infusion. In addition, we will describe existing implantable drug infusion devices, their origins, and current use status. We will address some special problems that must be considered in selecting or designing drugs for use in implantable pumps. Finally, we will speculate about the future therapeutic prospects for implantable infusion pumps.

II. PHARMACOKINETIC PRINCIPLES RELEVANT
TO IMPLANTABLE INFUSION PUMPS

Traditionally, drug development involved discovering, designing, or modifying molecules to maximize desirable therapeutic characteristics while minimizing untoward side effects. The range of circulating drug concentrations between beneficial and hazardous dosages is sometimes called the therapeutic window. This emphasis on chemical structure as a means of achieving drug concentrations within the therapeutic window was justified in the past because, until recently, means were not available to fully exploit the capabilities of drugs on the basis of their pharmacokinetic principles.

Because drug absorption and metabolism occur at varying rates, serum concentration is usually more indicative than dosage of the appropriateness of the amount given to achieve the desired effect. Where the therapeutic range is broad and the untoward effects of overdosage are not serious, serum drug levels may not be of much concern. However, in many instances, under- or overdosage can have serious consequences. For example, when warfarin and its derivatives are administered in the treatment of thromboembolic disease, underdosage increases the risk of life-threatening pulmonary embolism while overdosage can result in a fatal hemorrhage. A pharmaceutical compound with potential beneficial effects has little chance of being developed into a drug at this time if its therapeutic range of serum levels is too narrow to be maintained by current technology and techniques.

As shown in Fig. 1A, a peak in drug concentration generally occurs shortly after administration and then gradually declines until it reaches levels undetectable by available assay methods. The rate of disappearance from the blood is expressed as the half-life of the drug. If the half-life is short and the therapeutic range narrow, the drug will likely need to be administered at frequent intervals throughout the day, since large doses may cause toxic side effects. In certain instances, the therapeutic range may be so narrow that administration of the drug by oral means is impractical because of the frequency of administration required (Fig. 1B). Unfortunately, the half-life of a pharmaceutical agent given orally can only be estimated within a broad range, since it varies between persons and sometimes within the same individual due to variability within normal physiology.

Use of a totally implantable pump can improve the therapeutic effectiveness of pharmaceutical agents in several ways. It can (a) deliver the drug to the site where it will be most effective while minimizing contact with sites where it will cause side effects, (b) provide the drug continuously at constant or variable rates as appropriate to the needs of the patient, (c) maintain drug delivery rates within

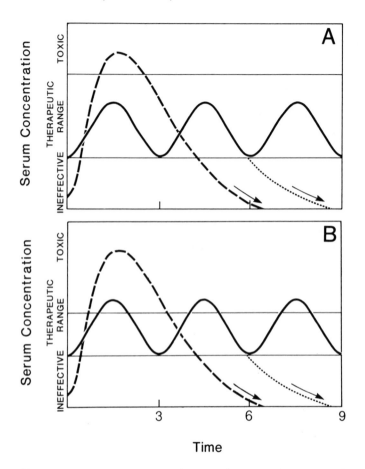

Fig. 1 Expected serum concentration patterns when drugs with (A) relatively wide and (B) relatively narrow therapeutic ranges are given in single large doses or multiple small doses.

precise limits, and (d) provide such delivery continuously on a protracted basis with minimal risk of infection or other complications. Most importantly, the pump permits the attainment of all these goals without significant risk to the patient or interference with his or her lifestyle.

III. EXISTING PUMP DESIGNS AND OPERATING PRINCIPLES

Currently, three basic types of implantable drug infusion device are in clinical use. They are the vapor-pressure-powered pump, which

is a simple mechanical device, and two types of electronically controlled
device utilizing peristaltic and solenoid pumping mechanisms. Of these,
the Infusaid implantable pump—a vapor-pressure-powered model developed at the University of Minnesota—has been approved since March
1982 by the Food & Drug Administration for commercial distribution.
Of the electronically controlled designs, the Medtronic DAS is in the
final stages of the FDA's premarket approval (PMA) process. In November 1986 an FDA panel completed their review of this product and recommended that it be approved for two chemotherapeutic applications.
It was not clear when final premarket approval would be granted, but
it was expected in the near future. Siemens AG has been conducting
clinical trials with pumps of their design since 1981. Beginning in
February 1986, clinical trials were initiated in four European medical
centers with a modified Siemens pump model. These pumps will likely
be marketed initially in Europe, where FDA approval is not required
for commercial distribution. The programmable implantable medication
system (PIMS), which was developed jointly by Johns Hopkins University and Pacesetter (now Minimed) Inc. initiated its first clinical trial
in November 1986. If all goes as planned, they expect to achieve FDA
approval within about 2 years.

A. Vapor-Pressure-Powered Devices

A vapor-pressure-powered pump was invented in August 1969 at the
University of Minnesota (Minneapolis) by Perry J. Blackshear, Frank
D. Dorman, Perry L. Blackshear, Jr., Richard L. Varco, and Henry
Buchwald. This dual-chambered, disk shaped device with an inex-
haustible volatile liquid power source is shown schematically in Fig.
2. Its principle of operation is the basic physicochemical concept that
at a given temperature, a liquid in equilibrium with its vapor phase
exerts a constant pressure that is independent of enclosing volume.
Charging fluid, selected to provide an appropriate vapor pressure
at physiological temperatures, is sealed in one chamber; the drug to

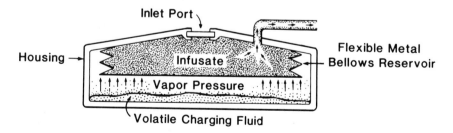

Fig. 2 Scheme of a vapor-pressure-driven pump in cross section.

be infused is placed in a second chamber accessible by a self-sealing septum. The two chambers are separated by a flexible metal bellows. Vapor pressure from the charging fluid compresses the bellows and expels the infusate through a bacterial filter, a capillary flow restrictor, and an infusion cannula into the desired body site. When the reservoir of the pump is refilled by percutaneous needle injection through the refill septum, the expansion of the bellows compresses and condenses the charging fluid vapor and simultaneously refills and recharges the pump. The pump is licensed by the University of Minnesota to Shiley-Infusaid Corporation of Norwood, Massachusetts, for manufacture and commercial distribution.

Infusaid pumps in the model 100 series (Fig. 3) are general-purpose pumps for applications that do not require an additional access port for adjuvant therapy. Characteristics of the model 100 series are shown in Table 1. The Infusaid model 400 pump is identical to the model 100 except that it has an auxiliary sideport septum that bypasses the pumping mechanism and allows the clinician to make bolus injections through the pump's catheter into the delivery site. The auxiliary sideport septum is particularly useful in organ-specific cancer chemotherapy, not only for drug bolusing, but when it is important to document by radionuclide imaging of the perfused organ that the chemotherapeutic agent is reaching the entire tumor. In some instances, the blood supply to the tumor is such that two catheters are needed to perfuse the entire tumor. For such situations a dual-catheter version of the model 400 pump is available. This unit has two side port septums that bypass the pumping mechanism (technical bulletins, Shiley-Infusaid Corp.).

B. Peristaltic Pumps

At the present time, the most popular design for an implantable programmable drug delivery system uses a peristaltic pumping mechanism, battery power, and electronic controls. Briefly, a peristaltic pump consists of a flexible tube placed in a U shaped chamber in contact with rollers that press against the tube with sufficient force to occlude its lumen (Fig. 4). The rollers are mounted on a rotor and rotated by a motor. As the rollers move and compress the lumen of the tube, fluid is moved toward the exit. The rollers and housing are arranged so that a second roller begins to squeeze the tube before the first disengages, preventing backflow of the infusate.

Currently, three groups have developed implantable pumps with peristaltic pumping mechanisms. They are Sandia Laboratories (Albuquerque, New Mexico), Siemens AG (Erlangen, West Germany), and Medtronic Inc. (Minneapolis). As indicated previously, the Siemens and Medtronic systems are currently in clinical trials and are described herein. The Sandia pump was evaluated in clinical trials that were initiated in 1981 but is not in clinical studies at this time and, thus, is not discussed in detail in this chapter.

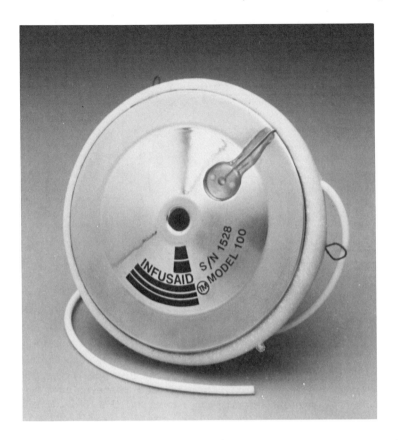

Fig. 3 An Infusaid model 100 series pump—a vapor-pressure-driven design. (Photo courtesy of Infusaid Corporation.)

TABLE 1 Dimensions and Reservoir Volumes of the Infusaid Model 100 Series

Model	Usable volume (ml)	Diameter (mm)	Depth (mm)	Empty weight (g)
100	47	87	28	187
200	32	87	23	172
500	22	87	20	165

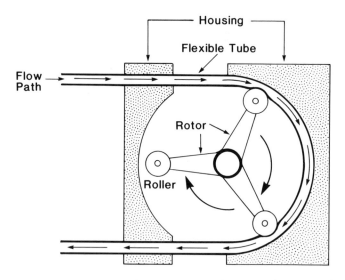

Fig. 4 Scheme showing a peristaltic pumping mechanism—the basic
mechanism used in the Siemens Promedos ID 1 and the Medtronic DAD.

The Siemens Pump

The Siemens implantable pump or dosing unit—the Promedos ID 1—is
driven by a stepper motor electronically controlled by means of an
external programming and monitoring unit, the Promedos IP 1. The
complete system, consisting of both the ID 1 and IP 1 is referred to
as the Promedos I 1. In addition to the peristaltic pump and the stepper
motor, components of the implantable dosing unit include two batteries,
control electronics, and a 10 ml drug reservoir that can be refilled
by percutaneous needle injection through a self-sealing septum. The
reservoir in the Promedos ID 1 has a capacity of 10 ml. All components,
including the reservoir, are hermetically encapsulated within a titanium
casing. The interior of the capsule is maintained at negative pressure
to prevent fluid loss into the body in the event of a leak. The pump
can provide 12 different programmable basal rates from 1 to 15 μl/hr
and 12 higher rates from 0 to 140 μl/hr, which can be superimposed
on each basal rate on demand. The demand rate is switched off automatically after one hour. Dimensions of the Promedos ID 1 are 85 ×
60 × 22 mm. Its weight is 170 g when the reservoir is empty. It has
an anticipated battery life of 3 years at an expected daily dose of 50
units of insulin. The Promedos IP 1 is a hand-held, external programming unit weighing 220 g. Its dimensions are 120 × 72 × 24 mm. It
is powered by a 5.6 V, 10 mA·hr battery with an anticipated performance lifetime of approximately 1 year. The external programming and

monitoring device has indicators for signaling successful completion of programming and low reservoir volume. Step frequency of the pump motor can be determined as desired by interrogating the implantable device with the external unit. This information can be used to calculate infusion rate (Promedos I 1 data sheet, provided by M. Franetzki, Siemens AG). Both the ID 1 and the IP 1 are shown in Fig. 5.

The Medtronic Pump

The Medtronic Drug Administration System (DAS) consists of three parts: a totally implantable programmable Drug Administration Device (DAD), a catheter specific for the delivery site, and an external physician programmer. The Medtronic DAD (Fig. 6) is a cylindrical device 70 mm in dimaeter and 27 mm high. It weighs 175 g. Components include reservoir, electronic module, battery, antenna, pump, suture pad, port for catheter connection, fill port with self-sealing septum, alarm mechanism, acoustic transducer, and needle stop. Certain models also include a filter for the retention of bacteria, which is used for intrathecal and epidural applications. The drug reservoir is a sealed collapsible titanium chamber, which can be filled or emptied by percutaneous needle puncture through a self-sealing septum. Reservoir capacity is 18 ml. The DAD utilizes a peristaltic pump driven by a stepper motor to deliver infusate. The accuracy of delivery is ±15%. The device is powered by a lithium thionyl chloride battery with an estimated functional lifetime of 2 years and is controlled by microprocessor-based hybrid electronic circuitry. The microprocessor can be programmed noninvasively by radiofrequency signals generated by an external physician programmer (Fig. 7).

Two-way communication between the DAD and the extracorporeal physician programmer is accomplished through an antenna, which is activated by the magnetic closure of a reed switch. Simultaneous presence of both a magnetic field and the recognized radiofrequency signal is necessary for programming of the pump. This is to avoid the possibility of pump reprogramming in the event of extraordinary environmental electronic interference. This programming concept is in common usage in programmable cardiac pacemaker designs. Programmable parameters in the system include: patient identification, date on which the current prescription was established, the prescription in current use, and alarm status. Parameters that can be entered in the prescription program include identification of the drug, concentraiton of the drug, infusion mode, the dose delivery rate (ranging from 0.025 to 0.9 ml/hr), and the volume of the drug remaining in the drug reservoir. Infusion modes that can be chosen include on/off bolus, multistep bolus, continuous, continuous-complex, and bolus delay.

The DAD has an alarm system to alert both the patient and the physician to the occurrence of certain events that may affect patient safety. One alarm is an audible buzzer on the implanted unit that can

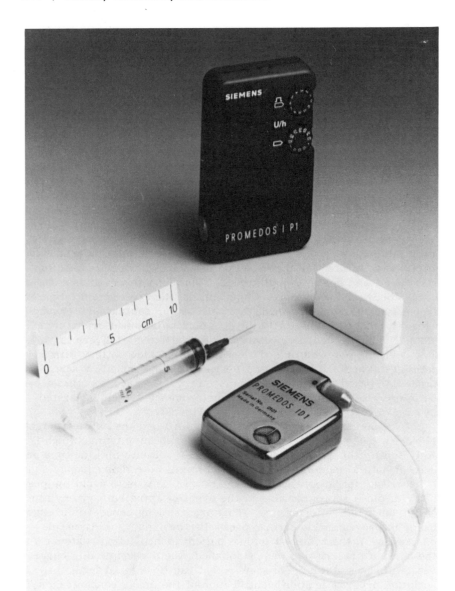

Fig. 5 A Siemens Promedos implantable dosing unit (ID 1)—a program-mable peristaltic pump. Also shown is the Promedos IP 1, the hand-held external programmer. (Photo courtesy of Siemens AG.)

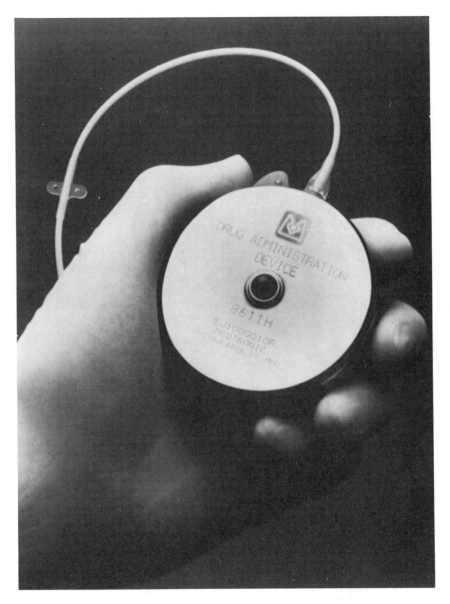

Fig. 6 A Medtronic Drug Administration Device (DAD)—an implantable peristaltic pump. (Photo courtesy of Medtronic Inc.)

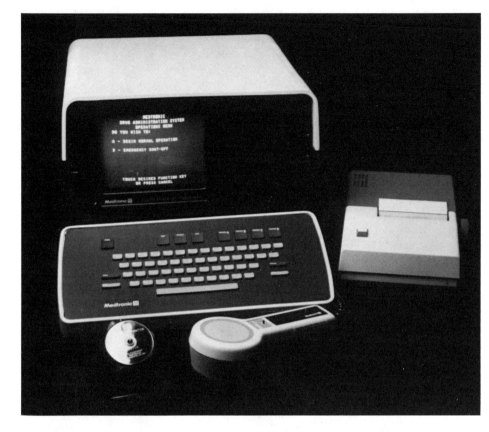

Fig. 7 A Medtronic external programmer. (Photo courtesy of Medtronic Inc.)

be heard or felt by the patient when it is activated. The other notifies the physician when he or she interrogates or attempts to program the pump. Both alarms are activated in the event of low battery power, low reservoir volume, or electronic malfunction (unpublished excerpts from a speech by J. Tremmel, provided by J. Pierce, Medtronic Inc.).

C. Solenoid Pumps

Fischell and colleagues at the Johns Hopkins University Applied Physics Laboratory in Laurel, Maryland, chose an alternative approach to fluid delivery of an infusate from a programmable implantable pump. Their PIMS system includes an implantable infusion device, an external physician's console, and a hand-held unit with which patients can initiate preprogrammed supplemental insulin doses at mealtimes. The device is manufactured by MiniMed Technologies (Sylmar, California). The implantable device—called the implantable programmable infusion pump (IPIP)—uses a solenoid-driven reciprocating chamber with attendant check valves to move infusate from the reservoir out through the delivery catheter (Fig. 8). This pulsatile pump delivers infusate in pulses of 2 µl utilizing less than 2 µW each. Infusate is stored in a 10 ml flexible diaphragm reservoir maintained at a pressure of -4 psi to preclude loss of drugs into the subcutaneous tissues in the event of a leak in the fluid path. The reservoir is filled through a refill septum located at the bottom of a ceramic cone. During refilling, the negative pressure in the reservoir sucks the insulin out of the vial, reducing the risk of inadvertent subcutaneous insulin spills. The reservoir holds a 3 month supply of concentrated insulin; refilling can be accomplished in approximately 2 min. The unit is powered by a 3.6 V lithium thionyl chloride battery. The batteries and implanted circuitry have provided more than 5 years of functional life in laboratory tests. New batteries, currently being tested, are calculated to provide more than 10 years of in vivo function. A system of complementary metal-oxide semiconductor (CMDS) microelectronics with a microprocessor and 8 kilobytes of random access memory controls the device. It can provide a programmable basal rate and any of six different insulin infusion wave forms in response to external commands. Insulin is delivered by means of a silicone rubber cannula with an insulin compatible lining.

An IPIP is shown in Fig. 9. The external dimensions of the pump are 81 mm (diameter) × 20 mm (thickness); its weight is 170 g. The physician's console is a conventional personal computer with appropriate software. Using the console, the physician can collect data stored

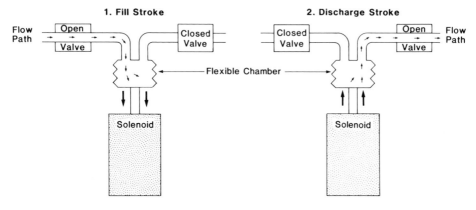

Fig. 8 Scheme of a solenoid pumping mechanism—the mechanism used in the Minimed IPIP.

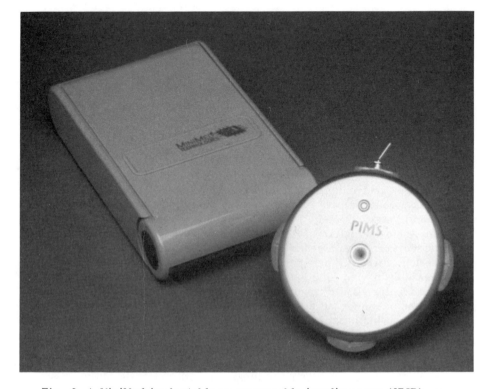

Fig. 9 A MiniMed implantable programmable insulin pump (IPIP)—a device that utilizes a solenoid pumping mechanism.

in the implantable unit and prescribe which insulin delivery profiles will be available to the patient. If desired, the physician can limit the amount of insulin the pump will deliver over a 3 hr or a 24 hr period. Programming and interrogation of the implantable unit can be accomplished via telephone when the patient is remotely located from the physician's console. The patient's hand-held unit can initiate any of up to six preprogrammed insulin delivery profiles prescribed by the physician. If an erroneous transmission is made of a command requesting a specific supplemental insulin delivery profile, it can be corrected or deleted. The hand-held unit can countermand or cancel any prior command or can shut off insulin delivery completely (Johns Hopkins Medical Institutions News Release, Nov. 18, 1986).

IV. CURRENT STATUS OF EXISTING DEVICES

A. Animal Studies

Heparin

Heparin was the first drug selected by our group at the University of Minnesota for investigation as an infusate for delivery by implantable pump because of its therapeutic potential and from pragmatic considerations. That it was anticoagulant of choice in the treatment of acute thromboembolic disorders suggested that long-term heparin anticoagulation might be superior to conventional means for the treatment of chronic refractory thromboembolism. Twenty-five dogs were successfully anticoagulated with heparin from implanted pumps for longer than 6 months and a cohort of these for more than a year [2]. Our results showed that the implantable infusion pump could perform predictably and reliably for periods of several months or years in dogs, which were selected as experimental animals because of their size. Surgical implantation of human-sized pump models was no problem in these animals and they tolerated the weight and the small bulge in the skin without restriction of activity. Furthermore, implantation of the pumps fabricated of titanium with stainless steel capillary flow restrictors and silicone rubber cannulae confirmed findings of other investigators concerning the implantability and biocompatibility of these materials.

Cancer Chemotherapy

In January 1975, prior to the initiation of the first clinical trial with heparin, studies were begun in laboratory animals to assess the feasibility of using the pump for 5-fluorodeoxyuridine (FUDR) infusion into the hepatic artery. One pump used in these studies was equipped with an auxiliary sideport intended for use in arteriography to ascertain the infusion pattern of a drug on a regular basis. This feature was not included on pumps used in the first clinical trial with FUDR because the bore of the catheter was too small to accommodate sufficient quantities of highly viscous radiopaque contrast medium for arteriography.

Insulin Infusion

When we began to consider the use of implantable pump technology in the treatment of diabetes, we initially viewed our device as the reservoir and pumping component of a totally artificial pancreas. Slow development of the implantable glucose sensor, in addition to our early experience with continuous insulin infusion, led us to conclude that continuous insulin infusion without feedback control might serve as a therapeutic alternative to conventional insulin therapy in insulin-requiring diabetes. Preivous glucose tolerance studies in laboratory animals indicated that near-normal glucose responses to an intravenous glucose challenge could be maintained using a continuous, single-rate, insulin infusion pump [3].

During insulin infusion experiments in laboratory animals, which began about 1977, we became acutely aware of the tendency of insulin solutions to clog the capillary flow restrictor of the pump (in contrast to heparin and FUDR). Insulin precipitated and occluded nine pumps implanted in dogs within 43 days. Attempts to overcome this difficulty included modifications of both the pump and the infusate. A Teflon capillary was substituted for stainless steel as the pump's flow restrictor to overcome a potential galvanic corrosion problem at the pump-flow restrictor junction and, thereby, prevent local pH shifts that could precipitate insulin. A variety of combinations of insulin, buffers, and chelating agents were also tested for their ability to resist insulin precipitation. These included both zinc and zinc-free insulin, buffers (0.02 and 0.2 M sodium acetate, 0.01 M sodium phosphate, and glycine), and a chelating agent, ethylenediaminetetraacetic acid (EDTA).

None of these methods prevented the precipitation of insulin in implantable pumps; plugging occurred despite maintenance of the pH of the insulin preparation in the pump within the soluble range [4]. Success in preventing insulin precipitation was finally achieved by the addition of 80% glycerol (v/v) to the infusate preparation. Glycerol is commonly added to peptide solutions to convey thermal stability. When implantable pump infusion studies in two dogs, with glycerol added to the insulin infusate, demonstrated continued patency for more than 250 days each [5], we decided to initiate clinical trials of continuous insulin infusion in man.

B. Clinical Studies

Heparin

The first human implantation of an implantable drug infusion device was performed on October 22, 1975, for continuous heparin infusion in the treatment of recurrent venous thromboembolism [6]. Our group at the University of Minnesota then studied long-term heparin infusion by implantable pump in 21 patients with recurrent venous thromboembolism, most of whom were failures on conventional forms of therapy. Marked reduction of pain and improvement of mobility were reported by several patients with vena caval ligature syndrome. Recurrences of thromboembolic events were prevented by this regimen in all except one patient. There were no spontaneous hemorrhagic episodes, but pump site hematomas occurred in several instances following pump refills (the refill technique has since been modified to eliminate this difficulty). Osteoporosis occurred in one subject after 1 year [7]; at 2 years, a 24% incidence of heparin-associated osteoporosis was noted [8]. While the population of individuals with refractory venous thromboembolism is small, it constitutes a group whose needs are not met by conventional medical techniques. In some cases, heparin infusion by pump has led to dramatic improvements in patient mobility and freedom from pain. The Infusaid pump was approved by the FDA in March 1982 for chronic heparin administration. Its use in the treatment of chronic thromboembolic disease, uncontrolled by other methods, has been designated an established procedure by Blue Cross and Blue Shield [9].

Cancer Chemotherapy

The implantable pump was first used for intra-arterial infusion chemotherapy in man by our group at the University of Minnesota in 1977. Four patients with nonresectable primary or secondary liver tumors were studied from 5 to 33 weeks. Beneficial responses occurred in two patients, but all subjects ultimately died of carcinomatosis. However, the study demonstrated that the devices were well tolerated by the patients and that continuous, organ-specific cancer chemotherapy could be performed in outpatients without significant risk and inconvenience [10]. Further demonstration of its safety and efficacy by other investigators [11-13], and approval by the FDA in March 1982, led to widespread use of the Infusaid implantable infusion pump for the infusion of cancer chemotherapeutic agents.

The role of the implantable pump in cancer chemotherapy remains controversial. Balch et al. [14] compared the survival rates of 81 patients who received regional FUDR infusion chemotherapy in the treatment of colorectal hepatic metastases with that of a historical control group of 129 patients with isolated liver metastases. Major prognostic indicators were similar for both groups. Carcinoembryonic antigen levels fell by one-third or more after two cycles of chemotherapy in 88% of patients receiving FUDR by pump. The pump group had improved one year (82% vs. 36%) and median survival (26 months vs. 8 months, p < 0.0001) when compared with the control group. An interesting finding of the study was that the natural course of development of the disease was changed by this treatment approach. Whereas, in the past, the major cause of death was tumor progression in the liver, hepatic metastases were effectively controlled by this treatment. Progression of disease in lung or bone was the cause of death in the majority of these patients.

These promising early results appear to be corroborated by the results of a similar study of 93 patients performed by Niederhuber and colleagues [15] at the University of Michigan. In their protocol, FUDR was infused into the hepatic artery at 0.3 mg/kg/day alternating with saline at 2 week intervals. Mitomycin C at 15 mg/m^2 was given to nonresponders. Results indicated a response rate of 83% with a median duration of response of 13 months. However, Schwartz et al.

[16], who studied 30 patients whose liver malignancies were treated
with hepatic arterial infusions of FUDR, found that only 3 of 20 patients
followed by sequential imaging studies showed a 50% decrease in size
of liver mass. No increase in duration of survival was found when
these patients were compared with 13 patients who received no chemotherapy. The pumps functioned well in all patients. However, 77%
showed signs of toxicity from FUDR. In a report of preliminary results
of a randomized, prospective trial of 100 patients, Kemeny and colleagues [17] reported that survival depended more on tumor burden
than on treatment method. Furthermore, they found a substantial
complication rate with FUDR, particularly sclerosing cholangitis, which
was sometimes fatal. Their study, which is still in progress, is designed to evaluate the effectiveness of hepatic resection and continuous intrahepatic arterial infusion of FUDR by implantable pump on metastatic liver disease from colorectal primaries. Thus, although the implantable pump has proven to be a safe and convenient means of delivering cancer chemotherapeutic agents, definition of its role in cancer
therapy awaits the results of randomized clinical trials that are now
in progress.

Clearly, there is a need for more effective chemotherapeutic agents
and methods for reducing toxicity. Kaplan et al. [18] suggest that
arteriovenous shunting within the liver allows the FUDR to evade de-
toxification by hepatocytes and reach toxic levels systemically. They
propose that slow infusion of technetium-labeled microaggregated albumin combined with monitoring of radionucleotide uptake by the lungs
can provide a method of identifying patients who are at risk of systemic
toxicity. In a pilot study, Roemeling et al. [19] studied the effect
of single rate versus time-modified FUDR infusion in the treatment of
primary and secondary liver tumors. They found no difference in
tumor response or survival, but toxicity was significantly reduced
in patients treated with time-modified delivery.

Intraspinal Morphine

Utilization of an implantable infusion pump to deliver analgesic agents
intraspinally has been described in case reports and in studies of small
series of patients, but controlled prospective trials have not yet been
reported. Onofrio et al. [20], who initiated this technique for intrathecal morphine delivery, found that they were able to achieve a pain-
free state in the single patient studied, while preserving motor and
sensory functions, which are usually suppressed by parenteral narcotics. Similar results were described in case reports by other authors
who administered morphine either intrathecally [21] or epidurally [22,
23]. Coombs et al. [24] studied a series of 13 patients who received
epidural morphine infusions from implantable pumps for periods of up
to 8 months. In this series, constant intraspinal flow rates of morphine
were observed without catheter or pump infection, respiratory depres-

sion, or pump failure. Another series of 10 patients with intractable pain (five cancer and five nonmalignant), were evaluated by psychometric examinations after 12 weeks of epidural morphine therapy. Both groups required significant serial increases in morphine dosage over time, indicating the development of opiate tolerance. Sustained analgesic response was maintained in the cancer patients but response in the nonmalignant-pain group was poor [25]. All the studies above were performed with Infusaid pumps.

Insulin

Clinical experience with implantable insulin pumps is reviewed in depth by Irsigler et al. [26]. Eight electronically controlled peristaltic pumps were implanted during the early 1980s. Of these, four were constructed by Sandia Laboratories and implanted by Eaton, Schade, and colleagues of the University of New Mexico in Albuquerque. These four pumps were implanted in three patients—one of the four pumps was replaced after 5 months when its battery became exhausted. In the report of early results from their first patient, Schade et al. [27] found that intraperitoneal insulin delivery from the unit normalized the patient's plasma glucose, plasma insulin, and glycosylated hemoglobin concentrations.

Four additional electronic pumps (Siemens PFA 1), manufactured by Siemens AG, were evaluated in clinical trials. One device was implanted by Irsigler et al. [28], who found that it achieved near normalization of glycemia. It ultimately had to be replaced because of electronic failure after 7 months, and its replacement also failed due to catheter damage after 2 months [29]. A Siemens pump implanted by Selam et al. [30] also achieved near normoglycemia and maintained it for 14 months with intraperitoneal insulin infusion. Insulin requirements were slightly reduced, although this may have been due to voluntary weight reduction by the patient. Although not entirely eliminated, hypoglycemic episodes were always minor. Dr. Walter's group in Munich implanted a Siemens programmable pump for intravenous delivery. The device was removed after 10 months due to deteriorating metabolic control in the patient. As indicated previously, clinical trials with a new version of the Siemens pump—the Promedos I 1—were initiated in 1986.

The vast majority of implantable devices that have been implanted for diabetes are Infusaid pumps. The largest series are those of Irsigler et al. in Vienna (69 patients), Buchwald and associates in Minneapolis (42 patients), Blackshear, Nathan, and colleagues at Harvard University (13 patients), and Pozza's group in Milan (8 patients) [International Study Group for Diabetes Treatment with Implantable Insulin Delivery Devices (ISGIID) Newsletter, November 1986].

The first successful implantation of an insulin pump in man was performed by Buchwald et al. [31] on October 25, 1980. The same

group [32] implanted pumps for insulin infusion in five type II diabetics. In this study, mean postprandial glucose and mean fasting
glucose values were improved on continuous insulin infusion by pump
when compared to values on their previous treatment regimens of insulin injections. Glycosylated hemoglobin (HbA1c) was normalized
and, interestingly, C peptide became elevated over the course of time.
Blackshear et al. [33] carefully studied two type II diabetics who received intravenous insulin from their implanted pumps. They found
that mean 24 hr plasma glucose levels decreased, glycosuria was eliminated, and HbA1c levels were in or near the normal range during the
3 year infusion periods. Improvements were also noted in serum triglycerides, serum anti-insulin antibody titers, and vitreous fluorescein
concentrations after intravenous fluorescein injections. Euglycemic
insulin clamp studies showed that no significant changes in glucose
disposal rate occurred after treatment. However, insulin secretion
was enhanced during hyperglycemic insulin clamps in both patients
after prolonged insulin infusion. Kritz et al. [29] reported the results of constant-rate insulin infusion in 21 type I subjects and one
pancreatectomized patient. They found that mean blood glucose levels
were significantly lower on constant-rate insulin infusion with supplemental injections than with insulin injections alone. Also HbA1c values
fell significantly. The frequency of hypoglycemic episodes decreased.
Interestingly, improvement was seen in four quantifiable parameters
of diabetic neuropathy.

A registry for clinical studies with implantable pumps has been
established by ISGIID. Currently 196 implantable pumps have been
implanted for insulin infusion in the treatment of diabetes. Mean pump
life (time from implantation to explantation) was 36 months. Eighty
percent of pumps implanted remained functional for at least one year
(ISGIID Newsletter, December 1986).

V. SPECIAL PROBLEMS WITH DRUG FORMULATIONS FOR IMPLANTABLE INFUSION PUMPS

Drugs delivered by implantable pumps often encounter more rigorous
environmental conditions than drugs administered by conventional means
These conditions include protracted storage at physiological temperatures, motion that can potentially cause breakage of surface films and
permit new films to form at infusate-air interfaces, exposure to shear
forces in capillary restrictors and peristaltic mechanisms in some implantable pump designs, possible contact with galvanic currents, contact with metal and polymeric surfaces, and contact with blood or other
body fluids. To some degree, the adverse effects on drug stability
brought about by these conditions can be mitigated by system design
and proper usage. This has already been accomplished to a great ex-

tent in existing designs. However, system design alone is often inadequate to achieve a suitable result. In many instances, drug formulation modification is also necessary. When protein drugs are infused, for example, minimizing the amount of gas dissolved in infusate is important regardless of pump type to prevent the scums of denatured protein that tend to form at the interfaces between protein solutions and air.

Thus, a pharmaceutical compound that is suitable for use in implantable pumps must include among its characteristics stability at physiological temperatures, compatibility with standard pump materials, and solubility allowing concentration sufficient to achieve a reasonable interval between refills. These criteria are met by heparin, FUDR, and morphine—the drugs initially approved by the FDA for the Infusaid implantable pump. Other drugs do not meet these criteria. For example, 5-fluorouracil (5-FU), an antitumor agent less expensive and more often chosen than FUDR for conventional administration, is not highly soluble in water and, thus, is available only in low concentrations that would require refilling every 1 to 2 days to achieve therapeutic drug levels. Such short intervals between refills, though achievable, are impractical for many patients and physicians. Thus, the majority of oncologists who use implantable pumps to treat nonresectable liver carcinoma select FUDR rather than 5-FU, thereby allowing a refill interval of several weeks.

Desferoxamine, a chelating agent used to treat iron overload, is indicated in disease states such as thalassemia in which frequent blood transfusions are required to sustain life. Since desferoxamine must be given parenterally at frequent intervals, delivery by implantable pump seemed to be a desirable administration technique. Indeed, it was selected at an early date for feasibility studies. Unfortunately, these pilot studies indicated that desferoxamine is heat labile and rapidly loses bioactivity at physiological temperatures. Thus, it was deemed unsuitable for delivery by implantable pump and means were devised to deliver it subcutaneously by portable infusion pump.

In both these cases, rather than attempt to find ways to make 5-FU more soluble or desferoxamine heat stable, therapeutic alternatives were found.

As described previously, insulin proved to be a particularly difficult drug to deliver by implantable pump. Commercially available insulins tended to clog implantable pumps within a few weeks. Our group and others have made progress toward an insulin formulation suitable for implantable pumps. After a series of investigations, we found that 80% (v/v) glycerol mixed with insulin infusates prevented pump occlusion in units implanted in dogs for more than 2 years. Insulin solutions containing 80% glycerol have been infused in more than 90% of the 196 pumps implanted in diabetic subjects. Although glycerol/insulin allowed clincial trails to proceed and the average functional lifetime of an implanted pump now exceeds 3 years, insulin/glycerol solutions tended to lose bioactivity in the pump, necessitating a 10 to 14 day interval between refills. This loss of bioactivity was associated with a time- and temperature-dependent tendency to form soluble, higher molecular weight insulin polymers, which apparently have lower biological activity than native insulin species [5].

After further investigation revealed that glycerol impurity was an important factor contributing to insulin instability, we replaced the USP grade glycerol, rendered from animal fat, with spectrographic grade synthetic glycerol. The glycerol was purified further by passing it through a mixed-bed ion-exchange column to remove both positively and negatively charged organic and inorganic contaminants. We then conducted experiments to determine optimum pH. When in vitro studies to optimize the glycerol/insulin formulation had been completed, we assessed its stability by conducting infusion studies in five diabetic dogs over periods from 3 to 8 months. No significant changes in flow rate occurred in four of the five dogs; one dog showed a slight increase in flow rate, which might have occurred as a result of reversal of the occlusive process that was occurring when the previous formulation was in the pump. Thus, there was no evidence of aggregation or precipitation, or any other indication of physical instability.

A study of insulin bioactivity was conducted as one indicator of chemical stability. Figure 10A is a plot of fasting blood glucose versus number of days postrefill for three dogs being maintained on the previous glycerol/insulin formulation (labeled "stock glycerol"); Fig. 10B is a plot of similar data for the new formulation (labeled "processed glycerol") collected from the same three dogs receiving the same daily insulin therapy. As comparison of the two graphs indicates, the relatively "flat" slopes of the plots for the new formulation indicate improved bioactivity. The improved glycerol/insulin formulation is now being evaluated in a clinical trial under an investigational new drug (IND) exemption. In addition to water, the modified formulation contains soluble (regular) purified porcine or human insulin at 60 U/ml, processed synthetic glycerol at 80% (v/v), and phosphate buffer (54 mM). The formulation has a pH of 6.7. Insulin concentrations for the pumps of individual patients are prepared by mixing the formulation above with an appropriate amount of diluent, which lacks insulin but is otherwise identical to the foregoing solution.

Aside from glycerol/insulin, perhaps the most successful of the insulin formulations for implantable pumps was developed by Hoechst AG (Frankfurt, West Germany). This insulin (Hoe PS 21) contains small quantities of polyethylene and polypropylene glycol. In a human clinical trial using an investigational implantable peristaltic pump developed by Siemens AG (the Siemens PFA 1), more than a year of continuous intraperitoneal infusion was achieved [30]. New clinical trials in which the Hoechst insulin formulation will be infused from the

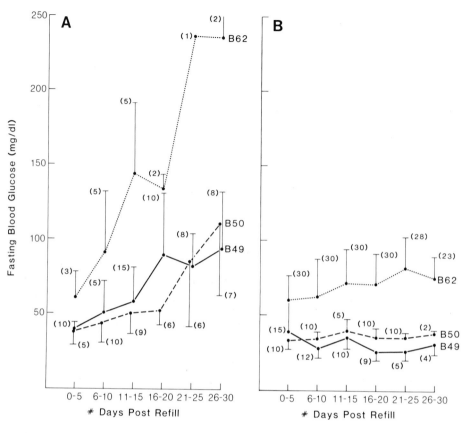

Fig. 10 (A) Mean fasting blood glucose (FBG) versus days after refill for three dogs (indicated as B 49, B 50 and B 62) being maintained on the standard glycerol/insulin formulation made with unpurified, rendered USP glycerol. (B) FBG versus days after refill for the same dogs while receiving the improved glycerol/insulin formulation made with purified synthetic spectrographic grade glycerol. (From Blackshear et al., American Society for Artificial Internal Organs 9:646-655, 1986.)

MiniMed (PIMS) implantable pump have been initiated at Baltimore. A higher viscosity version of the Hoechst formulation, for use in implantable peristaltic pumps, has also been developed. A cross-linked collagen product was added to this insulin as a viscosity enhancing agent. Clinical trials with this insulin in the Siemens (I 1) system were initiated in four European medical centers in February 1986. A formulation recently developed by Eli Lilly Company uses as its primary stabilizing agent poloxamer 188, which acts synergistically with m-cresol and phenol to improve the stability of insulin to thermomechanical stress (ISGIID Newsletter, December 1986).

VI. FUTURE PROSPECTS

The implantable infusion pump promises to be a versatile device especially well suited for long-term delivery of drugs in applications in which drug activity is enhanced by delivery directly into intravenous, intra-arterial, intrathecal, subdural, intraventricular, intraperitoneal, or other body locations with minimal risk of infection and interference in the patient's life. A list of several drugs that might be more effectively administered by pump is presented in Table 2. In several of these instances, the ability to accurately deliver therapeutic agents across the blood-brain barrier may permit the successful treatment of diseases that heretofore have lacked suitable therapeutic approaches. For example, Parkinson's disease is currently treated by L-DOPA. Upon passage through the blood-brain barrier, L-DOPA is converted into dopamine—the agent that is actually responsible for the therapeutic effect but cannot pass through the blood-brain barrier. Unfortunately, enzymes produced by bacteria in the gut also convert L-DOPA to dopamine at an uncontrollable rate, resulting in large fluc-

TABLE 2 Current Investigational and Probably Future Applications of Implantable Infusion Pumps

Disease	Drug	Route of delivery[a]
Clinical Investigational Applications		
Diabetes mellitus	Insulin	IV
Alzheimer's disease	Bethanechol chloride	IS
Probably Future Applications		
Prostate cancer	Luteinizing hormone releasing hormone	IV
Amyotropic lateral sclerosis (Lou Gehrig's disease)	Thyrotropin releasing hormone	IS
Organ failure and certain autoimmune disease)	Cyclosporine	IV
Parkinson's disease	Dopamine	IS
Parkinson's disease	L-Dopa	IV
Manic depressive psychosis	Lithium	IV

[a]IV = intravenous, IS = intraspinal.

tuations in dopamine concentrations in the brain. Implantable pumps can potentially be used to administer L-DOPA intravenously or to administer dopamine directly into the ventricles of the brain, thereby providing precise control of drug levels in the cerebrospinal fluid. This is one of many drugs that potentially can be administered more effectively by an implantable drug infusion device. The range of possible applications for implantable pump technology is limited only by the imagination.

REFERENCES

1. P. J. Blackshear, F. D. Dorman, P. L. Blackshear, Jr., R. L. Varco, and H. Buchwald, *Surg. Forum*, 21:136 (1970).

2. P. J. Blackshear, T. D. Rohde, R. L. Varco, and H. Buchwald, *Surg. Gynecol. Obstet.*, 141:176 (1975).

3. P. J. Blackshear, T. D. Rohde, J. C. Grotting, F. D. Dorman, P. R. Perkins, R. L. Varco, and H. Buchwald, *Diabetes*, 28:634 (1979).

4. H. Buchwald, T. D. Rohde, F. D. Dorman, J. H. Skakoon, B. C. Wigness, F. R. Prosl, E. M. Tucker, T. G. Rublein, P. J. Blackshear, and R. L. Varco, *Diabetes Care*, 3:351 (1980).

5. P. J. Blackshear, T. D. Rohde, J. L. Palmer, B. D. Wigness, W. M. Rupp, and H. Buchwald, *Diabetes Care*, 6:387 (1983).

6. T. D. Rohde, P. J. Blackshear, R. L. Varco, and H. Buchwald, *Minn. Med.*, 60:719 (1977).

7. H. Buchwald, T. D. Rohde, P. D. Schneider, R. L. Varco, and P. J. Blackshear, *Surgery*, 88:507 (1980).

8. W. M. Rupp, H. B. McCarthy, T. D. Rohde, P. J. Blackshear, F. J. Goldenberg, and H. Buchwald, *Curr. Surg.*, 39:419 (1982).

9. Diagnostic and therapeutic technology assessment (DATTA): Implantable infusion pump, *JAMA*, 250:1906 (1983).

10. H. Buchwald, T. B. Grage, P. P. Vassilopoulos, T. D. Rohde, R. L. Varco, and P. J. Blackshear, *Cancer*, 45:866 (1980).

11. A. M. Cohen, W. C. Wood, A. Greenfield, A. Waltman, C. Dedrick, and P. J. Blackshear, *Dis. Colon Rectum*, 23:223 (1980).

12. W. Ensminger, J. Niederhuber, S. Dakhil, J. Thrall, and R. Wheeler, *Cancer Treat. Rep.*, 65:393 (1981).

13. R. M. Barone, J. E. Byfeld, P. B. Goldfarb, S. Frankel, C. Ginn, and S. Greer, *Cancer*, 50:850 (1982).

14. C. M. Balch, M. M. Urist, S. Soong, and M. McGregor, *Ann. Surg.*, 198:567 (1983).

15. J. E. Niederhuber, W. Ensminger, J. Gyves, J. Thrall, S. Walker, and E. Cozzi, *Cancer*, 53:1336 (1984).

16. S. I. Schwartz, L. S. Jones, and C. S. McCune, *Ann. Surg.*, 201:560 (1985).

17. M. M. Kemeny, D. Goldberg, J. D. Beatty, D. Blayney, S. Browning, J. Doroshow, L. Ganteaume, R. L. Hill, W. Kokal, D. U. Riihimaki, and H. Terz, Cancer, 57:492 (1986).
18. W. D. Kaplan, S. E. Come, R. W. Takvorian, S. Laffin, R. S. Geleman, G. R. Weiss, and M. B. Garnick, J. Clin. Oncol., 11: 1266 (1984).
19. R. V. Roemeling, W. J. M. Hrushesky, B. J. Kennedy, and H. Buchwald, Surg. Forum, 37:400 (1986).
20. B. M. Onofrio, T. L. Yaksh, and P. G. Arnold, Mayo Clin. Proc., 56:516 (1981).
21. H. S. Greenberg, J. Taren, W. D. Ensminger, and K. Doan, J. Neurosurg., 57:360 (1982).
22. R. E. Harbaugh, D. W. Coombs, R. L. Saunders, M. Gaylor, and M. Pageau, J. Neurosurg., 56:803 (1982).
23. D. W. Coombs, R. L. Saunders, M. S. Gaylor, M. G. Pageau, M. G. Leith, and C. Schaiberger, Lancet, 425 (Aug. 22, 1981).
24. D. W. Coombs, R. L. Saunders, and M. G. Pageau, Reg. Anesthesiol., 7:110 (1982).
25. D. W. Coombs, R. L. Saunders, M. S. Gaylor, A. R. Block, T. Colon, R. Harbaugh, M. G. Pageau, and W. Mroz, JAMA, 250: 2336 (1983).
26. K. Irsigler, H. Kritz, and R. G. Lovett, CRC Crit. Rev. Ther. Drug Carrier Syst., 1:189 (1985).
27. D. S. Schade, R. P. Eaton, W. S. Edwards, R. C. Doberneck, W. J. Spencer, G. A. Carlson, R. E. Bair, J. T. Love, R. S. Urenda, and J. I. Gaona, JAMA, 247:1848 (1982).
28. K. Irsigler, H. Kritz, G. Hagmuller, M. Franetzki, K. Prestele, H. Thorow, and K. Geisen, Diabetes, 30:1072 (1981).
29. H. Kritz, C. Najemnik, G. Hagmueller, S. Leodolter, F. Olbert, A. Mostbeck, H. Denck, and K. Irsigler, in Diabetes Treatment with Implantable Insulin Infusion Systems (K. Irsigler, H. Kritz, and R. Lovett, eds.). Urban & Schwarzenberg, Vienna, 1983, p. 81.
30. J. L. Selam, A. Slingenmeyer, P. A. Chaptal, M. Franetzki, K. Prestele, and J. Mirouze, Artif. Organs, 6:315 (1982).
31. H. Buchwald, J. Barbosa, R. L. Varco, T. D. Rohde, W. M. Rupp, R. A. Schwartz, F. J. Goldenberg, T. G. Rublein, and P. J. Blackshear, Lancet, 1233 (June 6, 1981).
32. W. M. Rupp, J. J. Barbosa, P. J. Blackshear, H. B. McCarthy, T. D. Rohde, R. J. Goldenberg, T. G. Rublein, F. D. Dorman, and H. Buchwald, New Engl. J. Med., 307:265 (1982).
33. P. J. Blackshear, G. I. Shulman, A. M. Rousell, D. M. Nathan, K. L. Minaker, J. W. Rowe, D. C. Robbins, and A. M. Cohen, J. Clin. Endocrinol. Metab., 61:753 (1985).

8

A Programmable Implantable Medication System (PIMS) as a Means for Intracorporeal Drug Delivery

ROBERT E. FISCHELL / The Johns Hopkins University, Laurel, Maryland

Microcomputers, microsensors, micropumps, micropower sources, and micromedication dispensers, in the form of programmable systems, are being developed for implantation in humans. An implantable insulin pump system for the control of diabetes has been developed. An extension of this technique is discussed in the form of a microcomputer-controlled, closed-loop system by which medication is dispensed in specific response to a continuously measured physiological parameter. Particular stress is laid on the exquisite similarity between systems for orbiting spacecraft and implantable microcomputers.

I. INTRODUCTION

These are exciting times for the biomedical engineer whose career path involves work on the development of microcomputer-controlled devices that operate within the human body. The invention of the transistor in 1947 made possible the first electronic device to be implanted in a human subject: an artificial cardiac pacemaker [1]. That breakthrough resulted from three specific characteristics of the transistor as compared to the vacuum tube, namely: (a) an order of magnitude smaller size, (b) two orders of magnitude less electric power consumption, and (c) an indefinitely long life. Where the transistor made electronic medical implants possible, in the coming decade the integrated circuit chip will extend by orders of magnitude the capabilities of such devices. The result will be a revolution in the treatment of human disorders that until now have been treated only poorly if at all.

A first application of microcomputers implanted in humans is the programmable implantable medication system (PIMS), which has been developed at the Johns Hopkins University Applied Physics Laboratory (APL). This device has characteristics very similar to those of an orbiting spacecraft. The major similarities are that PIMS includes a command system, a telemetry system, a miniature, long-life power system, and very-large-scale integrated circuit chips. It also has been designed and fabricated using reliability and quality assurance techniques from the aerospace industry. Implantation in several diabetic humans occurred at the end of 1986. After PIMS, implantable microcomputers may be used for the closed-loop control of diseases such as hypertension; that is, blood pressure would be sensed in vivo and an antihypertensive medication released according to a programmed algorithm. This would be the first of a new generation of instruments that mimic the function of the human body by sensing a physiological parameter and make an appropriate response just as the body would do if it were functioning normally.

II. OUTER SPACE TO INNER SPACE

There is an unusual degree of similarity between spacecraft operating in outer space and electronic medical implants operating within the inner space of the human body. The major similarities occur in the command system, the telemetry system, the power system, microminiaturization, and reliability.

A. Command System

The first spacecraft (Sputnik, Explorer I) orbited the earth and merely emanated a steady radiofrequency output. The first electronic medical implant was a heart pacemaker whose output pulse rate was fixed. As space and implant technology developed, both spacecraft and implants required more flexibility and capability. Thus, command systems were developed that allow the spacecraft's mode of operation to be altered in orbit by a radio signal from a ground station. Examples of command functions that were used on APL (and other) spacecraft are those to turn various subsystems on or off, change the level of the radiofrequency output of a transmitter, replace a failed subsystem, and change a parameter of an orbiting experiment. Implanted electronic devices use command systems that operate from a radio signal originating in a physician's console that is, of course, exterior to the patient. Examples of control commands in modern pacemakers are those to change the stimulation pulse rate, pulse voltage, or pulse width; to enable or disable an electrical signal from the atrium; and to adjust the sensitivity for an electrical signal from the ventricle. The PIMS command system is used to change basal delivery rate, to turn the device on and off, and to set limits on medication usage. The command system permits the spacecraft to adapt to its environment and to the spacecraft's specific condition, thus maximizing its use for a variety of purposes. A command system for an implant allows it to adapt to the patient's changing needs.

B. Telemetry System

Telemetry involves the transmission of data from a remote location. In the case of a spacecraft, telemetry is accomplished via modulated radio waves sent down to ground receiving stations. Typical measurements from a spacecraft might be the confirmation of parameters that have been commanded into it, the battery voltage, and particle densities, both in real time and as stored data. Similarly, typical implant telemetered data might be the confirmation of the parameters that have been commanded into it, the battery voltage, and the rate of infusing medication, both in real time and as stored data.

264 / Fischell

C. Power System

Power systems for spacecraft and implants must be small and long-lived. Both spacecraft and implant systems have used rechargeable nickel-cadmium cells to store energy and operate the system between recharges. More recently, the power demands of implantable medical electronic devices have become so small that a single, AA size, lithium primary cell can operate some of these devices without recharging for more than 5 years. Such is the case with the PIMS implant.

D. Microminiaturization

Until the age of the space shuttle with its huge payload capability, it was a struggle for spacecraft designers to meet payload size and weight limitations. Thus, an extraordinary effort was made to reduce size and weight while, at the same time, striving to increase operating capabilities; therefore, microminiaturization of electronics became commonplace in spacecraft design. The ultimate striving for size reduction has been, and still is, a goal for the design of implantable electronic medical devices, while increased capability has also been demanded. The first pacemaker (circa 1960) [1] used only two transistors, measured 3 in. in diameter by 1 in. thick, and weighed approximately 250 g. Modern multiprogrammable pacemakers [2] (see Fig. 1 for a comparison) contain the equivalent of 100,000 transistors yet have one-tenth the volume and one-fifth the weight of the first pacemaker. Thus while demonstrating enormously better performance, their electronic components have been so miniaturized that they are now being comfortably implanted even in newborn babies.

E. Reliability

An often overlooked and sometimes unglamorous aspect of both spacecraft and implants is reliability. The failure of a spacecraft results in the loss of an extraordinarily expensive machine; therefore, a whole discipline of reliability was created to ensure long life in orbit. Early spacecraft frequently failed during launch or after a few days in orbit, but the careful application of reliability engineering has resulted in extended life. An excellent example is APL's Transit Navigation Satellites, whose lifetimes in orbit are now well beyond a decade [3]. The first pacemaker failed within 12 hr of human implantation. In early 1970, many pacemakers ceased to function in less than 2 years because of component failures. Because of the application of space-technology-derived reliability and quality assurance techniques to the design of the Johns Hopkins rechargeable pacemaker, hundreds of these devices are still functioning after more than 10 years of continuous operation in humans [4,5]. The lithium-battery-powered PIMS

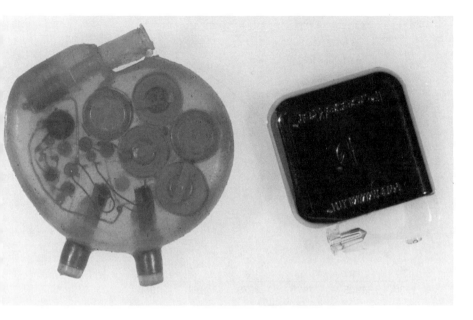

Fig. 1 Comparison of a fixed-rate pacemaker (circa 1970) (left) with a recent, multiprogrammable, demand pacemaker (right).

implant should demonstrate reliabilities that also will ensure at least a 5-year life in vivo.

III. DEVELOPMENT OF IMPLANTABLE MICROCOMPUTERS

The microelectronic chip has revolutionized hand-held computers. In only a few years the slide rule has become an antique. Although it will take longer, the chip as part of an implantable microcomputer system will revolutionize the treatment of a variety of human dysfunctions and will make the single transistor essentially obsolete.

The increased capability with time of integrated circuits (i.e., chips) is shown in Fig. 2. Whereas in 1959 there was only a single component on a single piece (or chip) of silicon, by 1982 chips were being made with 450,000 components. Although the number of components per chip may grow in the late 1980s to more than one million, even today the chips can provide extraordinary capability for implantable electronic devices.

Listed below are the parts of an implantable microcomputer. They are typically, but not always, on separate chips.

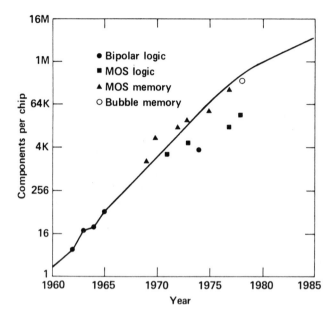

Fig. 2   The increase in the number of components on a chip since 1960.

1. The universal asynchronous receiver/transmitter is the means
    for interfacing the computer with the outside world; that is,
    it is the input/output interface of the microcomputer.
2. The microprocessor serves as the central processing unit of
    the microcomputer.
3. The read-only memory (ROM) is hard-wired (i.e., fixed) cir-
    cuitry that provides specific functionality for the microcompu-
    ter. Because ROMs are custom-made devices, a programmable
    ROM, a ROM erasable by ultraviolet light, or an electrically
    erasable, programmable ROM is frequently used in the early
    stage of microcomputer development because such a memory
    can be readily reprogrammed, as is often required during de-
    velopmental stages.
4. The random-access memory (RAM) serves as a recorder of
    any digitally encoded information, for example, programming
    instructions or the hourly use of medication.
5. Universal arrays are semicustom logic chips that can be pro-
    cured at reasonable cost ($10,000 for the first 100 chips) and
    in a reasonably short time (10 weeks). They provide a variety
    of AND gates, OR gates, and so on, required for a particular
    computer logic.

6. Custom very-large-scale integrated circuits offer the possibil-
    ity of 10 times the number of components per chip compared
    to universal arrays, but cost ($100,000 for the first 100 chips)
    and delivery time (6-12 months) preclude their use during
    developmental stages.

IV. THE STATE OF THE ART OF IMPLANTABLE MICROCOMPUTER SYSTEMS IN 1987

Not many computer-controlled implantable medication systems exist.
One, the programmable implantable medication system (PIMS), has been
developed at APL. Figure 3 is a block diagram that shows the various
parts of the system. At the left is equipment used by the patient,
and at the right is equipment used by the physician. The implantable
portion of PIMS, which contains the microcomputer subsystem is called
the implantable program infusion pump (IPIP).

The patient is provided with a hand-held device called a patient's
programming unit, by which he or she can initiate self-medication from
the IPIP within the constraints programmed into the IPIP by the physician. The main portion of the medicaiton programming system is a
computer terminal that is used for programming the IPIP. The device
for refilling the IPIP is called the medication injection unit. The last
major portion of PIMS is a telephone communication system, by means
of which the patient at a location remote from the medication programming system can have the IPIP reprogrammed with a new prescription
or can have stored telemetry data in the IPIP read out and displayed
by the medication programming system.

The potential advantages of PIMS or other implantable drug delivery systems are as follows:

1. A precise medication rate is available.

    (a) The medication level can be maintained within a very nar-
         row therapeutic range.
    (b) A medication level can be maintained that is at a minimum
         level within a broad therapeutic range. Thus, the de-
         sired physiological effect could be obtained while signifi-
         cantly reducing overdosage. This can decrease the
         buildup of tolerance and side effects.

2. Perfect compliance can be achieved. The physician can write
    a prescription into the electronics of the implanted device and
    medication will be delivered at that prescribed rate without
    requiring any effort from the patient.
3. Medication can be delivered by any desired time profile or
    periodicity.

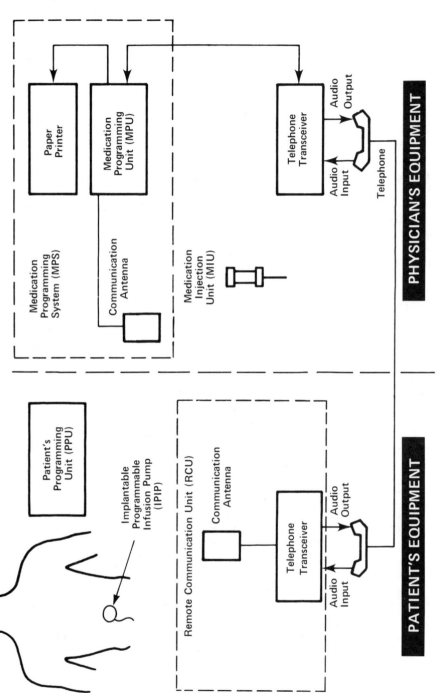

Fig. 3 Block diagram of the programmable implantable medication system (PIMS).

4. Accidental or deliberate overdose is prevented because the implanted device can be built with programmed limits that neither the patient nor the physician can violate.
5. Decreased use of medication is possible; for example, if a medication is more effectively delivered at a particular time of day, that can be accomplished by PIMS.
6. More appropriate medications can be used for the treatment of specific diseases. For example, if heparin therapy is more advantageous in the treatment of thrombotic disease as compared to another drug substance such as warfarin, then PIMS can be used to deliver intravenous heparin.
7. Closely related to the preceding advantage is that medications that normally would require the patient to be hospitalized can be safely given on an outpatient basis.
8. By placing the tip of the PIMS outflow catheter at an appropriate site in the body, one can deliver medications within a more confined boundary. Thus, one could enhance the action on the organ or cells that require the medication while decreasing the concentration of medications elsewhere in the body.
9. The physician can use PIMS to determine the precise medication level used by the patient on an hour-by-hour or daily basis.
10. An implanted system with a physiological sensor (not yet available with PIMS) could regulate medication delivery to exactly suit the patient's needs.
11. An implanted system can provide a patient-detectable alarm when a desired physiological effect is not being achieved or when the device functioning deviates from nominal performance.

The IPIP is disk shaped, with a diameter of 8.1 cm, a thickness at its center of 1.8 cm, a thickness at its edge of 1.3 cm, and a weight of 171 g. The IPIP can be programmed for a constant or a variable basal infusion of medication with a repetitive period of from 1 hr to 60 days. By far the most frequently used basal period is 24 hr. A period of 28 days is available, particularly for the infusion of sex hormones to mimic the female cycle. The medication programming system can be used to program six different supplemental infusion profiles that the IPIP can delivery, when such delivery is initiated by the patient's programming unit. The latter unit can also turn off the IPIP for an hour at the patient's request, countermand a prior command of the unit, or change the basal infusion rate to either half or full basal.

Figure 4 shows the IPIP with its outer cover removed to reveal the microcomputer electronics. At the center is the refill port. A hypodermic needle is placed through the skin, then through this port

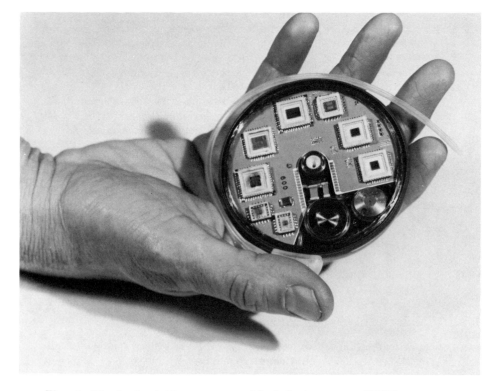

Fig. 4   The implantable programmable infusion pump (IPIP).

(which has a silicone rubber septum), for access to the IPIP reservoir. The chips (shown in ceramic chip carriers) are the microcircuits that make up the microcomputer controlling the IPIP. Toward the lower right in Fig. 4 are two circular metal parts; the smaller is the solenoid pump and the larger is the fluid-flow-smoothing network, which serves to smooth the pulsatile output of the pump so that the outflow simulates the flow of hormones from an endocrine gland.

Figure 5 shows a monolithic circuit on a chip mounted in a ceramic chip carrier. This construction is typical of the IPIP microcomputer. The wires connecting the pads of the chip to the chip carrier are gold alloy, 1 mil (0.0025 cm) in diameter. Thus, they are approximately one-third the diameter of a human blond hair.

The photomicrograph in Fig. 6 shows details of the universal asynchronous receiver/transmitter chip used in the IPIP. This particular chip is a RCA CMOS 1854. The line widths on the chip are approximately 0.2 mil (5 µm).

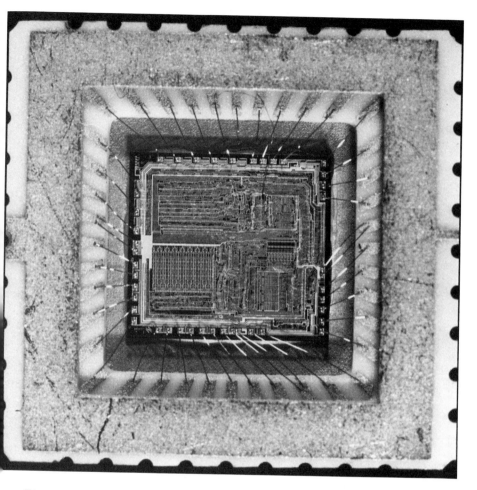

Fig. 5 Typical chip in a ceramic chip carrier.

Figure 7 is a block diagram of the IPIP. At the center is the fluid-handling system, to the right is the command system, and to the left are the power and telemetry systems. A noncoring (hole in the side) hypodermic needle is inserted through the skin, through a self-sealing septum, and into an antechamber, to permit filling the 10 ml reservoir with medication. The pressurant in back of the reservoir is a vapor-liquid system of Freon 113, which maintains a constant negative pressure of -4 psig. When the reservoir is filled, the Freon changes from mostly vapor to nearly entirely liquid. As the reservoir is emptied, the reverse is true while always maintaining a negative pressure.

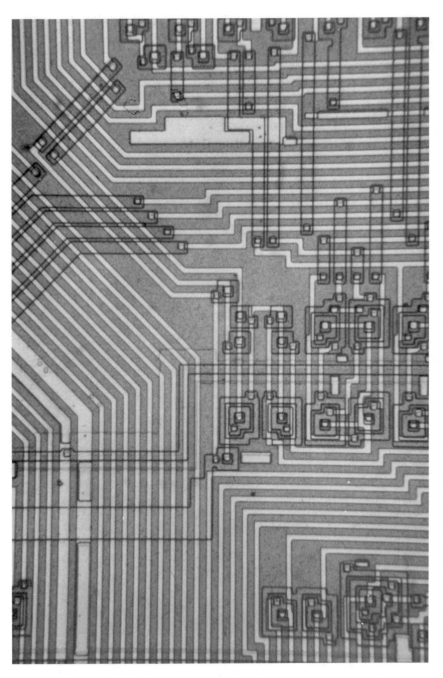

Fig. 6 Details of the IPIP universal asynchronous receiver/transmitter.

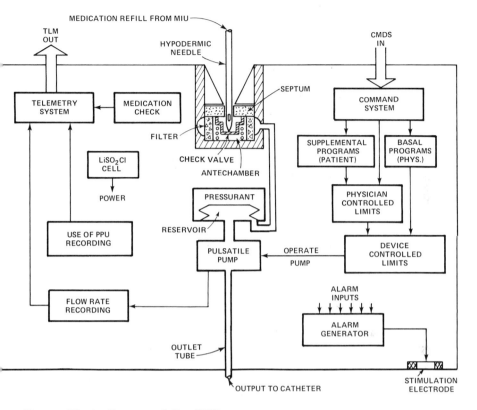

Fig. 7 Block diagram of the IPIP.

Thus, if there is a leak, body fluids will leak into IPIP and no medication will be forced out. The pulsatile pump sends 2 µl pulses of fluid
into the outlet tube which connects to a catheter through which the
medication is delivered into the body.

The command system operates by receiving commands from the
medication programming system or the patient's programming unit.
Satellites cannot function properly if "inadvertent commands" change
their operating state. Likewise, "phantom commands," as the analogous
anomalies in implanted devices are termed, would be disastrous for
users of such devices. That possibility is precluded by the "double-
handshake" secure command link shown in Fig. 8. From the external
medication programming system or the patient's programming unit,
a 12 bit command is sent to the IPIP, where it is stored in memory.
The data are then sent by telemetry back to the original source, where
a bit-by-bit correlation is carried out. If all bits check out correctly,
an "execute" command is sent that allows the IPIP to carry out the

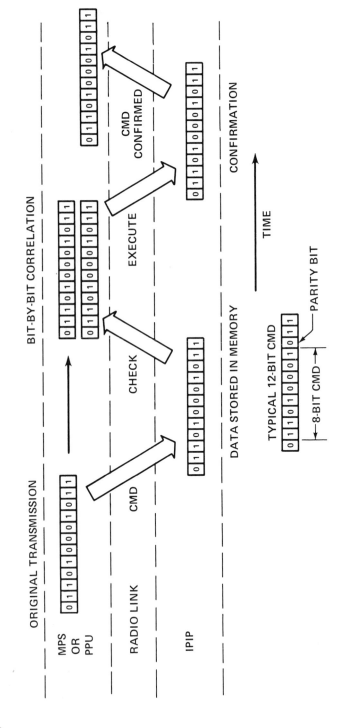

Fig. 8 "Double-handshake" signal format for secure communication.

274

command that has already been put in memory and therefore, since it was checked, is correct. This technique precludes the possibility of phantom commands.

Referring again to Fig. 7, by means of the command system, the patient uses the patient programming unit to request supplemental medication. Also, the physician can program basal programs with the medication programming system. There are limits, controlled by the physician, on the amount of supplemental medication the patient can request. There are also device-controlled limits that prevent the physician from prescribing too much medication.

To the right in Fig. 7 is the alarm system, consisting of many inputs into an alarm generator that, in turn, can alert the patient by means of a subcutaneous electrical stimulation or "tickle." Typical reasons for alarms are as follows.

1. Only a limited amount of medication is left in the reservoir.
2. Medication is leaking into the electronics chamber.
3. A basal program has inadvertently been changed.

On the left in Fig. 7 is the telemetry system. Probably its most important aspect is its ability to recall the hour-by-hour medication flow out of the IPIP. An example of such measured data is shown in Fig. 9. These data were sent from an IPIP implanted in a laboratory dog made diabetic by the removal of its pancreas. The data were recovered several days after the actual data of insulin infusion, which in this case was on May 23, 1982.

The last block in Fig. 7 is the lithium thionyl chloride ($LiSOCl_2$) cell. That cell, especially made for IPIP, can operate the first IPIPs for more than 6 years without recharging. New versions of the IPIP already in fabrication will have about 7 years of implant life.

Figure 10 shows how a patient might use a patient programming unit to self-medicate with insulin prior to eating a meal.

Figure 11 shows how a patient might have a new prescription "written" into her microcomputer without the IPIP by means of the telephone communication system. The patient could also have the stored data on medication useage telemetered back to the physician by telephone from her home.

V. MEDICAL APPLICATIONS OF PIMS

The microcomputer-controlled delivery of medication by PIMS will provide improved treatment for several diseases.

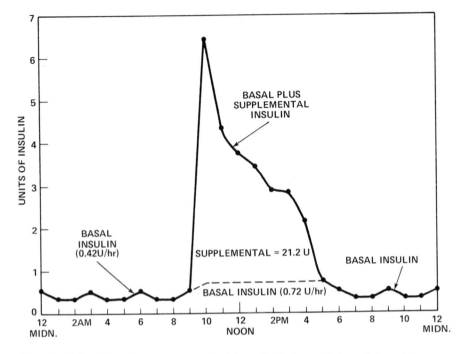

Fig. 9 Telemetered measurement of insulin infused into a laboratory animal on May 23, 1983.

A. Diabetes

The application of PIMS to diabetes by the controlled release of insulin is one such obvious medication application [6]. Preliminary data show that the continuous release of insulin from a pump with supplemental doses at mealtime provides dramatically better control of blood sugar. Furthermore, there have been reports of the reversal of diabetic retino-pathy [7] and of other improvements in the diabetic condition when the pump release of insulin has been used.

The first human application of PIMS was in a diabetic patient and took place at the Johns Hopkins Hospital on November 10, 1986. The IPIP utilized the intraperitoneal delivery route. Figure 12 shows the initial basal program commanded into the implanted portion of PIMS (the IPIP). Each pulse delivers a volume of 2 μl, which for 400 units of insulin provides 0.8 unit per pulse. The increased basal dosage between 3:00 A.M. and 5: A.M. was to counter the so-called dawn effect (i.e., increased blood sugars that occur in the early hours if increased insulin is not provided).

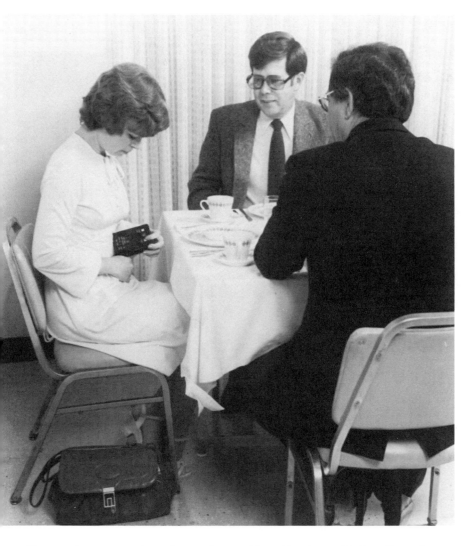

Fig. 10 Demonstration of a patient self-medicating with insulin prior to eating.

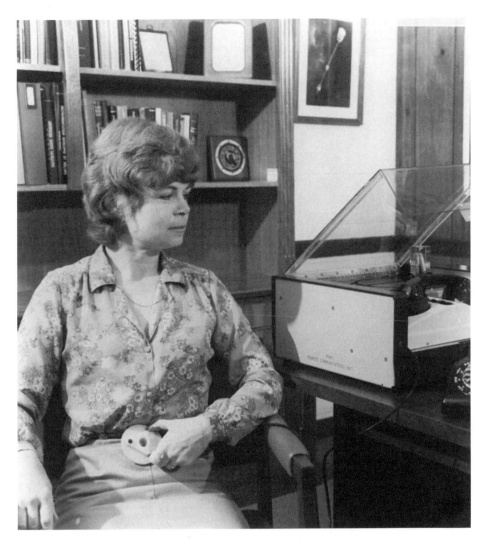

Fig. 11 Demonstration of a patient having a prescription "written" into her IPIP; data are being telemetered to the physician by telephone.

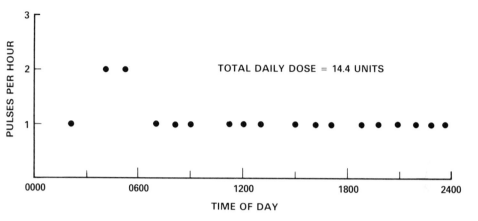

Fig. 12 Basal insulin infusion schedule for first patient.

Figure 13 shows how the first implanted IPIP responds to command
5 of the patient programming unit. The insulin is delivered with a
double exponential curve (first increasing then decreasing), which
mimics the action of a normal pancreas. The maximum delivery rate
is 1.0 unit per minute, the delivery time is 90 min, and the total integrated insulin dose for this command 5 is 12 units. The IPIP reservoir
contains approximately 12 ml of medication. For a patient using 50
units of insulin per day, the reservoir would typically be refilled four
times each year.

Figure 14 shows the first patient's blood sugar on days 1, 2, 17,
and 18. As with the case of laboratory animals, blood sugars immediately after surgical implant are quite high. However, by day 17, the
mean blood sugars are within the normal range.

Figure 15 shows the results of blood sugar measurements in the
first patient 30 days after implant. At 8:00 P.M. on December 9, the
patient ate a 900 calorie meal and inadvertently failed to request supplemental insulin. By 10:00 P.M., his blood sugar rose to nearly 400
mg/dl. He then immediately began a course of supplemental insulin
to lower his blood sugar. This inadvertent omission of supplemental
insulin indicates just how very sensitive such type I diabetic patients
are to lack of proper insulin infusion. By the next day, the patient
had a mean blood sugar level that was just at the center of the normal
range. Even though the patient did reach near 400 mg/dl for a short
time, it is believed that cellular damage is a result of the time integral
of the blood glucose and, therefore, a short duration at a high blood
sugar level, does not have a perceptible deleterious effect.

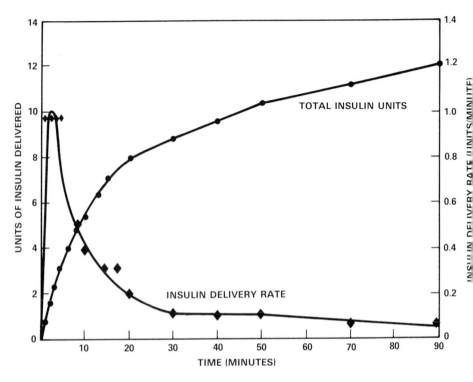

Fig. 13 Supplemental insulin delivery for patient's programming unit command 5. Total number of units = 12.

B. Relief of Chronic Pain

Another important PIMS application is for the spinal infusion of morphine for the treatment of chronic pain. Prior results with nonprogrammable, implantable medication delivery systems [8] have been shown to provide quite excellent pain relief without a great deal of tolerance buildup by the patient. The advantage of PIMS over nonprogrammable implants is that patients can elect (by means of the patient programming unit) to have the morphine delivered only when they have pain. Thus, pain relief would be maximized and tolerance buildup would be minimized.

C. Diseases of the Central Nervous System

There are several diseases of the central nervous system that might be ideally treated by PIMS using intrathecal (into the cerebrospinal fluid)

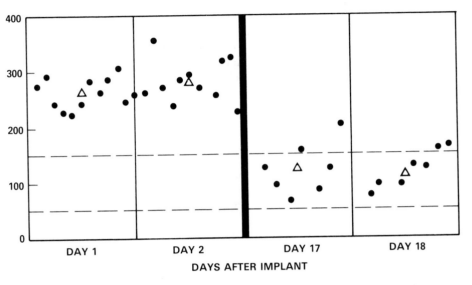

Fig. 14 PIMS results in first human subjects, implanted on November 10, 1986; Δ = daily mean value.

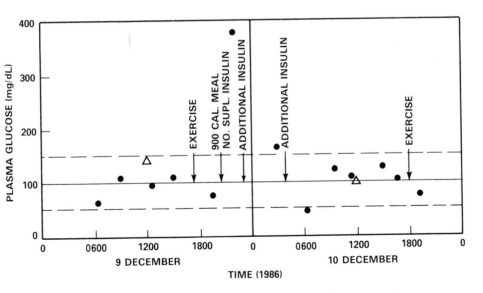

Fig. 15 PIMS results 30 days after implant; Δ = daily mean value.

infusion. Infusion directly into the cerebrospinal fluid bypasses the blood-brain barrier so that the medication can be delivered directly to the region where it is needed. The following subsections discuss some diseases that might be ideally treated by placing the IPIP subcutaneously in the abdomen while placing the catheter tip beneath the dura mater of the spine so that infusion is made directly into the cerebrospinal fluid.

Amyotrophic Lateral Sclerosis

From data obtained from Dr. T. Mansat of the New England Medical Center [9], the spinal infusion of the hormone TRH appears to decrease the rate at which patients with amyotrophic lateral sclerosis (Lou Gehrig's disease) lose their muscular strength. It is believed that TRH has a trophic effect on the deteriorating cells in the spinal cord. To date, these patients have used nonprogrammable pumps with a uniform rate of infusion. The pulsatile administration of TRH may offer some further advantage in that large boluses can be administered achieving very high TRH concentrations followed by a clearance of the drug so that the cells will "recover" to their normal state.

Parkinson's Disease

Parkinson's disease is a result of the lack of the neurotransmitter dopamine within the brain. Although the oral administration of L-DOPA is efficacious especially in the earliest years after onset, the later stages of the diseases are often poorly treated by this drug. Direct infusion of dopamine into the cerebrospinal fluid can have potentially great advantages in that the medication will be delivered to the site at which it is needed and any desired time profile as calculated to best control the manifestations of this disease may be chosen.

Alzheimer's Disease

Only recently has there been any progress in the treatment of Alzheimer's disease. Certain drugs (such as bethanechol) when taken orally have been reported in the news media to improve the patient's mental acuity. If there is some medication that can be beneficial in the treatment of Alzheimer's disease, it would undoubtedly be most effective if delivered into the cerebrospinal fluid so that it can reach the affected cells in the brain without passing through the blood-brain barrier. PIMS with a catheter tip placed beneath the dura of the spine, or actually within a ventricle of the brain, should be ideally suited for delivering such medication.

VI. CONCLUSIONS

Where do we go after PIMS? In the area of medication infusion, the next variation of PIMS is the sensor-actuated medication system (SAMS), a microcomputer-controlled, closed-loop system by which a physiological parameter will be sensed and medication will be released according to specific algorithms programmed into the IPIP. An example is the sensing of blood pressure within the body and the release of antihypertensive medication according to need for people with high blood pressure who do not readily respond to conventional therapy. The SAMS will be particularly valuable when the blood pressure not only is high but varies greatly from time to time. Another candidate application for the system is to sense the electroencephalogram precursor of an epileptic seizure and to release antiseizure medication in the brain so as to better control epilepsy with a minimum amount of medication.

Although closed-loop medication delivery systems will offer potentially great advantages in the somewhat distant future, in the coming decade, the extensive use of PIMS in an open-loop mode should find extensive applications to a large variety of diseases that have not been well treated in the past.

REFERENCES

1. R. Elmqvist and A. Senning, Implantable pacemaker for the heart. In *Medical Electronics* (Proc. 2nd Int. Conference on Medical Electronics, Paris, June 1959) (C. N. Smyth, ed.). Iliff & Son, London, 1960, p. 253.

2. S. Furman, Newer modes of cardiac pacing. Part I. Description of pacing modes, *Mod. Concepts Cardiovas. Dis.*, 1-5 (January 1983).

3. H. D. Black, The transit system, 1977: Performance plans and potential, *Phil. Trans. R. Soc. London*, A294:7 (1980).

4. R. E. Fischell, K. B. Lewis, J. H. Schulman, and J. W. Love, A long-lived, reliable, rechargeable cardiac pacemaker, in *Advances in Pacemaker Technology*, Vol. 1 (M. Schaldach and S. Furman, eds.). Springer-Verlag, New York, 1975.

5. J. W. Love, K. G. Lewis, and R. E. Fischell, The Johns Hopkins rechargeable pacemaker, *JAMA*, 234:64-66 (October 1975).

6. W. J. Spencer, For diabetes: An electronic pancreas, *IEEE Spectrum*, 15:38-42 (June 1978).

7. N. H. White, S. R. Waltman, T. Krupin, and J. V. Santiago, Reversal of abnormalities in ocular fluorophotometry in insulin dependent diabetics after 5 to 9 months of improved metabolic control, *Diabetes*, 31:80-85 (January 1982).

8. B. M. Onofrio, T. L. Yaksh, and P. G. Arnold, Continuous low-dose intrathecal morphine administration in the treatment of chronic pain of malignant origin, *Mayo Clin. Proc.*, 56:516-520 (1981).
9. T. L. Munsat, S. Reichlins, J. Taft, P. Andres, M. Kaplan, and D. Kasdon, Experience with long-term intrathecal infusion of TRH in ALS, *Muscle Nerve*, 9:103 (1986).

9

Direct Access Ports

LOUIS KOPITO / Shiley Infusaid Inc., Norwood, Massachusetts

I. BACKGROUND

Intravascular drug administration via indwelling catheters has gained rapid acceptance in recent years. Patients and medical providers alike have welcomed this alternative procedure replacing repeated venipunctures used in conventional drug therapy in cancer, hyperalimentation, infection control, pain management, and other treatments. An impressive record of therapeutic accomplishments has already accumulated and is steadily expanding for this technology.

The concept of "total implantation" of vascular access devices, substituting for the "percutaneous exit" catheters, has added appreciably to the range of applications and the safe duration of catheterization. New, highly biocompatible materials have extended the catheter indwelling time form a few days to a year or longer. The parallel development of small, lightweight, compact, and reliable infusion pumps, carried or worn by the patients, have provided mobility and relatively unrestricted patient activity. These important benefits have reduced significantly the frequency, duration, and cost of hospitalization associated with extended drug therapy in the treatment of selected chronic and transient diseases.

II. SCIENTIFIC RATIONALE

A. Intravascular Infusion

From the pioneering work of Ommaya [1], Hickman [2], and Broviac [3] evolved the concepts of drug infusion via catheters placed directly into blood vessels, major organs, and other relatively inaccessible body regions or compartments. These procedures have substituted for more conventional injections by repeated venipunctures. Patients undergoing long-term therapy (as in cancer) face frequent painful assaults on their progressively deteriorating vascular system. Early placement of totally sealed, implantable ports yields the following benefits for the patients as well as the medical staff.

Elimination of venipunctures.
Fewer infections: the infusion port is totally isolated from the
    outside environment except for the relatively short period
    of actual use.

Less physical trauma and skin sclerosis; fewer hematomas.
Painless and easier blood and blood product transfusion.
Safe access for nutrient infusion.

B. Time Factors in Protracted Drug Infusion

Cancer Chemotherapy: Cell Cycle Timing

The benefits of long-term or continuous drug administration with implanted ports differ with the drug and the condition treated. An important consideration in effective cancer therapy is the critical timing
of contact between a fresh, fully active drug and the malignant cells
during their drug-sensitive cyclic phase. Since these factors are highly variable, maximal tumor cell kill can be assured only by continuous
drug-tumor contact. In contrast, with bolus injections or other modes
of administration, this may not be possible [4].

Short Drug Half-Life

Certain valuable therapeutic agents have relatively short functional
half-lives. For example, the vinca alkaloids have half-lives on the
order of only a few minutes. Continuous infusion therapy may be more
effective with these drugs because it assures the presence of fully
active drugs through the entire course of therapy [4].

Anticipatory Therapy

Refractory congestive heart failure is difficult to treat with the dobutamine. Because of its very short half-life, this drug must be administered by continuous intravenous infusion. The successful use of an
implanted catheter and infusion pump in 11 patients with severe chronic
congestive heart failure was described by Roffman and associates [5].
Patients prone to cardiovascular accidents are suitable for this approach
because of the critical time factor from drug administration to the initiation of therapy. The long-term treatment (3-24 months in the study
above) justifies the implantation of a port system in preference to a
percutaneous exit catheter to minimize potentially dangerous infections
in these vulnerable patients.

Critical Chronopharmacology

The administration of hormones associated with puberty [6], reproduc-
tion, growth, and menstruation, and with diurnal, nocturnal, and other
cyclical of periodic events, is difficult in the clinical setting. Therapy
is usually protracted, discontinuous, and requires a great deal of individual attention. The use of relatively long-term implantable vascular
access devices with controllable or programmable pumps has considerable
logistic and monetary advantages in the following specialized treatments.

In the infuction of ovulation by cyclic infusion, gonadotropin releasing hormone (GnRH) must be delivered in pulsatile fashion
to mimic natural hypothalamic response in order to synthesize
and release follicle stimulating hormone (FSH) and luteinizing
hormone (LH).

In handling precocious puberty by means of constant infusion,
GnRH may be delivered for more than a year to correct hormonal imbalance [7].

Growth hormone treatment for adolescents of short stature [8] is
a nocturnal undertaking, requiring a year or longer.

Because these selected hormonal treatments have critical or unusual
requirements, including relatively long-duration therapy, dosing, and
timing, it is well worth the cost and effort to implant a vascular access
device early in the course of treatment. Since a considerable fraction
of patients requiring this therapy are children, adolescents, or young
adults, a totally implanted port will minimize interference with their
life and activities, including swimming and participation in vigorous
sports. The ports also enable the parents to administer therapy at
home, thus reducing the number and frequency of hospital visits.

III. FUNCTIONAL CONSIDERATIONS

A. Catheters

Advances in materials science and catheter fabrication technology have
created excellent catheters compatible with blood, other body fluids,
blood vessels, and other tissues.

Catheter-related complications, although rare, may occur due to
the following reasons:

Thrombophlebitis
Accidental dislodgement and migration
Plugging due to clot formation or accidental retrograde flow
Infections of internal or external origin
Faulty placement (surgeon's error)
Mechanical failure due to catheter rupture or breakage
Venipuncture by distal catheter end
Organ perforation

The frequency of catheter complications is related to type of usage,
indwelling time, and *particularly to the skill* and *experience of the
medical personnel involved* in the placement, care, and maintenance
of these devices. With increased experience, catheter/port complications are usually reduced to negligible levels.

B. Port Design

The totally implantable Infuse-A-Port evolved from the original Infusaid implantable pump's Sideport. The Sideport, an integral component of the pump, permits direct access to the drug discharge site by bypassing the main drug storage reservoir. Ensminger and Gyves [9] described its use for radionuclide angiography and as an auxiliary path for the administration of additional or different drugs. Because of its unique capability, this direct vascular access path was developed further into the separate, implantable Infuse-A-Port, consisting of two principal components without moving parts: a plastic disk with a centrally located septum for needle placement, and a radiopaque catheter leading to the desired drug discharge site (Fig. 1).

The Shiley Infusaid Infuse-A-Ports are made of highly biocompatible plastic materials. The design features include:

Relatively large base area for secure "anchoring"
Large-diameter recess septum for easier location and needle entry
Radiopaque catheter
Lightweight for maximum comfort

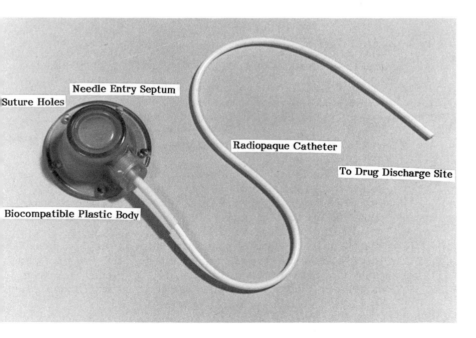

Fig. 1 The Shiley Infusaid Infuse-A-Port.

Noninterference with nuclear magnetic resonance (NMR) imaging
   or CAT scanning
One-piece design for greater safety and reliability
Availability of several port options and catheter configurations

   Selection of the optimal port design is based on the patient's size
and the site for selected implantation. The Shiley Infusaid Microport
is designed for pediatric patients and frail individuals. The large-
septum Macroport provides the most easy access in larger patients
whose subcutaneous tissues may obscure the smaller ports. Various
catheters are available for venous, arterial, and peritoneal catheter
placement.
   The port needle entry septum is the critical component of this device. It msut withstand numerous needle punctures, provide sufficient
"holding friction" to prevent the potentially serious consequences of
accidental withdrawal of the needle during infusion, and be able to
retain these properties over usage and time. The special silicone formulation used in this septum has withstood numerous punctures—many
times the expected lifetime use. The septum's needle retention properties are important during long-term infusions. Infusion ports are
usually implanted in the operating room (under local anesthesia), preferably by a surgeon familiar with this relatively simple procedure.

IV. APPLICATIONS

A. General Considerations

Prior to the implantation of temporary or permanent (life-long) drug
infusion devices, the physician must evaluate the patient's requirements on an individual basis considering the following variables.

   The nature of the disease, the drugs involved, and the location
      of the drug discharge site
   Patient characteristics: reliability, motivation, age, capacity for
      self-care, available family support, and assistance
   Requirement and/or preference for the infusion mode of therapy
   The expected duration of therapy and anticipated number of repe-
      titious drug infusion cycles
   Cost considerations, such as possible savings through outpatient
      therapy and earlier resumption of remunerative work activities
   Proximity to a primary health care facility, emergency care, con-
      tinuous drug supply, and other logistical considerations

B. Direct Access

At the time of port implantation, the drug discharge site is selected
or planned for the most advantageous delivery. Catheters are posi-

tioned to infuse drugs at, or near, most body compartments including relatively inaccessible locations such as the brain or spine. For purposes other than drug infusion—for example, for the periodic or continuous *removal* or drainage of fluids—catheters have been placed in the pleural space [10] or other locations.

The safe access for selective, direct drug infusion or fluid removal to and from anatomical regions or spaces made possible by this new technology has created certain advantageous therapies, as suggested in the research of Ommaya [1], Ensminger [9], Collins [11], Muchmore [12], and Lee [13]. In particular, cerebrospinal fluid space, the peritoneal cavity, and pleural and pericardial spaces are treated more efficiently in terms of increased local drug concentrations relative to systemic circulation. Ensminger stated [9]: "The future for regional chemotherapy appears exciting. There are many opportunities to apply therapeutic principles rationally with the potential of significant benefit to many patients."

C. Intravenous Access: Ports and Catheters

The most frequent applications for drug therapy via vascular access ports, implantable catheters, with pump infusion are the following.

Infections
Intractable pain—cancer origin
Postsurgical pain
Diabetes
Osteomyelitis
Chemotherapy
Thrombophlebitis
Transfusion
Cardiovascular diseases
Malignant ascites (fluid removal and drug infusion)
Hormonal imbalance
Clotting disorders
Nutrition (hyperalimentation)

These selected applications have a common requirement for long-term, repetitious, frequent, or cyclical drug administration. These features justify the implantation of a port for safety, cost reduction, functional treatment requirement logistics, and medical advantages.

Treatment of Infections

Patients with serious refractory infections or recurrent infections usually requiring prolonged hospitalization are the prime candidates for infusion therapy via implanted ports and external infusion pumps.

These conditions are readily adaptable to home therapy resulting in *substantial* financial advantages to the payors and patients alike. Infection management, treatment, and prophylaxis accounts for more than 30% of all current therapy by drug infusion lasting 5 days or longer per course of therapy.

Patients with osteomyelitis, septic arthritis, and cystic fibrosis requiring continuous attention for weeks, months, or longer, are excellent candidates for Infuse-A-Port implantation. This approach reduces the need for frequent dressing changes and physician visits and lessens the opportunity for developing secondary infections and other complications. The totally implanted port provides easier and more effective self-care and permits the patients to resume productive lives earlier than is possible with conventional therapy.

A growing number of hospitals offer extension services from their pharmacies for reliable home drug infusion as well as emergency back-up services [14]. Patient preference is high for this alternative therapy substituting for costly hospitalization.

Diabetes

Insulin infusion pumps and related devices account for the largest single use of drug infusion technology. Among the contraversial topics that dominate present research as well as clinical applications are the following.

Mode of delivery: continuous, intermittent "on-demand," with or without feedback (blood glucose or other variables)
Site of administration: intravenous, intramuscular, subcutaneous, intraperitoneal, or other
Patient profile: Who should receive this therapy and who should be excluded?
Means for monitoring effectiveness of therapy and establishing duration limits

Both implanted and external pumps are gaining acceptance for treating selected groups comprised of elderly, unstable insulin-resistant patients, and incapacitated individuals in whom other means of self-therapy are difficult, more expensive, or impossible.

Continuous infusion of insulin without patient involvement is attractive for children, adolescents, and young adults [15]. However, the use of percutaneous exit catheters results in a 25% infection rate. Insulin infusion via a totally implanted port with an external pump has the advantages of minimal care and attention and it does not interfere with the patient's physical activities, including swimming and other sports.

The relative merits of various routes of insulin delivery (with and without glucose feedback) were explored by Irsigler and Kritz [16]

using two types of mechanized pump. Insulin was infused via intravenous, intraperitoneal, and subcutaneous routes. The authors preferred the intraperitoneal route.

Pain Control

Severe pain, secondary to terminal cancer, occurs in the majority of
patients. In view of the current palliative nature of most cancer treatment modalities, the humane therapeutic approach in this condition
is to provide maximal patient comfort via effective pain control. Patients who cease to respond to conventional pain control measures beginning with oral opiates and parenteral administration usually respond
to direct intraspinal administration using lower concentrations via ports
and catheters. Cousins and Mather reviewed this subject extensively,
supporting this modality of pain control [17]. The use of the totally
implanted port provides an added measure of safety by isolating the
spinal region to the outside environment during the therapy.

Postsurgical Pain Control

Frequently, the limiting factor in the postoperative patient's ability
to return to useful pursuits is the lingering or residual pain associated
with the surgery. Patients equipped with portable opiate infusion
systems are able to resume most activities one to several days earlier
than with conventional treatment. In some cases, the infusion devices
and catheters are installed prior to the surgery, providing for conti-
nuity in the analgesia during and following the surgical procedures.

Use of patient-controlled analgesia (PCA) postsurgically via these
portable-catheter-accessed systems is gaining in popularity. PCA is
based on the premise that the patients themselves are the best judges
of the severity of their pain and the quantitative treatment required
to obtain adequate relief [29]. Accidental or deliberate overdosing
is prevented by certain design features incorporated by the device
manufacturers.

Prolonged Therapy in Children

Pegelow [18] described the Infuse-A-Port implanted in 15 children
with cancer. Their cumulative experience of 4094 days, with catheters
in place from 28 to 251 days, showed a high degree of acceptance by
the patients, their parents, and physicians. The major benefits of
this approach were:

Freedom from daily changes of dressings conventionally used with
    percutaneous exit catheters
Unrestricted bathing of the children
Low complication rate

Intravenous Cancer Chemotherapy

Results form the use of 826 vascular access devices (from several manufacturers) were reported by Raaf [30] in the treatment of 681 patients with neoplastic diseases over a period of 7 years. This represents, perhaps, the most comprehensive and longest study in this field. While only 12 ports with an indwelling time of 2 ot 6 months were included in this study, none of these had any complications.

Bland and Woodcock [31] described the use of the Infuse-A-Port in cyclic or continuous chemotherapy as well as blood withdrawal. The authors suggested that the totally implanted port presented certain advantages over the percutaneous access catheters in lower complications and infection.

D. Intra-Arterial Access

The intra-arterial drug infusion route is used primarily in the treatment of selected localized malignant disease. This is based on the premise that in certain body compartments the concentration of drug in the target compartment will exceed, by a significant ratio, the concentration of drug going into systemic circulation. This provides a local "tumor kill" advantage.

Hepatic artery infusion was reviewed by Sterchi [19]. High-pressure external pumps are required for this therapy. The totally implanted Infusaid pump is preferred for hepatic artery infusional chemotherapy. Various infusion techniques and devices for arterial access were described by Lokich and Ensminger [20].

E. Intraperitoneal Access

Cytotoxic agents administered intravascularly do not penetrate into the peritoneal cavity at sufficiently high concentrations to destroy microscopic residual tumor fragments. With the development of adequate catheters and infusion technology, it is now possible to administer intraperitoneal chemotherapy on an outpatient basis to individuals with abdominal, gynecological, and other tumors located in the peritoneal cavity. In prolonged treatment, use of temporary or more permanent catheter systems is advisable. The Infuse-A-Port has been used advantageously by Markman [21] for high-volume (1.5-2 liters) fluid infusions

Nursing management guidelines for peritoneal cavity access via ports and catheters may be found in the report by Swenson and Ericksson [22]. In this application the Infuse-A-Port carries the following considerable advantages over conventional catheters.

The port is totally implantable, eliminating the common danger of infection at the skin penetration site with conventional catheters.

The port reduces requirements for dressing changes and maintenance.
Compared with other alternatives, the port is aesthetically pleasing
to the patient and family, since it is only palpable, not visible,
when not in use (i.e., the majority of the time).

F. Fluid Removal

Infusion technology via special access devices is generally envisioned
as a means for discharging into the body various drugs, fluids, nutrients, and so on. The removal of fluids from bodily cavities or the
vascular system also is possible as well as practical. The important
reported applications in this category include the following.

    Ascites
    Pleural fluid
    Hydrocephalus
    Spinal fluid
    Blood sampling

The accumulation of malignant or nonmalignant fluids in the pleural
space is frequently a consequence of the progressive neoplastic disease
as well as its treatment. Common management of this condition involves
periodic drainage via syringe aspiration or a thoracostomy tube placed
in the pleural space. Pleural fluid accumulation is continuous; hence,
this treatment must be repeated as required. This may be accomplished
advantageously via an implanted port.
    Markman [23] reported on the use of indwelling catheters inserted
into the pleural space for administration of chemotherapy. These catheters were also used for the temporary drainage of the chest cavity.
Fuhrman [24] developed a special catheter for the chronic drainage of
pleural fluids and for pericardial effusions. Leff [25] used an implanted port for this purpose.
    Approximately 1 million Americans per year develop pleural effu-
sions due to malignant disease, congestive heart failure, pneumonia,
and other causes. The management of fluid accumulation, a common
problem, is substantially safer and easier with the new access devices
[25].

G. Blood Sampling

With an Infuse-A-Port already in place for drug infusion or fluid removal, blood may also be drawn for analytical purposes without additional discomfort to the patient. Blood samples drawn in this manner
are relatively free of hemolysis, since no needle punctures are involved.
A small loss of blood occurs in cleaning the "heparin-lock" and dis-
carding the residual blood in the catheter lumen.

V. COMPLICATIONS

Fewer, and less severe complications are associated with totally implanted ports than with percutaneous exit catheters. This is a major
factor in favor of the use of implanted ports for therapy expected to
last for a week or longer, to be repeated for several cycles in the
course of treatment, or to be kept in place for emergency use for relatively long periods (weeks to months). In comparison, percutaneous
exit catheters have a less favorable record as shown in the following
reports.

Schwartz-Fulton and Tischenko [26] described 24 oncology patients
with a total experience of 3872 catheter days; 83% of these patients
were intolerant to the frequent disinfection procedures employed in
central catheter line care. Skin irritation, itching, sensitivity to touch
or blistering due to iodophor ointment and Elastoplast dressing were
noted within 30 days of catheter insertion. In a "collective review",
Bozzetti [27] reported that despite vigorous disinfection procedures,
contamination from the skin was the primary route for the initiation of
infections in percutaneous exit catheters. With the use of totally implantable catheters these serious complications were eliminated. Brickner and Saeter [28] reported that in 78 patients with implantable ports
with a median indwelling duration of 16 months, the complication rate
was only 1 in 990 days of use. The authors noted that the implanted
ports functioned adequately fof 4.4 to 12 times longer than conventional catheters. Gyves et al. [29] used the Infuse-A-Port for chemotherapy infusion in cancer patients who lacked adequate peripheral
venous access sites due to excessive previous drug treatments. The
median period of new therapy for the port was 63 days with a range
of 5 to 203 days.

VI. SUMMARY

Totally implantable vascular access devices have added considerably
to the treatment and management of patients requiring protracted or
frequent drug therapy. This technology has the following advantages.

It is safer than percutaneous catheterization and has significantly
    lower infection rates [26,27].
It permits considerably longer indwelling catheter time.
It requires less frequent skilled nursing attention.
It is much more convenient for the patient because it permits un-
    restricted patient mobility.
It enables the patient to bathe and swim without use of protective
    measures.

It is suitable for treatment by the parents of active young children and infants.
It is easier to care for in a home setting.
It is readily available for a multiplicity of applications: drug infusion, hyperalimentation, blood sampling, fluid withdrawal, and transfusions.

VII. COMMERCIALLY AVAILABLE IMPLANTABLE VASCULAR ACCESS DEVICES

Implantable vascular access devices are available from various sources, as indicated in the following (partial) list.

Alfred Cook Inc.: a subcutaneous implanted vascular access device
Cormed, Inc. (Mediport): a metal/plastic totally implantable vascular access port
Norfolk Medical Products, Inc.: a stainless steel vascular access port
Pharmacia, Inc. (Port-A-Cath): a metallic vascular access device
Strato Medical Corporation: a metallic totally implantable port
American Hospital Supply Company (Ommaya Capsule Catheter): an all-plastic, totally implantable access device
HDC Corporation (Chemo-Port): a metal/plastic totally implantable vascular access device
Similar devices from several European companies

REFERENCES

1. A. K. Ommaya, Implantable devices for chronic access and drug delivery to the central nervous system, *Cancer Drug Delivery*, 1(2):169-179 (1984).
2. J. Bjeletich and R. D. Hickman, The Hickman indwelling catheter, *Am. J. Nurs.*, 80:62-65 (1980).
3. J. W. Broviac, A Silicone rubber atrial catheter for prolonged parenteral alimentation, *Surg. Gynecol. Obstet.*, 136:602-606 (1973).
4. N. J. Vogelzang, Continuous infusion chemotherapy: A critical review, *J. Clin. Oncol.*, 2(11):1289-1304 (1984).
5. D. S. Roffman, M. M. Applefeld, W. R. Grove, B. S. Talesnick, F. J. Sutton, K. A. Newman, and W. P. Reed, Intermittent dobutamine hydrochloride infusions in outpatients with chronic congestive heart failure, *Clin. Pharm.*, 4:195-199 (1985).
6. A. R. Hoffman and W. F. Crowley, Induction of puberty in men by long-term pulsatile administration of low-dose gonadotropin-

releasing hormone, *New Engl. J. Med.*, 307:1237-1241 (1982).

7. H. M. Fraser, GnRH and its analogues, *Drugs*, 27:187-193 (1984).
8. G. Van Vliet, D. M. Styne, S. L. Kaplan, and M. M. Grumbach, Growth hormone treatment for short stature, *New Engl. J. Med.*, 309:1016-1022 (1983).
9. W. E. Ensminger and J. W. Gyves, Regional chemotherapy of neoplastic diseases, *Pharm. Ther.*, 21:277-293 (1983).
10. R. S. Leff, B. Eisenberg, C. E. Baisden, K. R. Mosley, and G. L. Messerschmidt, Drainage of recurrent pleural effusions via an implanted port and interpleural catheter, *Ann. Intern. Med.*, 104(2):208-209 (1986).
11. J. M. Collins, Pharmacologic rationale for regional drug delivery, *J. Clin. Oncol.*, 2(5):498-504 (1984).
12. J. H. Muchmore, R. D. Carter, and E. T. Krementz, Regional perfusion for malignant melanoma and soft tissue sarcoma: A review, *Cancer Invest.*, 3(2):129-143 (1985).
13. N. Lee Yeu-tsu, Regional management of liver metastases, Parts I and II, *Cancer Invest.*, 1(3):237-257 (1983), 1(4):321-332 (1983).
14. H. G. Stiver, G. O. Telford, J. M. Mossey, D. D. Cote, E. J. Van Middlesworth, S. K. Trosky, N. L. McKay, and W. L. Mossey, Intravenous antibiotic therapy at home, *Ann. Intern. Med.*, 89:690-693 (1978).
15. S. J. Brink and C. Stewart, Insulin pump treatment in insulin-dependent diabetes mellitus, *JAMA*, 255(5):617-621 (1986).
16. K. Irsigler and H. Kritz, Alternate routes of insulin delivery, *Diabetes Care*, 3(2):219-228 (1980).
17. M. J. Cousins and L. E. Mather, Intrathecal and epidural administration of opioids, *Anesthesiology*, 61:276-310 (1984).
18. C. H. Pegelow, M. Narvaez, S. R. Toledano, J. Davis, C. Oiticica, and D. Buckner, Experience with a totally implantable venous device in children, *Am. J. Dis. Child.*, 140:69-71 (1986).
19. J. M. Sterchi, Hepatic artery infusion for metastatic neoplastic disease, *Surg. Gynecol. Obstet.*, 160:477-489 (1985).
20. J. Lokich and W. Ensminger, Ambulatory pump infusion devices for hepatic artery infusion, *Semin. Oncol.*, 10(2):183-190 (1983).
21. M. Markman, Review: Cytotoxic intracavitary chemotherapy, *Am. J. Med. Sci.*, 291:175-179 (1986).
22. K. K. Swenson and J. H. Eriksson, Nursing management of intraperitoneal chemotherapy, *Oncol. Nurs. Forum*, 13(5):33-39 (1986).
23. M. Markman, S. B. Howell, and M. R. Green, Combination intracavitary chemotherapy for malignant pleural disease, *Cancer Drug Delivery*, 1(4):333-336 (1983).
24. B. P. Fuhrman, B. G. Landrum, T. B. Ferrara, D. M. Steinhorn, A. P. Connell, D. L. Smith-Wright, and T. P. Green, Pleural drainage using modified pigtail catheters, *Crit. Care Med.*, 14(6):575-576 (1986).

25. R. S. Leff, B. Eisenberg, C. E. Baisden, K. R. Mosley, and G. L. Messerschmidt, Drainage of recurrent pleural effusion via an implanted port and intrapleural catheter, *Ann. Intern. Med.*, 104(2):208-209 (1986).

26. J. Schwartz-Fulton and M. M. Tischenko, Hickman catheter exit site skin sensitivities in an oncology patient population, *J. National Intravenous Ther. Assoc.*, 8:63-68 (1985).

27. F. Bozzetti, Central venous catheter sepsis, *Surg. Gynecol. Obstet.*, 161:298-301 (1985).

28. H. Brickner and G. Saeter, Fifty-five patient years' experience with a totally implanted system for intravenous chemotherapy, *JAMA*, 251(19):2538-2541 (1984).

29. J. W. Gyves, W. D. Ensminger, J. E. Niederhuber, J. Dent, S. Walker, S. Gilbertson, E. Cozzi, and P. Saran, A totally implanted injection port system for blood sampling and chemotherapy applications, *JAMA*, 251:2538-2541 (1984).

30. J. H. Raaf, Results from use of 826 vascular access devices in cancer patients, *Cancer*, 55:1312-1321 (1985).

31. K. I. Bland and T. Woodcock, Totally implantable venous access device system for cyclic administration of cytotoxic chemotherapy, *Am. J. Surg.*, 147:815-816 (1984).

32. R. E. S. Bullingham, O. L. R. Jacobs, H. J. McQuay, and R. A. Moore, The Oxford system of patient controlled analgesia, In *Advances in Pain and Research and Therapy*, Vol. 8 (K. M. Foley and C. E. Inturrisi, eds.). Raven Press, New York, 1986, pp. 319-324.

10

Delivery of Contraceptive Drug by Subdermal Implants

BRIJ B. SAXENA and MUKUL SINGH / Cornell University Medical
College, New York, New York

I. INTRODUCTION

The population explosion, particularly in some parts of the world, continues to be a problem in spite of the availability of a variety of contraceptive methods. There is, therefore, a need for the development of
simpler and newer delivery systems of contraceptive drugs that have
greater safety, availability, and acceptability in terms of a variety of
religious, socioeconomic, and cultural backgrounds. Currently oral
contraceptives and intrauterine devices are most popular and each are
used by 60 million to 100 million women. Devices to enhance their convenience and acceptability have included intramuscular depot injections
and subdermal steroid-polymeric implants, as well as intravaginal,
intracervical, and intrauterine delivery systems. Capsules releasing
ST-1435 and progresterone implants are currently under clinical trials
as contraceptives during postpartum and nursing periods. Similarly,
the injectable and implantable long-acting delivery systems are under
clinical trials and have the potential for improved contraception. Long-
acting contraceptive vaccines are the targets of the future [1-3].
    Among the subdermal implants for the delivery of contraceptive
agents for long-term use, the most promising ones are Norplant, bioabsorbable Capronor, and fused pellets [2,3]. Steroids have so far
been the most effective contraceptive agents for the control of fertility.
Administration of 19-norprogesterone derivatives prevents ovulation
and corpus luteum function, and these substances have been used to
induce reversible protracted infertility in mammals and in humans [4].
Steroids administered by the oral route first dissolve in the gastrointestinal fluid, then are transferred into the mesenteric blood system
via the gastrointestinal mucosa. The drug then passes through the
liver. The first pass through the gastrointestinal mucosa and liver
enzyme metabolizes almost 80% of the orally ingested steroids before
the drug reaches the target site. It is, therefore, necessary to ingest
higher doses of the drug to achieve effective contraceptive levels.
Intake of steroid hormones for contraception by the oral route has
resulted in a variety of side effects such as migraine headaches, vomiting, fatigue, nausea, hypertension, and higher risk of cardiovascular
disease. These adverse effects have been dose related. The paradox
is that higher doses of steroids, required for greater contraceptive
efficacy, are accompanied by higher risks of adverse side effects,
whereas lower doses minimize side effects but the risk of pregnancy is
greater. The present chapter deals with the current status of subdermal implants as delivery systems for sex steroids for contraception.
    In 1936 M. J. Shear [5] first used implants of fused cholesterol
and a carcinogen to produce tumors in animals. Much later, Bishop
[6] described the use of a pellet of estrone in an ovariectomized woman.
Gambrell [7] in 1976 described how Salmon had treated menopausal
women as early as 1939 with estradiol benzoate implants. Greenblatt

studied the effect of androgen implants in women with functional menstrual disorders [8]. The implants used in the early experiments were made according to Shear [5] and Shimkin and White [9]. Subsequently, subcutaneous implants have been used for the administration of steroid sex hormones [10,11].

Subdermal implants of various types, namely pellets, rods, and fibers of biodegradable and nonbiodegradable polymers containing steroid hormones, are currently being developed. Subdermal implants have provided the alternative that serves to avoid the first gastrointestinal and liver bypass and to deliver sustained release of steroids in relatively smaller and safer quantities. The contraceptive effectiveness of subdermal implants is due to the cumulative effect of the drug at the target site, which equals the concentration of the steroid produced by daily oral pills containing substantially higher quantities of the drug. A subdermal delivery system, however, can provide constant, but low and efficacious, blood levels of contraceptive steroids for a desired length of time with little likelihood of either drug insufficiency or accumulation due to lack of congruence between drug availability and drug depletion. Such a system would be easily administered, would eliminate patient intervention, and would be effective for extended periods. Subdermal delivery systems provide the mechanism by which controlled release of a contraceptive drug can be achieved.

An approach to steroidal contraception by the use of subdermal implants makes use of biologically compatible polymers in the creation of systems for delivering contraceptive agents at an optimum rate and concentraiton. Segal and Croxatto [12] first suggested utilizing a subcutaneous, nonbiodegradable, polymeric Silastic capsule (Norplant) for prolonged and constant delivery of contraceptive steroids. A subcutaneous implant, Capronor, composed of a new bioerodible polymeric poly-ε-caprolactone (PCL), which disappears from the site of implantation by the time drug depletion is complete, has also been developed [13]. The direct use of the fused pellets of norethindrone without a polymeric capsule has also shown a potential subdermal delivery system for the release of the drug at a constant and sustained concentration [14,15].

II. MECHANISM OF RELEASE OF CONTRACEPTIVE STEROIDS FROM SUBDERMAL IMPLANTS

The ideal system for drug release should approach zero-order kinetics. The device should be biocompatible, nontoxic, nonmutagenic, nonteratogenic, nonimmunogenic, and noncarcinogenic. In general, subdermal implants should possess a high drug-to-polymer ratio, have good mechanical strength, be free of drug leakage, be easy and inexpensive to manufacture, be easily sterilizable, and be stable and safe. Table 1

TABLE 1 Mechanisms of Contraceptive Steroid Release from
Subdermal Implants

Mechanism	Devices
Diffusion	
Reservoir	Membrane, capsules, liposomes and hollow fibers, fused implants
Matrix	Slabs, cylinders
Chemical	
Biodegradable	Slabs, spheres, cylinders
Polymer bound	Spheres, cylinders
Solution	
Swelling	Spheres, rods, fused implants
Osmosis	Spheres, rods, fused implants
Magnetic	
Diffusion	Beads

and Figure 1 summarize various mechanisms that control the release of
drugs from various types of subdermal implants containing the contraceptive drug. The rate of release of steroids from the implants into
the peripheral circulation is dependent on the total surface area of
the implant, the polymer, and the pore size, which in turn is dependent
on concentration gradient and physical hindrances, such as the formation of a tissue barrier in response to foreign body. The rate of drug
release can be regulated by the shape and size of the implants, as
well as the use of materials to reduce fibrosis to achieve the desired
levels. The mechanism of drug release from the implants can be classified as described below.

A. Diffusion

Reservoir

In the reservoir system (Fig. 1a) a core of drug is surrounded by a
polymer and diffusion of the drug through the polymer is the rate-
limiting step. Reservoir systems can be engineered easily to produce
zero-order release kinetics. However, these systems are generally
nonbiodegradable; therefore subcutaneous implants must be surgically
removed. They are expensive and can leak to provide large amounts
of drug, which could be toxic. The release rates form the membranes
are determined by the steady state Fick's diffusion equation:

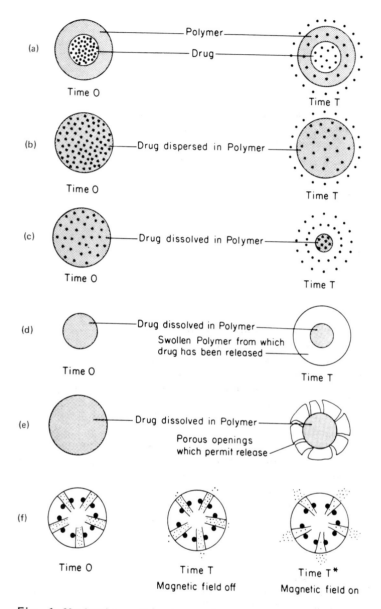

Fig. 1 Mechanisms of contraceptive drug release from subdermal implants of nonbiodegradable and biodegradable polymers as well as from implants of steroids (norethindrone) fused with cholesterol: (a) Diffusion—reservoir; (b) diffusion—matrix (nonbiodegradable polymers or fused drug implants); (c) chemical; (d) solution, solvent-activated systems (biodegradable polymers); (e) osmotically controlled systems (biodegradable polymers); and (f) magnetic systems. (Adapted from: G. I. Zatuchni, A. Goldsmith, J. D. Shelton, and J. J. Sciarra, eds., *Long-Acting Contraceptive Delivery System*, Harper & Row, New York, 1984.)

$$J_i = D_{im} \frac{dc_i}{dx}$$

where J_i is the drug molar flux and D_{im} is the concentration-independent drug diffusion coefficient in the membrane and dc_i/dx is the drug concentration gradient within the membrane [16]. This equation can be rewritten for a zero-order release as follows:

$$J_i = D_m \frac{c_i}{\delta}$$

where Δ is the membrane thickness. Δc_i is kept constant by maintaining a high drug concentration at the internal wall of the membrane. Such systems, for example, Norplant, are nonbiodegradable and have to be removed surgically [17].

Matrix

Matrix systems (Fig. 1b) do not generally yield zero-order release rate, which can be achieved by compensating for the increase diffusional distance with an increasing area of the drug. For example, a cylinder sector that releases drug only from the inside surface can be used in conjunction with a hemisphere that is laminated with an impermeable coating in all places except a small cavity in the center face. Applications include cases of a drug that is distributed uniformly in the matrix or chemically bound to a polymer (soluble or insoluble) backbone chain. The release rate is governed by Fick's law as described above. Hopfenberg and Hsu [16] found that if the kinetics of the biodegradation of the polymer is known, a zero-order release can be maintained by a geometery where the surface area did not change as a function of time (e.g., a slab). The most commonly used biodegradable polymer is polylactic acid or lactic-glycolic copolymers.

B. Chemical

Chemical systems (Fig. 1c) are the same as the diffusion type except that the drug is distributed throughout the polymer and the bioerodible polymer also decreases with time to allow the drug to escape. One has to be careful that the degradation products of the polymer are not toxic. A zero-order release can be obtained by using a geometry in which the surface area does not change as a function of time. Heller [18] has considered three dissolution mechanisms: (a) water-soluble polymers insolubilized by degradable cross links, (b) water-insoluble polymers solubilized by hydrolysis, ionization, or protonation of the side groups, and (c) water-insoluble polymers solubilized by backbone chain cleavage to small water-soluble molecules.

C. Solution (Solvent-Activated Systems)

In case of a swelling-controlled polymeric system (Fig. 1d) the rate of release is equal to the product of the surface area and a rate constant corresponding to rate of advance of the boundary separating the outer shell (swollen and containing no drug) from the central core (unswollen and containing drug). If the absorption rate of the environmental fluid is constant, the release rate should also be constant. The advantages are that the matrix design using simple shapes could be used to provide constant release rates and the rate-limiting step is confined to ingression of an external agent and is not dependent on the diffusive or physicochemical properties of the incorporated drug. In osmotically controlled systems in the form of matrix (Fig. 1e), where the core is surrounded by a semipermeable film, it is difficult to achieve zero-order release. However, if the system is designed in the form of a pump with a laser-drilled hole at the outlet, zero-order release is readily achievable.

D. Magnetic

In magnetically controlled systems (Fig. 1f) the drug and small magnetic beads are uniformly dispersed within a polymer matrix. On exposure to aqueous media, the drug is released in a diffusion-controlled fashion, and the rate can be increased on exposure to a oscillating external magnetic field. These systems may be useful when drug delivery is designed to correspond to the changes in steroid secretion during the menstrual cycle.

III. CONTRACEPTIVE STATUS OF SUBDERMAL STEROID IMPLANTS

A. Nonbiodegradable Subdermal Implant: Norplant

The Norplant devices are Silatic implants containing levonorgestrel (LNG). The capsules are placed beneath the skin of the forearm and must be removed surgically. Initially a 2 year study resulted in only 0.4% pregnancy rate, and a subsequent 5 year study indicated 0% pregnancy rate [17]. Norplant users have experienced frequent irregular bleeding, prolonged bleeding, and prolonged amenorrhea both during treatment and following removal of the Norplant; however, hemoglobin levels were not affected. Other complaints included visibility of the implant, headaches, nervousness, depression, general discomfort, acne, and infection at the site of implant, though rarely. The acceptability rate has been reported to be as high as 96%.

B. Nonbiodegradable Implantable Rods

There has been a need to develop a low-dose, progestin-only, long-acting implant system with as few implants as possible. Hence the development of subdermal implants continued with the aim of increasing the total load of drug per unit length of implant while maintaining the dose delivery by multiple implants. Toward this goal two systems were developed, namely the homogeneous rod system and the covered rod system. The homogeneous rods, 2.44 mm in diameter and 3 cm long, contain 25% of LNG dispersed in Silastic. The covered rods contain a core of LNG sealed inside thin-walled Silastic tubing. The core rods are 2.44 mm in diameter and 3 to 4 cm long. The release rates range from 136 μg/day in the first 100 days to 30 μg/day from 801 to 1316 days.

C. Biodegradable Capronor

In 1973 the concept of subdermal drug delivery using permeable polymers to control release rates was well documented [19-21]. Since the nonbiodegradable polymer implants were visible and required surgical removal, a search for a biodegradable polymer was initiated; it was desired to develop reservoir devices (capsules) to provide sustained and constant drug release by a diffusion mechanism, with the polymer eroding only after the drug had been exhausted. The erosion could be controlled by choosing the polymers of an appropriate molecular weight and the drug release rate could be controlled by the dimensions of the capsule. The material selected for manufacturing biodegradable subdermal implants (Capronor) was poly-ε-caprolactone, because of its availability, permeability, biodegradability, and biocompatibility. The polymer is conveniently sterilized by γ-irradiation. The biodegradation of PCL is due to continuous decrease in the molecular weight due to the cleavage of the ester linkages. Bioabsorption of the polymer occurred by intracellular degradation in phagosomes of macrophages, giant cells, and fibroblasts. Capronor revealed no toxic effects when implanted subdermally. The capsules evoked a bland response at the implant site and a minimal inflammatory or tissue-encapsulating response. Clinical evaluation indicated side effects normally associated with minidoses of a progesterone, for example, mood swings, breast tenderness, and increased appetite. Anovulation occurred at a plasma level exceeding 300 pg of LNG per milliliter.

D. Biodegradable Norethindrone and Cholesterol-Fused Implants

The fused pellets contain norethindrone (NET: 17α-ethynyl-19-nortestosterone) in lipoid carrier (cholesterol) in a ratio of 85:15 (w/w) dispersed uniformly in a matrix. The NET was purified by recrystalli-

zation. Pellets were prepared by a fusion method [13]. Each NET
pellet is ellipsoidal, with dimensions of 5.5 mm × 3 mm × 2.6 mm, yield-
ing a surface area of 58.0 mm^2, and weighs 34.4 ±0.6 mg. NET pellets
were packaged in Teflon tubes and stored individually in sterile glass
vials with a screw cap (Fig. 2). The pellets remained intact and did
not increase in weight after boiling in water, suggesting little absorption of moisture. The NET pellets dissolved completely in chloroform
without leaving any insoluble residue. These observations attest that
fused pellets were made of only pure crystalline mass of NET and cholesterol. Average tensile strength calculated from six pellets by a
formula developed by Fell and Newton [22] was 0.0883 ±0.0069.

Gas chromatography and mass spectrometry demonstrated little
noticeable hydrolysis, oxidation, decomposition, or polymerization of
NET or cholesterol after fusion. A physical mixture of NET and cholesterol and the pellets after fusion showed no loss in weight when
heated up to 210°C, suggesting absence of any volatile materials in the
pellets. When a physical mixture of NET and cholesterol in the ratio
of 85:15 (w/w) and fused pellets was analyzed by X-ray diffraction,
the patterns obtained were similar and, to a great extent, representative of NET, indicating that after fusion the crystal structure of NET
remained unchanged [14].

The differential scanning calorimetric thermograms (DSCTs) obtained for the samples of cholesterol and NET yielded sharp endotherms,

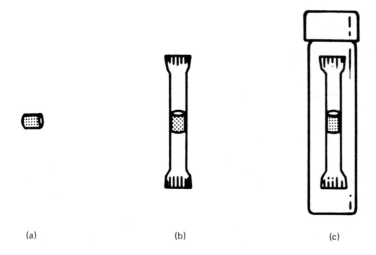

(a)   (b)   (c)

Fig. 2 (a) NET-cholesterol implant, (b) Sterile NET-cholesterol fused
implant sealed in Teflon tube, (c) Teflon tube containing NET-cholesterol implant in a sterile screw-top glass jar for transport and long-
term storage.

which confirm the purity of the pellet components. The melting points obtained from the thermograms were 422 and 482 K, respectively. Thermograms of the physical mixture and fused pellets showed typical patterns for binary mixtures exhibiting eutectic formation. In this case, cholesterol and NET melted at 415 K to form a eutectic mixture. The endotherm at the eutectic temperature was followed by another, much broader endotherm. The second endotherm was at 466 K in the 85:15 mixture of NET and cholesterol. There was no evidence of polymorphism. A small droplet of water was placed on the flat surface of a fused pellet and monitored under a light microscope more than 4 hr. The water droplet did not spread at all and evaporated gradually from the surface at the end of the fourth hour. This test indicated that the fused pellets had a nonwetting surface. Characterization of fused NET-cholesterol pellets by gas chromatography, gas chromatography-mass spectrometry, DSCT, and X-ray diffraction provided substantial evidence that both compounds remained in their native form and showed little signs of oxidation, polymerization, or decomposition after fusion.

The NET-cholesterol pellets have the advantages of small size, bioabsorbability, retrievability, high degree of acceptability, and ease of preparation, sterilization, packaging, and storage, as well as stability and low cost. Since the drug release from a pellet is directly proportional to its surface area, the release of NET could be precisely regulated for a given period by controlling its surface area. The fused pellets release a sustained and constant level, at near zero order, of [3H]NET and [3H]LNG in rats, rabbits, and monkeys over an extended period. In human, the NET pellets also provide a sustained release of NET that is more constant and higher per unit surface area than that provided by Silastic capsules, Silastic rods, or polylactic polymeric preparations. Among subdermal delivery systems, NET fused pellets showed promise of a simpler alternative for long-term and safe contraception at a lower dose of medicaiton.

Both NET and d-norgestrel (d-NG: 17α-ethynyl-18-homo-19-nortestosterone) are used as contraceptives in oral pills in humans. Initially NET-cholesterol fused implants containing progestin and cholesterol in a ratio of 85:15 (w/w), 7 mm × 3.1 mm × 2.4 mm in size, and 40 mg in weight were used to determine long-term daily release rates of [3H]NET and [3H]-d-NG in monkeys based on excretory activities in urine and feces [23]. In case of [3H]NET, each of the two monkeys received two implants having length and weight of 11 mm and 63 mg and 9.3 mm and 55.7 mg, respectively. Average release rate was initially 250 μg/day for a 3 month period. For the [3H]d-NG study each of the two monkeys received a single pellet, one having length and weight of 5.7 mm and 33.6 mg and the other with dimensions of 5.1 mm and 30.3 mg. The [3H]d-NG showed an initial burst effect of 600 to 500 μg/day for 5 to 60 days. The release rate declined to a steady level of 125 μg/day within 20 days and continued at a sustained rate at a level of 30 µg/day for a 3 month period. Plasma levels also remained fairly constant.

In another study the NET-cholesterol fused implants were placed subdermally in four cycling bonnet monkeys (*Macaca radiata*) [24]. No skin reaction or inflammation was observed at the site of implantation. In the first month, samples were analyzed weekly for plasma concentrations of NET by radioimmunoassay, and subsequently at monthly intervals for 14 to 16 months. NET was released into circulation within 24 hr after insertion of the implant. In all the monkeys except one, a sharp rise in NET (1.9-20 ng/ml) occurred immediately after insertion. Levels then remained between 1.7 and 0.6 ng/ml for about 4 months. Thereafter, the NET levels remained steady up to about 9 months in two monkeys and gradually declined to approximately 0.4 ng/ml in the remaining two. In all the monkeys except one, there was a sudden burst of NET release between the tenth and eleventh months. By months 14 to 16, the hormone was almost cleared out of circulation. Initial menstrual cycles after pellet insertion were accompanied by spotting and irregular bleeding. Five to eight months after the insertion of the implant, menstrual cycles returned to normal and became ovulatory, as indicated by the progesterone levels. These studies suggested that one or two pellets may provide more sustained and effective progestin levels than Silastic capsules, biodegradable devices, and the injectable depot method used for the human contraception.

A phase I clinical study in women [25] with one subdermal NET or LNG pellet fused with cholesterol in a ratio of 85:15 (w/w) and weighing 30 mg revealed that the NET levels reached a maximum concentration within 48 hr, gradually declined within 2 weeks, and thereafter ranged between 200 to 700 ng/ml up to 90 days postinsertion. Cycle lengths during NET implant were of 25 to 37 days' duration except one cycle of 55 days. All cycles during treatment were ovulatory, and no consistent effect was observed either on cervical mucus of postcoital test (PCT). Similarly, with one LNG pellet the maximum levels were reached within 24 hr and declined in a week's time; thereafter the serum LNG levels ranged between 100 and 400 pg/ml up to 8 months. Cycle length varied between 21 and 42 days. The pellet did not show a consistent effect on ovulation inhibition, cervical mucus, or PCT. Thus a single NET of LNG pellet did not seem to have a reliable contraceptive potential. The pellets were otherwise well tolerated, and the women did not experience any headache or nausea. There was little reaction at the implant site, and no lymphadenopathy. Histopathology of the tissue around the pellet revealed a normal foreign body reaction with mononuclear infiltration and an absence of any neoplastic changes. There were no changes in the blood pressure and metabolic parameters, such as glucose tolerance test, liver function test, plasma proteins, and lipid components in any of the women.

In another phase I clinical study, 50 female volunteers at five centers were studied for 6 to 12 months with two subdermal NET-cholesterol implants [14,26,27]. Two blood samples of 10 ml each were drawn every week for two consecutive control cycles prior to the implantation of the pellets to determine pituitary and gonadal hormonal levels in the serum. Between days 1 and 7 of the third cycle, two NET-cholesterol implants were implanted subcutaneously in the ventral forearm by the aid of a trocar (Fig. 3). The pellets were left in place for 6 months. During the postimplantation period, blood samples were drawn at weekly intervals for the determination of NET, follicle stimulating hormone (FSH), luteinizing hormone (LH), estradiol (E_2), and progesterone (P) levels by radioimmunoassays.

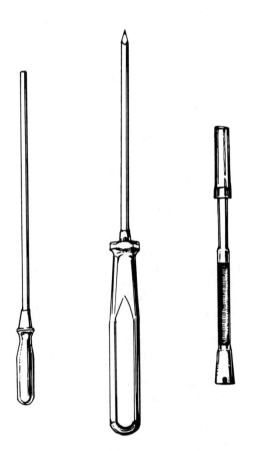

Fig. 3 Diagram of trocar: (left) cannula, (middle) stylet, and (right) plunger.

The mean daily NET releases per pellet surface areas of 58 and 100 mm^2 were 36.9 ±2.6 and 63.6 ±4.5 µg, respectively. The mean (± SEM) NET level at the five centers was 0.74 ±0.12 ng/ml during the first 2 months after the pellet implantation and remained relatively sustained at levels of 0.54 ±0.12 ng/ml up to 330 days of the study (Fig. 4). No burst effect was observed following implantation of pellets. The NET serum levels rapidly decreased and disappeared after pellet removal.

Urinary pregnanediol and LH were measured daily during the fifth cycle following pellet implantation. The results showed that in 50% of cases, a sporadic pregnanediol secretion was delayed from the initial LH peak and in 10% of the cases a normal ovulatory pattern was observed with s subsequent short luteal phase. From these results, even in the case of ovulatory cycles, luteal phase insufficiency was a common feature that may be attributed to the presence of circulating NET levels. The incidence of ovulation was decreased to 20% to 50% of controls in the first three cycles and gradually returned to a normal pattern thereafter. After removal of the pellets, the ovulatory rate was restored completely. Generally, the subjects experienced a marked increase in bleeding days during first cycles following pellet implantation but returned to a normal, pretreatment pattern 3 months post-implantation. There was no major adverse local reaction at the site of the implants following either implantation or removal of the NET-cholesterol implants. No serious systemic side effects were observed at any of the centers (Table 2). Concentrations of lipoproteins–namely the high density (HDL), low density (LDL), and very low density (VLDL) types–and cholesterol in the blood did not alter during the entire preimplant and postimplant periods in the volunteers. The blood levels of LDH and of the enzymes serum glutomic-oxaloacetic transaminase (SGOT) and serum glutamid-pyruvic transaminase (SGPT) were not significantly affected by the pellets during the postimplant period. The presence of the NET-cholesterol fused implants was associated with a disappearance or amelioration of the severity of menstrual cramps [12,26,27].

The continuous subdermal mean (± SEM) dose of 110.6 ±20 µg of NET per day, about one-third of oral minipill dose, from the two pellets provided ovulatory patterns and bleeding days similar to those of 300 µg of NET per day of the minipills. This finding confirmed the earlier observation of Chang and Kincl [28] that the biological potency of progestins through the subdermal route was severalfold higher than by the oral route. This study provides evidence that the ovarian effect of 300 µg of NET in oral dose is equivalent to that produced by the much lower dose of 110.6 ± 20 µg of NET/day administered subdermally from the two NET-cholesterol fused implants. Furthermore, the suppression of ovulation appeared to be a dose-dependent phenomenon.

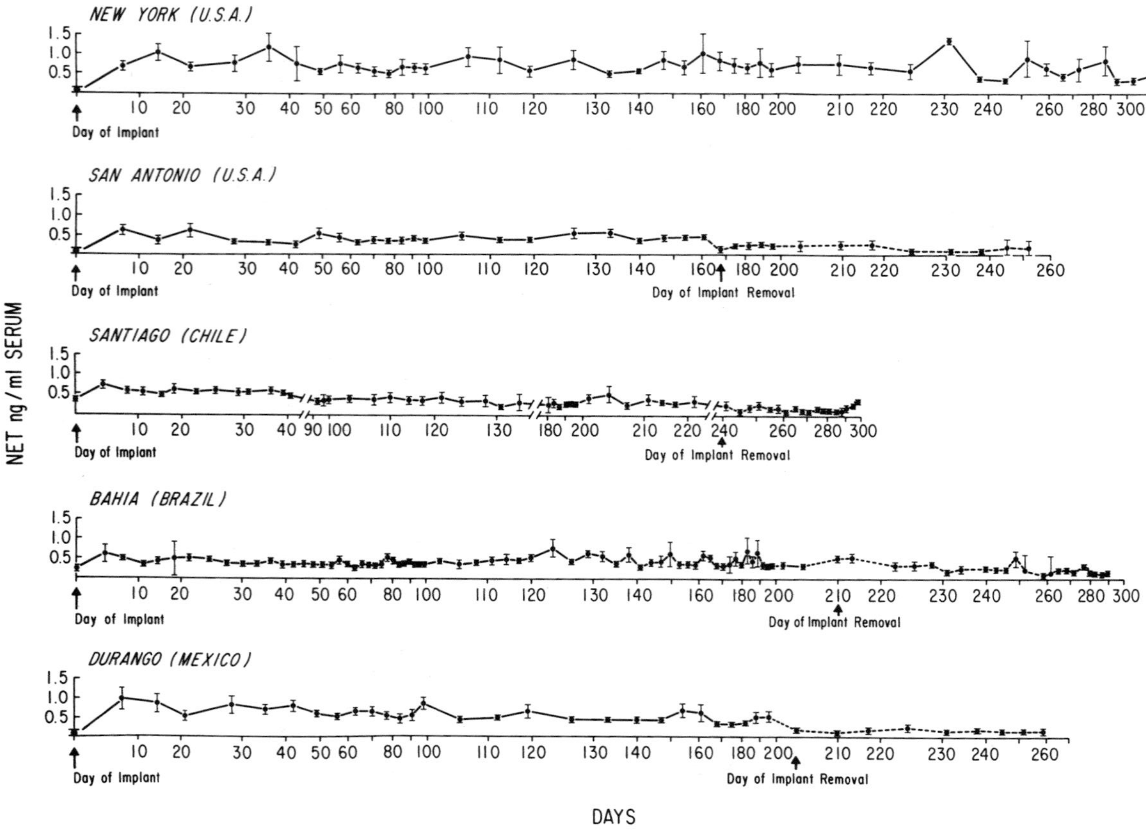

314

Fig. 4 Mean serum NET levels during phase I clinical clinical study in 50 women with two subdermal NET-choles-

TABLE 2 Effects Observed in Women with Norethindrone (NET)-Cholesterol Fused Implants

Number of pellets (women)	Local reaction	Transitory effects				Uterine cramps	Dysmenorrhea (%)		Premenstrual syndrome (%)	
		Nausea	Headache	Mastaglia			Appearance	Disappearance	Appearance	Disappearance
Two (50)	0	0	0	0		0	0	100	0	100
Three (51)	0	5	0	1		1	0	100	0	100
Four (30)	0	0	1	1		0	0	100	0	100

The results of the phase I clinical study with two pellets suggested that NET-cholesterol fused implants may provide a simple and acceptable approach to long-term contraception in women. However, there were two pregnancies, suggesting higher dose of norethindrone for a rate of contraception better than 99%.

Hence, in a phase II clinical study 81 healthy, fertile, sexually active female volunteers at three centers were studied for contraceptive efficacy of three and four NET-cholesterol implants, each implant containing 35 mg of NET, for 12 months. The release rates of NET from three and four pellets, respectively, were 150.3 ±7.2 and 212.5 ±8.6 μg NET/day. Following the implantation of NET pellets, serum NET levels did not show any burst effect and were sustained at levels between 0.4 and 0.6 ng NET per milliliter of serum with three pellets and 0.6 to 0.7 ng NET per milliliter of serum with four pellets (Fig. 5). With three and four pellets, respectively, 40% and 27% of the women had normal menstrual cycles, 20% and 14% were amenorrheic, 27% and 37% had midmenstrual spotting or bleeding, and 13% and 22% had prolonged episodes of bleeding. Cardiovascular, hepatic, and renal functions were normal throughout the study (Fig. 6). Ovulation was inhibited in 85% and 92% of the cycles with three and four pellets, respectively. In women using three pellets, two pregnancies occurred, one at the sixth cycle and another at the twelfth cycle. In women using four pellets, no pregnancies occurred during the entire period of study [15].

IV. CONCLUSION

In conclusion, among the long-acting subdermal contraceptive drug delivery devices, NET-cholesterol fused implants were relatively easy to manufacture, sterilize, and store at relatively low cost and effort. Because the NET-cholesterol implants are relatively small, implantation and removal are simple and minor outpatient procedures. The NET-cholesterol fused subdermal implants created low and sustained levels of NET in the circulation; there were no significant side effects, and the contraceptive efficacy was high. For example, NET-cholesterol fused implants caused neither any significant changes in serum LDL:HDL ratio nor in serum metabolites and liver enzymes during the entire period of contraception. A marginal increase in daily serum NET level with four NET-cholesterol fused implants, over that of three implants (Fig. 5) caused significant increase of the ovarian response and contraceptive efficacy, which may be attributed to the cumulative effect of NET at the target site. Studies have demonstrated that four NET-cholesterol fused implants of 35 mg each (i.e., a total dose of 140 mg NET) provided greater than 99% contraception for a year or more. To obtain similar results, the amount of drug in the form of oral pills would be significantly higher. In addition, the drug delivered by the

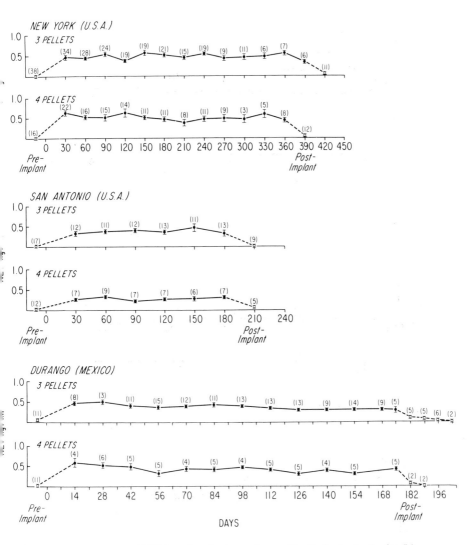

Fig. 5 Mean serum NET levels during phase II clinical study in 51 women and with three and in 30 women with four subdermal NET-cholesterol fused implants at three centers.

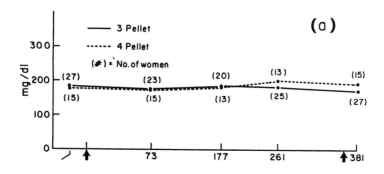

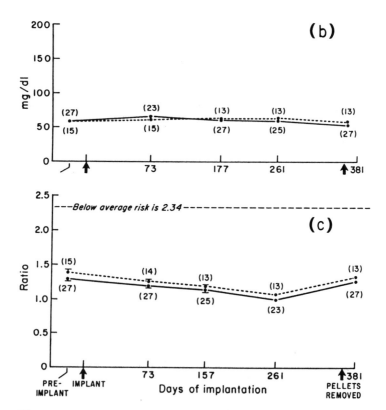

Fig. 6 Mean serum levels in 51 women with three and in 30 women with four NET-cholesterol fused implants during phase II clinical study of levels of (a) cholesterol and (b) triglycerides, (c) LDL:HDL ratio, (d) and levels of glucose, (e) LDH, and (f) SGOT.

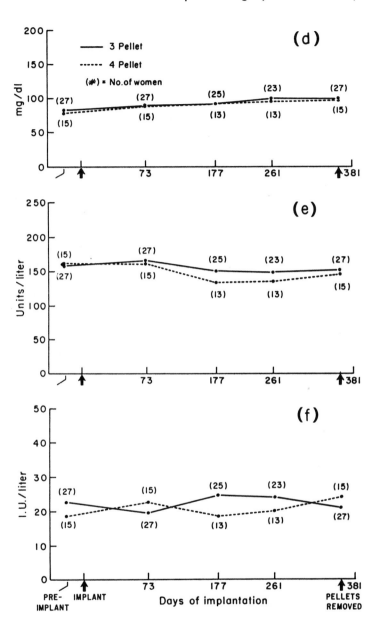

Fig. 6 (*continued*)

subdermal implants bypasses gastrointestinal tract and liver. The state of contraception with NET-cholesterol fused implants was completely and quickly reversible as and when desired. An additional benefit of subdermal NET-cholesterol fused implants was the amelioration of dysmenorrhea and premenstrual syndrome in women. All women in the study, in spite of menstrual disturbances, indicated a high degree of acceptability and considered NET-cholesterol fused implants the first choice of long-term contraception as an alternative to the "pill."

ACKNOWLEDGMENTS

These studies reported in this chapter were supported by PARFR 330 Subagreement DPE-0546-A-00-1003-00, Endocon, Inc., the Rockefeller Foundation, and the Robert Wood Johnson Charitable Trust.

The authors thank Miss Jane E. McLoughlin for her patience in the typing of this manuscript.

REFERENCES

1. B. B. Saxena, R. Landesman, G. N. Gupta, M. Singh, P. Rath-nam, and B. Dattatreyamurty, *J. Obstet. Gynecol.*, 4(Suppl. 1): PS 16 (1984).
2. G. I. Zatuchni, A. Goldsmith, J. D. Shelton, and J. J. Sciarra, eds., *Long-Acting Contraceptive Delivery Systems*. Harper & Row, New York, 1984.
3. E. Diczfalusy, *Contraception*, 33(1):7-22 (1986).
4. G. Pincus, M. C. Chang, M. X. Zarron, E. S. E. Hafez, and A. Merrill, *Endocrinology*, 59:694 (1956).
5. M. J. Shear, *Am. J. Cancer*, 26:322-332 (1936).
6. P. M. Bishop, *Lancet*, 229-232 (Aug. 11, 1951).
7. R. D. Gambrell, Jr., *Obstet. Gynecol.*, 47:569-576 (1976).
8. R. B. Greenblatt, *J. Clin. Endocrinol. Metab.*, 14:1564 (1954).
9. M. B. Shimkin and J. White, *Endocrinology*, 29:1020-1025 (1941).
10. C. D. Kochakian, *Am. J. Physiol.*, 145:549 (1945).
11. H. W. Rudel and F. A. Kincl, *Acta Endocrinol.*, 64:253-264 (1970).
12. S. J. Segal and H. Croxatto, Single administration of hormones for long-term control of reproductive function, presented at the 23rd meeting of the American Fertility Society, Washington, DC, April 14-16, 1967.
13. A. Schindler, Y. M. Hibionada, and G. G. Pitt, *J. Polym. Sci. Chem. Educ.*, 20:319 (1982).
14. G. Gupta, B. B. Saxena, R. Landesman, and W. J. Ledger, *Fertil. Steril.*, 41:726-731 (1984).

15. M. Singh, B. B. Saxena, R. Landesman, and W. J. Ledger, *Adv. Contraception*, 1:131-149 (1985).
16. H. Hopfenberg and K. C. Hsu, *Polym. Eng. Sci.*, 18:1186-1191 (1978).
17. R. N. Shain and M. Potts, in *Long-Acting Contraceptive Delivery Systems* (G. I. Zatuchni, A. Goldsmith, J. D. Shelton, and J. J. Sciarra, eds.). Harper & Row, New York, 1984, pp. 1-19.
18. J. Heller, *Biomaterials*, 1:51-58 (1980).
19. E. J. Frazza and E. E. Schmitt, *J. Biomed. Mater. Res. Symp.*, 1:43 (1971).
20. A. C. Tanquary and R. E. Lacey (eds.), *Advances in Experimental Medicine and Biology*, Plenum Press, New York, Vol. 47 (1974).
21. H. J. Tatum, *Contraception*, 1:253 (1963).
22. J. T. Fell and J. M. Newton, *J. Pharm. Sci.*, 59:688-691 (1968).
23. G. Gupta, B. B. Saxena, D. V. Amin, and S. J. Segal, New bioabsorbable contraceptive pellet implants: Sustained release of H-Norethindrone and ^{3}H-d-Norgestrel in rhesus monkeys, American Chemical Society Abstract No. O13 (1980).
24. A. Maitra, U. M. Joshi, S. D. Kholkute, S. M. Munshi, G. N. Gupta, and S. Tejuja, *Contraception*, 21(2):165-173 (1980).
25. U. M. Joshi, J. V. Joshi, U. M. Donde, G. M. Sankoli, K. D. Virkar, and B. N. Saxena, *Contraception*, 31(1):71-82 (1985).
26. R. H. Asch, in *Long-Acting Contraceptive Delivery Systems* (G. I. Zatuchni, A. Goldsmith, J. D. Shelton, and J. J. Sciarra, eds.). Harper & Row, New York, 1984, pp. 431-440.
27. Program for Applied Research on Fertility Regulation, *Contraception*, 1:295-304 (1985).
28. C. C. Chang and F. A. Kinel, *Fertil. Steril.*, 21:134-139 (1970).

Part Three
SPECIALIZED DEVICES

11
Magnetically Controlled Devices and Biomodulation

DAVID F. RANNEY / The University of Texas Health Science Center,
Dallas, Texas

I. INTRODUCTION

A. Objectives and Agents

Magnetic control of drugs and devices addresses three major issues in experimental and clinical pharmaceutics: high-efficiency targeting of transvascular drug carriers, external guidance of magnetic catheters, and magnetic modulation of internally implanted devices (e.g., drug-polymer slabs and infusion pumps) for which a complete skin seal is required.

Drug Targeting

The definition of targeting most widely accepted by the pharmaceutical industry is tissue or cellular localization that increases the therapeutic index by at least half an order of magnitude. Hence, targeting generally causes drug levels in liver, spleen, bone marrow, kidney, and other major sites of toxicity to rise by less than 0.3 to 0.1 of the increment achieved in target organs (tissues). There are three exceptions to this. The first is "site avoidance" targeting, in which drug is allowed to reach therapeutic levels in multiple nontarget sites, provided it avoids the major organ(s) of toxicity. A second exception occurs when the objective is to localize a nontoxic drug for reasons of rapid plasma clearance, biodegradation, high production costs, or limited commercial availability. The third occurs when a carrier targets the drug "effect" but not the drug itself. Examples include the new liposomal and microemulsion forms of amphotericin B [1-5]. These have antifungal efficacy that is equal on a dose basis, to standard amphotericin B deoxycholate (Fungizone). However, the new formulations have an 8- to 20-fold lower acute toxicity toward normal host cells. Therefore, much higher total doses are tolerated and this results in improved host survival. A greatly increased fraction of the injected dose is delivered to reticuloendothelial organs (liver, spleen, and bone marrow) relative to primary sites of infection. Hence, the drug is not actually targeted, just the drug effect. One consequence of this approach is that it results in hepatic and adipose sequestration of drug at high levels for weeks to months [1,5]. Intercurrent diseases that cause acute hepatocellular necrosis or fat breakdown can potentially release active drug at toxic levels. From a regulatory standpoint, these sequellae require extensive investigation for each drug-carrier combination before a formulation is deemed safe. Hence, it is important to remember that targeting drugs and drug effects are not biologically equivalent.

Magnetic Drug Targeting

Magnetic drug targeting is a highly efficient method of site-specific delivery that is appropriate for a select group of agents and diseases [6,7]. In qualifying agents for magnetic targeting, four questions must be asked. Is this drug so dangerous or labile that you cannot allow it to circulate freely in the bloodstream? Is the agent so expensive that you cannot afford to waste 99.9% of it? Must you achieve a selective, regional effect (e.g., abscess-directed inflammation or transplant-specific immunosuppression) to meet your therapeutic objective? Do you require an alternative formulation of an essential agent (e.g., amphotericin B, doxorubicin, or bleomycin) to continue treatment in patients whose systemic therapy must be temporarily discontinued due to life-threatening toxicity directed at selected organs (e.g., kidney, heart, or lung, respectively)? In these situations, magnetic targeting has the four advantages of crossing microvascular barriers independent of endothelial status, protecting drug, blood cells, and endothelium during transit, delivering up to 60% of the injected dose to target tissues, and making drug available in a controlled fashion within the tissue [6]. This reduces circulating concentrations of free drug by a factor of 100 or more [8], minimizes damage to normal tissue cells [6], and allows effective treatment of regionalized disease at 0.1 the free-drug dose or less [6-8]. These advantages are achieved at significant cost [6,9]:

1. Magnetic targeting is an expensive, technical approach limited to universities and research centers.
2. It requires specialized microspheres and magnets.
3. It demands new methods for noninvasive, localized monitoring of drug levels in target tissues.
4. Treatment of multiple body regions requires sequential targetings.
5. Tissue localization of microspheres results in long-term deposition of magnetite (Fe_3O_4) at levels of approximately 3.5 mg/1000 g (wet weight) [7].

The last effect is nontoxic as assessed epidemiologically in miners of hematite (magnetite), who exhibit neither inflammatory sequellae nor increased tumor incidence over occupational lifetimes, even at lung concentrations 100 to 1000 times above those produced by drug targeting [10]. However, due to the preceding constraints, magnetic targeting will be limited to agents that are highly toxic, labile, or cleared rapidly from plasma, and agents that experience impeded access to target tissues (e.g., brain) or required regional distribution to meet localized therapeutic objectives [6]. Specific examples are: adriamycin, amphotericin B and other membrane-active agents, white cell chemoattractants such as f-met-leu-phe, interleukin 2, tumor necrosis factor, prostaglandins, immunosuppressives, neuropeptides, and potentially in the future, magnetized white blood cells, labile gene vectors for high-efficiency organ reconstitution, and diagnostic agents for experimental studies of brain metabolism.

B. Barriers and Transport

The problem of targeting drugs with macromolecular and supramolecular carriers (monoclonal antibodies, drug-receptor conjugates, polymeric drugs, liposomes, and standard microspheres) is that the body comprises not one, but four major test tubes: (a) the external compartment (including the gastrointestinal tract, buccal and bladder mucosa, respiratory epithelium, and skin), (b) the blood pool, (c) extracellular space (including lesional glycocalyx, loose and dense connective tissue, and extracellular matrix of cartilage and bone), and (d) multiple intracellular compartments [11]. For intravascularly administered drugs, the initial biological barrier is endothelium [6-9]. This represents both a metabolic barrier (degradative enzymes) and physical barrier (cell and basement membranes) [12]. Endothelial enzymes can partially degrade prodrugs, drugs, peptides, and proteins when these agents attempt to cross in a physically and chemically exposed form [6,12]. Moreover, except for reticuloendothelial organs, which have highly porous sinusoidal endothelium, the remaining body organs exhibit physical barriers that severely restrict transendothelial migration of most drug carriers above a molecular size of 3 to 5 nm [13,14]. This means that most carriers large enough to encode receptor-binding information are excluded from the extravascular compartment of normal target organs other than liver and spleen, and variably, bone marrow and kidney. Regions of disease (e.g., infarcts, infections, and tumors) exhibit selective barrier breakdown [15-18]. Experimental tumors, whose vascular filtration properties have been sized with fluoresceinated dextrans, display intermediate and lower permeabilities, respectively, to 150,000 and 3,000,000 MW species [18]. However, even with partial barrier breakdown, macromolecular and particulate carriers experience rates of lesional accumulation that are generally too slow to compete with faster rates of active hepatic clearance [1,4-6,11,15,19]. This highlights the major challenges facing intravascular drug targeting, namely, that the initial (organ) distribution of carrier, its transport across target endothelium, and penetration of tissue gel (e.g., lesional glycocalyx) [6,18,20] are the principal bioengineering problems that must be solved before receptor-mediated uptake by target cells [21] or microorganisms can be meaningfully addressed.

In devising efficient methods of targeting drugs, it is valuable to observe how the body localizes its own macromolecular drugs (biopharmaceuticals) in diseased tissue. This is accomplished by inducing targeted extravascular migration of particulate drug carriers in the form of white blood cells, which produce controlled release of proteolytic enzymes, potent toxins (such as interleukins 1 and 2, lymphotoxin, and tumor necrosis factor) and oxygen free radicals [6,8,11,22,23]. Long-lived lipid peroxides are formed. These mediators plus elevated tissue metabolites and coagulation proteins [24] induce partial opening of endothelial junctions. Microvascular filtration is increased nonspecifically for plasma macromolecules, such as albumin, α-globulins, γ-globulins (including antibodies) [19], polymeric drugs, and diagnostic polymers [6,15,18]. Both release and degradation of white cell toxins occur locally within the tissues. Those that diffuse into the bloodstream are cleared extremely rapidly ($t_{1/2}$ = 3-6 min) [25]. Normal bystander cells in the microenvironment of disease are frequently damaged and occasionally killed; however, these effects are minimized by the controlled manner in which the most potent toxins are released [6,8,23,26]. Hence, uninvolved portions of the organ and body are relatively protected except in very severe disease. It is also instructive to note that most of the naturally occurring mediators are immunologically nonspecific in relation to surface receptors on microorganisms and tumors. Immunological specificity may also be undesirable in the design of drug carriers due to heterogeneity and loss of target antigens caused by mutation, cell cycle modulation, and antibody-induced shedding [27]. Moreover, recent in vivo evidence on human lymphomas indicates that high-affinity monoclonal antibodies are bound predominantly in the outer few millimeters of each tumor nodule [28]. The outer antigen "sponge" acts as a functional barrier to prevent permeation of antibody into the central regions of tumor, even though viable, antigen-positive cells are located there. Such results indicate that an immunologically nonspecific carrier that becomes widely distributed in the anatomic subregions of target lesions ("magic shotgun pellet") may be superior to a antigen-specific carrier ("magic bullet").

Given these biological barriers and responses, our present knowledge about pharmaceutical design, and regulatory constraints on drug devices, the major objectives of drug targeting must be to produce localized, controlled release of penetrating, broad-spectrum agents in the extravascular compartments of selected organs and tissues. The most immediate "targets" for circulating carriers are endothelial cells [6,9,12,29]. The first objective is to achieve selective endothelial transport. Ways to meet this objective will arise from viewing the microvascular *barrier* as a *bridge*. This bridge can be crossed in five ways:

1. Magnetic dragging of ferromagnetic microparticles directly through the endothelium and basement membrane [6-9,30-32]

2. Transient regional opening of endothelial junctions combined with vascular infusion of drug-carrier formulations, which become sequestered in the tissue compartment [9,33]
3. Biochemical transport of specific drug-ligand conjugates by binding to endothelial receptors [9,29,34,35]
4. Bioadhesion transport of microparticulate drugs by multivalent binding of surface coatings to endothelial antigens [9,36]
5. Equilibrium partitioning of noncharged prodrugs across microvessels followed by generation of charged (tissue-locked) drugs by enzymes specific to the target tissue (e.g., brain, lung, and ciliary body of the eye) [37]

For each of these approaches, it is important to decide if the objective is to traverse (or permeabilize) normal endothelium—the requisite target for delivering physiological mediators—or to traverse (or permeabilize) structurally altered endothelium—the requisite target for treating tumors and infections that induce biochemical, antigenic, and physical changes in their endothelium [6,9]. In this context, magnetic targeting is the only method that achieves transcapillary migration by a mechanism independent of endothelial status. Until more is learned about endothelial changes in specific classes of disease, methods 2 to 5 above will be reliable only for targeting drugs across *normal* endothelium. Hence they are best suited for localizing physiological mediators. During endothelial transit and once in the tissues, it is necessary to protect drugs from degradative enzymes and to protect normal tissue cells from the immediate bioavailability of toxic drugs [6,9,12,38]. Hence, carriers with a stabilized controlled-release matrix, such as microspheres, are preferable to free and polymeric drugs, which make portions of the agent bioavailable as they interact with the first cells encountered in vivo: red cells, white cells, and endothelium. The two methods that provide nearly complete physical and chemical sequestration of agents during blood and endothelial transport are magnetic and bioadhesion targeting (Fig. 1). As has been appreciated recently [6] and will be described below, bioadhesion is involved as an adjunctive transport mechanism in all cases of magnetic drug targeting. The remainder of this chapter will focus on magnetic microspheres and devices.

II. HISTORY OF MAGNETIC GUIDANCE

The earliest applications of magnets to the delivery of clinical agents involved guidance of catheters for selective angiography [39-41] and intravascular localization of carbonyl iron for selective arterial thrombosis [42]. The feasibility of targeting small particles to tissues by arterial injection was first reported by Meyers et al. [43]. His group showed that strong magnetic fields would retain 1 to 3 μm particles of

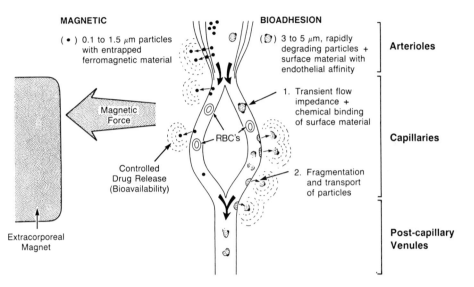

MAGNETIC

(•) 0.1 to 1.5 μm particles
with entrapped
ferromagnetic material

Magnetic
Force

Extracorporeal
Magnet

Controlled
Drug Release
(Bioavailability)

RBC's

BIOADHESION

(🌑) 3 to 5 μm, rapidly
degrading particles +
surface material with
endothelial affinity ⎤ Arterioles

1. Transient flow
impedance +
chemical binding
of surface material

Capillaries

2. Fragmentation
and transport
of particles

Post-capillary
Venules

Fig. 1 Methods of microsphere targeting. (From Ref. 9.)

carbonyl iron at selected intravascular sites in the presence of arterial
flow forces. A portion of the iron remained at the site for at least 7
days. This suggested that some of the particles had migrated out of
vessels into the arterial walls and tissues. Initially, it was thought
that drugs could be grafted onto the surface of native magnetite particles; however, two problems were encountered. Loading capacities
were too low (by a factor of 100-1000) for acceptable dosing of recipients
with magnetite, and irreversible particle aggregation occurred when
native magnetite was exposed to clinically useful magnetic fields [44].
This caused emoblization of large (arterial) vessels and prevented homogeneous particle distribution at the capillary level. Irreversible aggregation was reduced by coating ferromagnetic materials with albumin
and other charged polymers [44]. This provided the basis for recent
approaches in which albumin is emulsified to form small microspheres,
which completely microencapsulate the ferromagnetic material [30-32].

III. TRANSVASCULAR MAGNETIC MICROCARRIERS

A. Carriers and Methods of Formulation

Magnetic microcarriers are supramolecular particles that are small
enough to circulate through capillaries without producing embolic occlusion (<4 μm), but are sufficiently susceptible (ferromagnetic) to become

captured in microvessels and dragged into the adjacent tissues by magnetic fields of 0.5 to 0.8 tesla (T) [7,9]. They include microspheres,
liposomes, and cells. Magnetic liposomes have been prepared by the
Eli Lilly Drug Targeting Group (R. Morris, personnal communication).
To date, they have not been extensively tested in vivo. The author
and co-workers have prepared magnetic neutrophils that remained functional after targeting to mouse lungs [6] (see Magnetic Neutrophils,
under Section III.F). The carriers most extensively studied are magnetic microspheres. These are made by preparing an aqueous mixture
of water-soluble drug (or lipophilic drug plus water-soluble adducting
agent) [6], matrix material (typically albumin [7,30-32], but alternatively carbohydrate [45] and 10 nm Fe_3O_4 particles, emulsifying the
mixture in biodegradable oil, sonicating or shearing to produce sub-
micrometer spheres, stabilizing the matrix by heating or chemical cross-
linking [7], extracting the oil with a volatile organic solvent (typically
hexane or ether), and lyophilizing the preparation to dryness. The
usual magnetite content is 20% (by dry weight) [8,30-32]. In the absence of detergents, magnetite particles cluster to form multiple aggregates within each sphere [7,32]. By electron microscopy, most of
these aggregates are larger than a single magnetic domain (50 nm).
Stabilized microspheres have a shelf life of greater than 1 year at 22°C,
and no burst release of drug occurs with storage [6]. An electron
micrograph of the original magnetic microspheres (containing adriamycin) is shown in Fig. 2.

B. Routes of Injection and Mechanisms of Targeting

Most of the microspheres that become captured in target vessels are
caught during the first circulatory pass through a strong magnetic
field. Consequently, to obtain high-efficiency targeting (e.g., 60%
of spheres) at a systemic site, injection is performed intra-arterially
[30-32,46,47]. When targeting is to the lungs, similar efficiency can
be achieved by intravenous injection [8,9]. Lower efficiencies [ca.
20-25% of spheres) can be achieved at systemic sites by intravenous
administration. The reason for reduced targeting in this last case is
that microspheres are diluted in the entire blood pool, and standard
(uncoated) spheres are cleared by the liver at a half-time of 10 to 20
min [8]. Consequently, reduced numbers of spheres remain available
to circulate past the magnet. Particle coatings, such as the block
copolymers, tetronic 908 and pluronic F108, prolong the circulation
times of 60 to 100 nm spheres (nanospheres) from minutes to hours
or even days [4,48]. This may allow high-efficiency systemic targeting
by the intravenous route. Limiting factors would be the rate of drug
release (typically 4-8 hr) and the length of time that relatively ill subjects could remain in the magnet. (Only 10-15 min is required for irreversible localization of spheres following arterial injection.) These

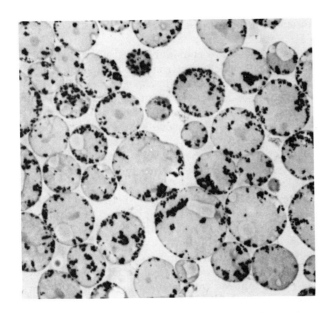

Fig. 2 Transmission electron micrograph (magnified ×50,000) of albumin microspheres containing entrapped Fe_3O_4 and adriamycin. Spheres range in diameter from about 0.35 to 1.6 μm. Small black particles are microaggregates of 10 nm Fe_3O_4. Albumin matrix appears gray; adriamycin is not visualized by this method. (Adapted from Refs. 7 and 32.)

new coatings may also allow the operator to vary the fraction of spheres that biodistributes to primary (target) and secondary (reticuloendothelial) sites.

Three additional factors affect the efficiency of targeting: the extent of venous shunting that occurs before spheres reach a strong magnetic field [8,30-32], the homogeneity of the magnetic field gradient throughout the target volume [6,9] (see Section III.C), and anatomic heterogeneity within the target tissue [6,46]. As an example of the last point, gamma camera images obtained from canine limb sarcomas have shown that arterial injection plus magnetic capture gives efficient targeting to soft tissue components of tumor but not to ossified components [46]. Targeting to bony components of the sarcomas required intramedullary administration of microspheres (intravenous injection with a tourniquet to reverse blood flow). These results emphasize two important factors in treating complex lesions: (a) anatomic subregions must be recognized in advance if one is to successfully treat all components of a lesion, and (b) high resolution imaging with tracer spheres is necessary to monitor the subregion distribution of carrier and drug (see Section III.E). Because magnetic microspheres are considerably smaller than the 4 μm diameter that separates nonembolizing from embolizing particles, they would normally pass through target capillaries and be cleared by the liver. However, in the presence of a gradient magnetic field, they are captured in small arterioles and capillaries enveloped by the field. The targeting achieved in two separate rat models is as follows:

1. Approximately 55% of injected spheres were localized in the magnetic segment of rat tails (0.8 T field; ventral caudal arterial injections) [7,30-32].

2. Of the injected spheres, 40% were localized in the magnetic segments of thoracic viscera: 35% in lungs and 5% in heart (0.55 T field; intravenous injections) [8,9].

Microsphere localization occurred within seconds of injection [8]. At linear flow rates below about 0.75 cm/sec, the magnetic force exceeded microvascular flow force, and spheres were caused to impinge on the microvascular endothelium in pairs and short chains [7-9,30-32]. It has recently been reported that endothelial cells have albumin receptors on their luminal surfaces [49]. Hence, although it was not appreciated initially, the combined effects of magnetic drag and albumin adhesion to endothelial receptors [6,49] resulted in migration of microsheres both between and through endothelial cells into the adjacent interstitium [6,8,32]. As assessed by electron microscopy, intravascular capture and extravascular migration were complete within 2 and 15 min, respectively [8].

C. Magnet Design

Microsphere targeting results from the force exerted by a gradient magnetic field. The relationship of magnetic force to field gradient and magnetic moment of particles is expressed in the following general equation [50]:

$$F = M \nabla H$$

where

F   = force on particles
M   = magnetic moment of particles after saturation magnetization
∇H = magnetic field gradient

This equation indicates that spheres with increased magnetic moments will experience forces sufficient for extravascular migration at proportionately lower field gradients. The magnetic moments of microsphere magnetite can be increased in three ways: by magnetizing the spheres to saturation levels prior to vascular targeting, by clustering magnetite at the center of each sphere to produce larger macrodomains, and by substituting one of the newer ferromagnetic materials that has higher susceptibility than Fe_3O_4 [6,51]. Before the last alternative can be employed, the acute and chronic toxicities of several new magnetic alloys must be assessed.

Small-animal experiments indicated that satisfactory targeting of microspheres (with 20% magnetite) could be achieved using magnets of 0.55 to 0.80 T field strength, 0.01 T/mm field gradient, and 0.4 to 0.8 cm (diameter) pole pieces positioned adjacent to normal lungs [8,9] and tail tumors [7,30-32,47]. In recent attempts to treat larger animals (canine limb sarcomas), a 1.8 T electromagnet was used which had a single, chisel shaped, 10 cm pole piece [46]. Initially, technical problems were encountered due to field inhomogeneity created by the increased magnetic flux at each point of the chisel. This caused focal overcapture of microspheres. Subsequently, the magnet was repositioned to minimize this problem. A preferred, general solution lies in designing a magnet whose gradient is nearly constant throughout the targeting volume. This is achieved with a quadripolar field configuration [6] (Fig. 3). As tested by computer modeling, it produces a gradient whose magnitude varies by less than 15% across the targeting volume. A 2 T electromagnet of this configuration would provide the required gradient of 0.01 T/mm over the 40 cm pole gap required for targeting within human thoracic, abdominal, and cranial cavities [6]. Such magnets could be constructed for one-fifth to one-tenth the cost of a magnetic resonance imager.

D. Biodistribution and Tissue Concentration of Microspheres

Aggregation in target vessels is minimized by injecting microspheres in a physiological solution containing 0.1% (w/v) Tween 80 or a viscosity-enhancing agent, such as 50% (w/v) dextran [6,32]. For spheres smaller than 3 μm, initial (5-30 min) biodistribution is a function of (a) the dose relative to the capacity of target capillaries, (b) the degree to which the magnetic field overlaps microvessels supplied by the injection vessel, (c) the extent of venous shunting before microspheres reach the field, and (d) the flow rates in target vessels. In an early study, 1 mg/kg of ^{125}I-labeled microspheres (sufficient to produce therapeutic tissue levels of adriamycin) was infused at a native arterial rate of 0.6 ml/min into the ventral caudal arteries of rats at the bases of their tails and captured in the third of four, 4 cm, distal tail segments by an 0.8 T field [30-32]. At 30 min postinjection, the following tissue concentrations of spheres were measured (in micrograms per gram of tissue, wet weight): target tail segment, 215 ±18; other tail

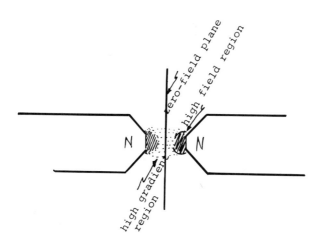

Fig. 3 Diagram of quadripolar magnetic field for improved homogeneity of microsphere localization. Uniform gradient region is shown as dotted and high-field region as cross-hatched. A zero-field region exists at the midplane between pole pieces. Other arrangements are made possible by introducing additional magnetic elements. To avoid microsphere aggregation in the infusion syringe, injections are performed near the zero-field region. (From Ref. 6.)

segments, < 1; liver, 25 ±2; spleen, 40 ±2; lung 27 ±2; kidney and remainder of the carcass < 1 (limits of detection = 1 μg/g) [7,32]. In the absence of magnetic capture, only the liver, spleen, and lung had detectable levels of carrier, at 40 ±2, 50 ±2, and 31 ±2 μg/g, respectively. Hence, magnetic localization produced a target-to-liver ratio of 8.6:1 and slightly reduced the uptake of microspheres by lung and reticuloendothelial organs relative to that observed without magnetic capture.

In a recent study, larger doses of trace-labeled spheres (6.6 mg/kg--sufficient to produce effective tissue levels of f-met-leu-phe) were infused intravenously into rats over a 3 min interval, allowed to travel at native flow rates into the central venous system through the right heart into both lungs, and captured by an 0.55 T magnetic field (gradient of 0.01 T/mm), which enveloped the right thorax and the middle half of the left thorax [8]. At 5 min postinjection, the biodistribution of spheres, as percentage of injected dose, was as follows: right lung, 15.9%; left lung, 11.2%; heart, 3.3%; liver, 45%; spleen, 7.6%; kidneys, 11.3%; blood plasma, 3.4%; circulating white blood cells, < 0.1% (% of total dose recovered, 97.8%). The corresponding tissue concentrations of spheres were (μg/g wet weight): right lung, 195; left lung, 135; spleen, 67; kidneys, 37; liver, 27; heart, 24; blood plasma, 3; and circulating white blood cells, < 0.004 (limits of detection 0.004 µg/g). The splenic and renal concentrations of spheres in the latter study were slightly higher because there was greater vascular shunting due to incomplete magnetic envelopment of the left lung. Still, pulmonary targeting was sufficient to allow transvascular delivery of an otherwise lethal inflammatory peptide, f-met-leu-phe. Tissue drug levels are described under Chemoattractant Microspheres in Section III.F.

When injecting microspheres into normal tissues, it is important to infuse them over a 3 to 5 min interval, rather than inject them as a bolus. This is because the arterioles that feed each 50 to 200 µm segment of tissue undergo cyclical constriction and dilatation. Hence, to obtain homogeneous distribution in all capillaries, spheres must be infused over at least one vasomotor cycle (D. F. Ranney, unpublished studies). By contrast, the small vessels supplying most malignant tumors are relatively unresponsive to circulating vasoconstrictors and therefore, are chronically vasodilated compared to surrounding normal vessels. Cineangiograms have documented that magnetic microspheres are shunted selectively into tumor arterioles and capillaries (R. Morris; R. Richardson, personal communications). This effect further enhances the therapeutic index of microsphere-delivered drugs. It may be possible to exploit this phenomenon by injecting vasoconstrictors into the regional circulation just ahead of spheres.

E. Noninvasive Monitoring

Carrier Localization

To avoid injuring normal regions of a target circulation, washed and sized microspheres should be infused at moderate rates. Blood flow and tissue perfusion should be monitored. It is also important to monitor the mass of microspheres that becomes localized in a given mass of tissue. Based on the pattern of targeting obtained with trace-labeled spheres, it may be necessary to modify or supplement the delivery regimen. For example, magnetic shielding may be required to prevent microsphere capture in adjacent body parts (e.g., head versus upper arm); or intramedullary administration may be required to treat the bony subregions of a multicomponent sarcoma or a carcinoma invading mineralized bone.

Carrier localization can be quantified by gamma dosimetry and gamma camera imaging at a resolution of about 0.5 to 1.0 cm [46,52]. Alternatively, high-frequency ultrasound or magnetic resonance (MR) techniques may be used to evaluate targeting at much higher, submillimeter resolutions. The latter two methods have the advantage of assessing microsphere distribution within critical anatomic subregions of the target. Small collections of untreated tumor cells or microorganisms can be detected that might be missed by lower resolution gamma isotopic techniques and positron emission tomography (PET). Magnetic resonance assessment of carrier localization is based on the capacity of ferromagnetic materials to decrease the apparent T2 relaxation time (T2*) of water protons positioned near localized spheres. This effect results from microinhomogeneities of the externally applied magnetic field, which are introduced by the magnetic dipoles of ferromagnetite particles. These dipoles act across distances of at least 1 to 3 μm. Table 1 shows the MR spectral effects of targeting Fe_3O_4 microspheres to the right lung of a rat and allowing the escaping spheres to be cleared by liver [6]. This early study was performed on freshly excised organs (ex vivo); however, recent reports indicate that a related change, image darkening, is observed in vivo by standard proton MR imaging [53]. This makes it feasible to determine whether microspheres have distributed evenly throughout anatomic subregions of normal or lesional soft tissues. One apparent disadvantage of MR analysis is that it may not allow quantitative assessment of microsphere localization in mineralized bone (versus bone marrow). The reason for this is that the diffusion and relaxation rates of water protons are restricted in mineralized bone. Studies are in progress to determine the extent of this problem. Assessment of microsphere localization by ultrasound techniques is just beginning to be evaluated (P. Antich and D. F. Ranney, work in progress).

TABLE 1 Effect of Albumin Microspheres[a] on NMR Proton Spin-spin (T2*) Relaxation[b] in Rat Target Organs

Organ	Fe_3O_4 in spheres[c]	Tissue Fe_3O_4[d] (μg/g wet wt)	Line width at half peak height (1/π·T2) (Hz)
Lung	-	0.0	454
	+	54.8	1395
Liver	-	0.0	120
	+	17.6	330

[a]Dose of spheres = 2 mg/kg.
[b]300 MHz NMR spectrometer
[c]Fe_3O_4 content = 20% (w/w).
[d]Tissue iron measured by acidic oxidation of tissues and graphite furnace photometry; Fe_3O_4 calculated from lattice formula for the mixed oxide.
Source: From Ref. 6.

Drug Release

Because magnetic targeting reduces circulating free drug levels by a factor exceeding 100, it is frequently difficult to use classical methods for drug monitoring [8]. Even when blood monitoring is feasible, the results do not correlate with tissue levels. Estimates of free tissue drug can be made at various posttargeting intervals from the combined determinations of carrier localization in tissue and the drug release rate in vitro. Such estimates are crude because additional processes take place in vivo that are ignored by this method. Specifically, enzymatic digestion of microspheres accelerates drug release, and back-diffusion of drug into microvessels accelerates drug clearance. Hence, if one wishes to obtain precise results, levels must be determined by measurements on the target tissue per se. This can be approached by MR methods.

For example, free tissue drug may be detected by attaching a paramagnetic label to the drug. A paramagnetic substance is one that becomes aligned in an external magnetic field but loses its alignment when the field is removed. By contrast to ferromagnetic materials (e.g., Fe_3O_4), paramagnetic ions and ion chelates have the following properties. They act on susceptible nuclei (water protons) at distances of angstroms rather than micrometers, give preferential T1-type rather than T2-type relaxation at the doses employed in vivo, and induce brightening rather than darkening of standard, T1-weighted images [54,55]. A paramagnetically tagged drug must be fully dissolved (hydrated) before adjacent water protons can diffuse to within the very short distances required to accelerate their magnetic relaxation [56]. Consequently, only the fraction of drug that has been released from spheres should be capable of detection. As an initial test of this hypothesis, the author prepared heat-stablized dextran microspheres that contained the paramagnetic metal chelate, Gd-DTPA (gadolinium diethylenetriamine pentaacetic acid) [15]. These spheres were designed to remain physically intact for 20 to 30 min postinjection. This is long enough for them to become cleared as particles by the liver, but short enough that Gd-DTPA is released rapidly in the liver. The effect of these spheres is shown in Fig. 4. Marked image brightening of the liver was observed at 30 min with therapeutically relevant doses. By comparison, microspheres containing the same quantity of Gd-DTPA entrapped in a very slowly releasing albumin matrix ($t_{1/2}$ = 8 hr) gave no MR enhancement at 30 min [6].

These results indicate that paramagnetic tagging of drugs provides a workable method for quantifying tissue levels of free drug, provided the microspheres have moderate to rapid release kinetics, and tissue Gd^{3+} remains below levels at which T2 effects begin to predominate and image brightening reverses. This method should also allow non-invasive monitoring of drug washout from tissues. Dextran Gd-DTPA

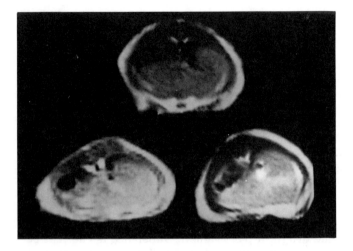

Fig. 4 Magnetic resonance images at mid-liver of prone Sprague-Dawley
rats, performed to demonstrate hydration and release of the gadolinium
chelate, Gd-DTPA, from dextran microspheres. Images are oriented
transaxially and acquired at 5 mm thickness using a T1-weighted, spin-
echo pulse sequence (TR = 0.5 sec; TE = 26 msec). Experimental rats
(lower panels) were imaged at postinjection times optimized for their
respective agents. Upper image, uninjected control; lower left image,
15 min after intravenous injection of soluble Gd-DTPA (0.3 mmol Gd/kg);
lower right image, 40 min after intravenous injection of Gd-DTPA-
dextran microspheres (0.06 mmol Gd/kg). Both experimental rats
(lower panels) had prominent liver brightening due to paramagnetic
T1 relaxation of water protons by hydrated (released) Gd-DTPA. As
assessed by image intensity analyses, microsphere Gd-DTPA was 11
times more potent than soluble Gd-DTPA, reflecting the selective uptake of microspheres by liver. Also, image enhancement by soluble
Gd-DTPA had faded almost completely by 40 min, reflecting Gd washout. (From Ref. 15.)

microspheres are nontoxic and also clear from the livers of test rats
within 3 weeks of injection (by [153]Gd radioisotopic methods) [6,15].
Hence, they may be of value as a new MR contrast agent for selective
enhancement of liver tumors. Due to the relative insensitivity of MR
spectroscopy as a monitoring technique, it is unlikely that paramagnetic tags will provide adequate sensitivity for quantifying conventionally administered drugs. However, higher sensitivities may be
achieved by tagging with ^{19}F because the natural abundance of this
isotope in body tissues is nearly zero [57]. The drawback of fluorine
imaging is that it requires special instruments with ^{19}F capabilities.

Such instruments are not widely available for clinical use and may not become so. This does not detract from the merits of acquiring experimental animal data that can be used to optimize drug distribution in patients.

Tissue Effects

MR spectroscopy of naturally occurring ^{31}P metabolites and ^{13}C-labeled metabolic precursors may provide a way to monitor tissue responses to localized drugs. Because this field is still in its infancy, it is uncertain whether reliable correlations can be drawn between therapeutic or toxic effects and MR spectral changes. For human melanomas grown in nude mice, acute, reversible decreases have been observed in the spectral peaks of high-energy phosphates (ATP and phosphocreatine) after treating the tumors with diphtheria toxin (P. Antich, personal communication). Also, as assessed by spectral shift, a more prolonged (24 hr) decrease has been observed in the pH of inorganic phosphates. This latter change is also reversible; however, it recovers more slowly and corresponds in time to the major tissue damage (D. F. Ranney and P. Antich, unpublished studies). One disadvantage of phosphorus spectroscopy in vivo is that signal averaging must be carried out over volumes of 1 to 2 cm^3 to obtain acceptable signal-to-noise ratios. This precludes assessment of anatomic subregions within centimeter-sized tumors. It has also proved difficult to verify the exact position and depth of tissues monitored by surface-coil spectroscopy. Hence, at present, phosphorus spectroscopy has been limited to relatively superficial lesions and has been compromised by the inability to employ labeled precursors or to acquire data in an imaging mode. Finally, although relatively good correlations exist between the disappearance of high-energy phosphate peaks and irreversible damage to a working tissue such as heart muscle, this correlation does not appear to hold for a "nonworking" tissue such as brain [58]. Hence, additional studies are needed to determine whether phosphorus spectroscopy can provide reliable inter-organ data. Spectroscopic drug monitoring with ^{13}C-labeled metabolites is even less well characterized but may hold greater promise for the future because of the large number of compounds that can be used as metabolic probes [59,60].

A third approach to tissue monitoring by MR techniques is based on the observation that acute broadening of spectral peaks occurs in rat organs that were exicsed and measured shortly after the induction of acute inflammation in vivo (D. F. Ranney and R. Nunnally, unpublished studies). Peak broadening indicates shortened tissue T2 relaxation times and appears to result from generation of long-lived free radicals within the inflamed tissue. Reversal of this spectral change provides a basis for monitoring the treatment effects of anti-inflammatory and antimicrobial agents. The usefulness of MR spectro-

scopy as a noninvasive tool for in situ drug monitoring should become
clearer within the next 2 years.

F. Prototype Systems

Magnetic microcarriers fall into four categories with respect to the
type of agent targeted: *standard drugs,* which act directly (e.g., on
tumor cells or microorganisms); *biomodulators* (biological response
modifiers or BRMs), which act either indirectly or directly to recruit
host cells, activate cellular or soluble host enzymes, or affect gene
structure or function; *biophysical agents,* such as radioisotopes for
brachytherapy and magnetic macrodomain materials for enhancing local
hyperthermia by hysteresis mechanisms; and *diagnostic agents.* The
most extensively tested prototype systems are described below.

Standard Drugs

Antitumor Microspheres

Adriamycin was the first agent chosen for magnetic targeting because it is active against a wide variety of human solid tumors, but its
efficacy is compromised by a major, organ-directed side effect of irreversible, dose-dependent cardiomyopathy [61]. The original spheres
were made of albumin and contained 9% adriamycin (with 4.5% available
for controlled release) and 20% Fe_3O_4 [7,30-32]. Adriamycin was
released according to modified first-order kinetics [62]. By employing
various temperatures for matrix stabilization, three formulations were
prepared having release half-times of 15 min, 4 hr, and 8 hr [62]. The
ratios of biological to chemical activity of spontaneously released drug
were 80% or more for all three formulations. The most highly stabilized
formulation ($t_{1/2}$ = 8 hr) was used in subsequent studies. Transarterial targeting was performed using the rat tail model described in
Section III.D. Drug release was documented in vivo by the histological
appearance of diffuse adriamycin fluorescence in tissues surrounding
the localized spheres [7]. Drug concentrations were monitored by
fluorescence measurements performed on acid-alcohol extracts of the
tail and body organs (Table 2). These results indicate that at 30 min,
the tumor-to-liver ratios of adriamycin were improved by a multiple
of 17.7 or more for magnetic versus simple arterial delivery. This
reflects the general finding that magnetic targeting improves the therapeutic index by a factor of 10 or more.

Microspheres with a polyglutaraldehyde matrix have been reported
to alter the in vitro targeting of adriamycin such that it acts preferentially at the surfaces of L1210 leukemia cells rather than intracellularly [63]. This has decreased the ED_{50} concentration of adriamycin
by a factor of 12.5 for one drug-resistant line. Hence, microspheres
may have an additional advantage of increasing the cytotoxicity of

TABLE 2 Localization of Microsphere-Targeted and Free Adriamycin

| Form of drug | Dose (mg/kg)[a] | Magnet[b] | Tissue concentrations (μg/g wet weight)[c] | |
			Target tail skin	Liver
Microsphere	0.05	-	<1	<1
	0.05	+	3.9	<1
Free	0.05	-	<1	<1
	5.00	-	3.3	15.0

[a]Drug and microspheres infused into the ventral caudal artery of the tail.
[b]0.8 T field.
[c]At 30 min after infusion; limits of detection 1 μg/g.
Source: Adapted from Refs. 7 and 32.

surface active drugs. In the study just cited, adriamycin was covalently linked to the glutaraldehyde. It remains to be determined whether comparable effects would be achieved for simple drug entrapment in alternative matrix materials.

Initial studies of antitumor efficacy were carried out in Holtzman rats with malignant Yoshida sarcomas grown subcutaneously in the tails [64]. These tumors exhibited complete remission in 75% of the animals following a single arterial targeting of microsphere adriamycin at 0.5 mg/kg administered 6 to 8 days after tumor inoculation (n = 12). By contrast, no remissions were observed with free adriamycin at 10 times the microsphere dose (5 mg/kg) administered either intraarterially or intravenously on days 1, 5, and 9 (n = 10). In a second efficacy study performed on Yoshida sarcomas, microsphere-targeted vindesine sulfate produced complete remission of tail tumors in 85% of the rats at doses of 0.5 and 2.5 mg/kg [47]. Free vindesine was ineffective at 0.5 mg/kg and lethal due to toxicity at 2.5 mg/kg. The third efficacy study was performed on a larger animal model, spontaneous canine limb sarcomas [46]. These were expected to mimic the tumor biology and magnetic field requirements of subsequent human studies. Unfortunately, the canine sarcomas were relatively insensitive to adriamycin vis-à-vis alternative drugs, such as cisplatinum, which would have been the drug of choice, had it been available in microsphere form (R. C. Richardson, personal communication). Inappropriate drug susceptibility together with poor magnetic localization of arterially administered spheres in the bony subregions of tumor led to an overall

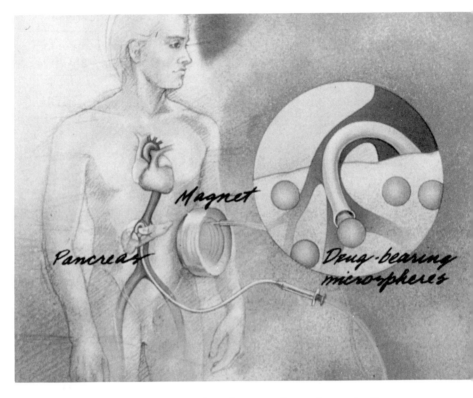

Fig. 5 Magnetic targeting of antitumor microspheres to the pancreas.
(Drawing by Narda Lebo, courtesy of University of Texas Health
Science Center at Dallas.)

failure of tumor response. Additional agents and combined targeting
regimens await testing in this model. Figure 5 is a schematic diagram
showing how magnetic microspheres would be administered by the arterial route to treat pancreatic carcinoma involving the organ and adjacent structures supplied by common regional vessels (superior and
inferior pancreaticoduodenal arteries).

In CBA mice, the LD_{50} of 1 μm albumin-magnetite (placebo) spheres
is 1250 mg/kg [6]. Based on an available adriamycin content of 4.5%
and an effective dose of 0.5 mg/kg in rat sarcomas (above), the ratio
of the toxic dose of placebo spheres to the effective dose of adriamycin
spheres is 111:1. This emphasizes the safety of albumin microspheres
as drug carriers. Albumin is also safe from the standpoint of allergic
reactions. None of the 50 patients who received serial injections of
larger (embolizing) spheres over a course of 3 weeks to 12 months

experienced acute allergic reactions [65]. However, one property of
albumin makes it suboptimal as a matrix material, namely its tendency
to become phagocytized and cleared from target sites within 8 to 16 hr
of localization [7,65-67]. This functionally limits the interval of controlled drug release that can be achieved in vivo. A reasonable means
of overcoming this problem is to use more inert materials, such as the
biodegradable polymeric metabolites, poly-L-lactic and polyglycolic
acids. When injected subcutaneously in appropriate crystalline forms,
these materials remain at the original site for months to years [68].

Although magnetic adriamycin spheres have reached an advanced
stage of animal testing, they have not yet progressed to human trials.
Hesitancy has resulted from a number of considerations: suboptimal
magnetic field design; difficulty in obtaining large quantities of human
serum albumin that are free of viral biohazards and have uniform drug
loading capacities from batch to batch; practical problems of mass producing the microspheres, controlling particle diameters, and quality
controlling the multiple (apparently artifactual) adriamycin metabolites
generated by the in vitro digestion of spheres used in drug balance
studies (see Section III.G); problems of moderate aggregation encountered with hydrophobic spheres; unattractiveness of long-term magnetite deposition at target sites; inappropriateness of the first large-
animal model with respect to drug susceptibility and microsphere accessibility to subregions of tumor; local tissue toxicities observed in dogs
but not observed in rats—apparently resulting from greater heterogeneity of microsphere size and failure to wash away the surface (burst
release) drug prior to injection; the general perception (common to
all new drug evaluations) that arterially targeted adriamycin must be
effective on its own (i.e., without supplementation by other indicated
routes of administration); and the recognition that commercial returns
would be limited for such a high-technology approach to drug targeting. All these objections except for the limited deposition of ferromagnetite and the technical nature of the approach can be resolved by
appropriate magnet design, microsphere materials, scaleup procedures,
and administration protocols. The incentive for proceeding is that a
major improvement in drug localization can be achieved relative to other
methods of delivery, and life-threatening malignancies may be cured
by existing but toxic agents.

Amphotericin B Microspheres

Invasive pulmonary aspergillosis is a life-threatening condition
in neutropenic and immunocompromised patients. The spread of *Aspergillus* fungi from primary sites of deep infection (principally lung) to
the brain, liver, spleen, and other organs causes the death of several
patients each year in most major medical centers. Amphotericin B
(AMB) remains the treatment of choice [69], however, it produces

frequent, serious side effects. The major one, nephrotoxicity, requires occasional interruption of systemic therapy [70]. Since alternative drugs are less effective, the result is compromised patient survival. Because of the clinical need for an AMB formulation that spares the kidney, the author and co-workers have entrapped AMB in albumin-magnetite spheres for targeting to lung (or brain) and reticuloendothelial organs [6]. This was accomplished by complexing AMB to the water-soluble adductor, γ-cyclodextrin (CD), entrapping AMB-CD in fatty-acid-free alubmin-magnetite spheres, and heating them briefly to 135°C. To test for drug entrapment and controlled release, spheres were suspended at 10 mg/ml in phosphate-buffered saline and washed once (with magnetic separation) to remove a minor surface component of AMB. Spheres were resuspended in fresh buffered saline and either bioassayed immediately or incubated in saline, washed, and resuspended for delayed bioassay, to determine how much AMB remained entrapped at various times. Bioassays were performed with an AMB-sensitive strain of *Candida albicans*. This gave reliable quantificaiton of growth inhibition at 24 hr (Fig. 6). Although microspheres were restricted to the precut wells, they were surrounded by large zones of growth inhibition. This indicates that AMB-CD (or AMB-CD-albumin) is released in a diffusible form that penetrates into the 1.7% agar for distances of greater than 7 mm. This has important implications for clinical treatment because it indicates that when AMB-CD is released in vivo, it should be capable of penetrating into the microthrombi induced by *Aspergillus* organisms [71].

To compare the gel penetration of AMB-CD to that of native AMB and Fungizone (AMB deoxycholate), each formulation was plated at a supramaximal concentration of 200 µg per well and the areas of growth inhibition quantified (Table 3). These results show that AMB-CD penetrates substantially farther than AMB or Fungizone. Hence, microsphere AMB-CD should have the additional therapeutic advantage of penetrating lesional gels. The general importance of this property is emphasized by a recent report indicating that the second major barrier for intravenously administered antimicrobials is lesional glycocalyx produced by microorganisms [20]. The present approach of modifying "sticky" drugs to form "slippery" drug adducts is gaining substantial attention in new drug formulations. AMB is released from the present microspheres at a half-time exceeding 24 hr (see Fig. 6). Bioactive drug is detectable in the spheres for up to 5 days of incubation. Hence, controlled bioavailability is compatible with potent antifungal activity.

Pilot experiments were conducted to test the acute pulmonary toxicity of AMB-CD microspheres in CBA mice [6]. The spheres were injected intravenously and captured magnetically (0.55 T field) in target lung at numbers designed to deliver a supratherapeutic dose to lung tissue (equivalent to 5 mg/kg of free AMB). To put this in perspective, the effective dose of magnetically targeted AMB is 0.2 mg/kg.

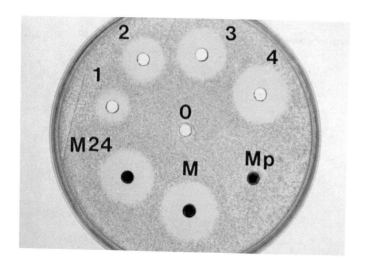

Fig. 6 Bacteriological plate (Mueller-Hinton, 1.7% agar) showing inhibition of *Candida albicans* growth by amphotericin B microspheres. Plates were incubated for 24 hr at 37°C. Samples 1-4, standards of 1:1 γ-cyclodextrin-AMB, added as follows (μg/well): 1.3×10^{-2}, 3.5×10^{-2}, 7×10^{-2}, 1.4×10^{-1}; sample 0, cyclodextrin alone at a concentration equal to that in the top cyclodextrin-AMB standard; sample M, Fe_3O_4 fatty-acid-free human albumin microspheres containing 1:1 γ-cyclodextrin-AMB, plated immediately after rapid washing and magnetic recovery of the controlled release spheres; sample M24, same as M, except that the washed spheres were incubated in phosphate-buffered saline for 24 hr at 37°C, recovered by centrifugation at 1750 g for 15 min, and plated at the same concentration as M. Placebo microspheres (Mp) were formulated as in M, except without AMB. Drug values for M and M24 were read from a standard curve (not shown) of areas generated by inhibition standards 1 to 4, above. The ratio of M24/M = $(1.2 \times 10^{-1} \mu g/1.8 \times 10^{-1} \mu g) = 0.67$. Hence, the $t_{1/2}$ for release of AMB release in physiological saline is greater than 24 hr. (From Ref. 6.)

Mice were sacrificed at 70 min, based on the time required for endothelial toxicity to develop after administering f-met-leu-phe (see Chemoattractant Microspheres, below). Light microscopic analysis revealed homogeneous lung targeting and showed no evidence of septal edema, inflammation, or hemorrhage. At 70 min, the majority of spheres had migrated through endothelial cells into the interstitium. However, in isolated foci, clusters of spheres remained in the capillary walls. Electron micrographs representative of these foci are shown in Fig. 7. The

TABLE 3 Penetration of Amphotericin B and Amphotericin B Adducts into Mueller-Hinton Bacteriological Agar[a]

Group[b]	Area of growth inhibition (mean ± 1 SD)[c]	P value[d]
Amphotericin B	4.91 ± 0.34	(> 0.50)
Amphotericin B- deoxycholate (Fungizone)	4.97 ± 0.24	< 0.001
Amphotericin B- cyclodextrin (1:1)	6.65 ± 0.22	< 0.001

[a]Agar content 1.7% (w/v).
[b]Quantity of amphotericin B = 200 µg added in 20 µl per well.
[c]Of Candida albicans.
[d]Newman-Keuls multiple comparison test (n = 7).

endothelium containing AMB-CD spheres revealed no evidence of the vesiculation, membrane redundancy, vacuolation, or white cell adherence characteristic of acute toxicity. Hence, controlled release of AMB is sufficient to protect host cells from the acute toxic effects of a supratherapeutic dose. Efficacy studies are pending on immunosuppressed mice with experimental pulmonary aspergillosis. If developed for human use, AMB microspheres could also have an important application in cancer treatment because of AMB's membrane-directed potentiation of standard chemotherapeutic agents [72].

Biomodulators

As summarized by Herberman [73], biological response modifiers (BRMs) alter host, tumor, and microbial responses in a wide variety of ways, which include augmenting host effector mechanisms directed against tumor cells (or microorganisms), decreasing host responses that interfere with tumor resistance, adding to the quantity of endogenous effector molecules or redirecting their sites and duration of action, augmenting tumor sensitivity to host cells, redifferentiating tumor cells, and increasing host tolerance of conventional cancer treatments (especially chemotherapy and radiotherapy). This section focuses on the BRMs involved in white cell function.

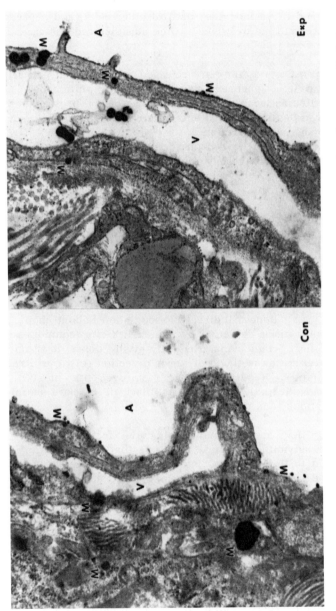

Fig. 7 Electron micrograph (magnified ×15,000) of CBA mouse lung 70 min after magnetic intravenous targeting of microspheres (M); V = vascular space, A = airspace. In the experimental group (Exp), targeted Fe_3O_4 fatty-acid-free human albumin microspheres contained 1:1 γ-cyclodextrin-AMB (see text for injected dose). In the control group (Con), targeted placebo microspheres were formulated as in Exp, except without AMB. (From Ref. 6.)

There are two major classes of agents, indirect and direct [73]. Indirect agents are immunomodulators, such as the interferons (α, β, and γ), interleukins (1 to 4), and white cell chemoattractant/activator peptides. Indirect BRMs act by enhancing the responses of monocytes, macrophages, T and B lymphocytes, natural killer cells, and neutrophils. These agents have multiple drawbacks when administered systemically [6,73].

1. In the natural state, they are released and degraded primarily within the local tissue compartment or by immigrating white cells. Hence, they function as local hormones, much as do the prostaglandins.
2. Being large peptides or proteins, their tissue access is poor following intravenous administration.
3. The two agents that have been adequately studied (interleukins 1 and 2) are cleared extremely rapidly from the plasma ($t_{1/2}$ <5 min) [25]. Consequently, very high doses are required, and these result in severe side effects (see Section on Interleukin 2 Microspheres, below).
4. Indirect BRMs have pleotropic effects because many cell types exhibit receptors or respond secondarily to mediators produced by receptor-positive cells.
5. There is an upper limit to the number of host cells that can be recruited by indirect BRMs. For muramyl peptides this limit is such that if the entire body store of monocytes were recruited under optimal conditions, it could eradicate only about 1 to 2 g of a typical malignant tumor [74]. Hence, indirect biomodulation fails at about the limits of present tumor detection by standard X-ray techniques. Of course, these limits could be improved by giving monocyte transfusions or using higher resolution methods of tumor detection (e.g., contrast-enhanced MR imaging). Regardless of such improvements, inherent biological limits make it likely that indirect BRMs will be more useful for treating infections than tumors [74].

Direct-acting BRMs are the final lymphocyte effector molecules [73]. A potential advantage of these agents is that there is no inherent upper limit to their pharmacological effects. Three major examples of direct BRMs are antibodies, lymphotoxin, and tumor necrosis factor (TNF, also called cachetin) [75]. TNF is highly effective at reducing human tumor growth in nude (athymic) mice [76-77]. However, when administered systemically in rats, TNF is exceedingly toxic and pleotropic. It is thought to be the common effector molecule in endotoxin shock [78]. In this role, TNF stimulates endothelial secretion of procoagulant factor, activates polymorphonuclear leukocytes, induces diffuse pulmonary inflammation and hemorrhage, causes ischemic and hemorrhagic lesions of the gastrointestinal tract, and produces acute renal tubular necrosis. Minute doses are lethal in rats within hours of intravenous injection. Hence, despite its efficacy, TNF is so toxic that it is extremely difficult to carry out clinical trials with systemically administered agent.

Based on discussions between the author and scientific represen-tatives of several biotechnology firms, the present consensus is that, due to the lability, toxicity, and unfavorable biodistribution of the newly developed recombinant BRMs, approximately 40 to 60% of them will require microencapsulation, site-specific targeting, and controlled release in target tissues. This provides a strong rationale for the continued development of magnetic drug targeting. An important ex-ception to this general problem is erythropoietin. It gains access to the bone marrow by passing through sinusoidal endothelium and acts directly to stimulate erythropoiesis. Even though it induces the circu-lation of nucleated erythrocytes, this appears to have no untoward side effects.

Chemoattractant Microspheres

Neutrophil chemoattractant, f-met-leu-phe, was selected as the first biomodulator for magnetic targeting [8] because it is lethal when administered freely in the circulation at concentrations above 2×10^{-7} M, it requires local delivery to modulate local inflammation, and it is a small, bacterially derived peptide that is stable to microsphere en-trapment. For optimal effects in vivo, the f-met-leu-phe content and release rates of spheres were designed to be 0.65% (by weight) and 20 min ($t_{1/2}$), respectively. Animal testing was carried out in the recently developed rat lung model of Section III.D [8]. Due to the low total dose of microsphere f-met-leu-phe (15.7 μg/kg), high efficiency of pulmonary targeting (25% of the injected dose), and rapid reticuloendo-thelial clearance of untargeted agent (10 min), free blood levels re-mained below 1.9×10^{-8} M [8]. This is 10 times lower than the acute LD_{50} concentration. Within target lung, the controlled release and hy-drophobic nature of f-met-leu-phe combined to facilitate cell-membrane binding. This formed a second tissue reservoir of peptide as it was released from the spheres. Consequently, total tissue levels remained nearly constant over the posttargeting interval of 5 to 70 min, at 2.9 $\times 10^{-6}$ M and 2.7×10^{-6} M, respectively [8] (150 times higher than the peak free plasma concentration). These results illustrate the gen-eral finding that free plasma levels of microsphere-entrapped agents are kept at least 100 times lower than the total levels in target tissues.

Locally released f-met-leu-phe broadcasts an attractant signal to circulating neutrophils that migrate out of adjacent arterioles and capil-laries into lung interstitium. When the peptide dose is adjusted to produce tissue levels above about 3.3×10^{-8} M, localized neutrophils are activated to release O_2^- and lysosomal enzymes [8,9,23]. This produces targeted acute inflammation and edema. When the injected dose is lowered by half an order of magnitude, chemoattraction occurs without widespread neutrophil activation [6]. This transition correlates with in vitro findings, which indicate that neutrophils undergo directional movement in the presence of low peptide concentrations but cease to move and initiate effector functions in the presence of low peptide concentrations but cease to move and initiate effector functions in the presence of higher concentrations [23]. Targeted f-met-leu-phe also attracts alveolar macrophages [6,9]. These cells engulf almost all the excess microsphere material that has passed across alveolar septa into the small air spaces. By this means, excess peptide is detoxified and removed in the sputum.

Microsphere f-met-leu-phe has potential uses both in disease modeling and clinical therapy. In pulmonary medicine, it could be used as (a) an experimental method to test new agents that block neutrophil degradation of lung elastin in smokers, (b) a means to study the contribution of acute alveolar damage to adult-type respiratory distress syndrome (ARDS), and (c) an adjuvant method to treat patients with invasive pulmonary aspergillosis. The last use is based on the rationale that hyphal forms of *Aspergillus fumigatus*, which predominate in established pulmonary infections, are killed by locally generated neutrophil products [79]. Nonpulmonary applications of f-met-leu-phe spheres include the induction of acute arthritis, nephritis, and other organ-specific models of inflammation, in which it is important to avoid the systemic effects of circulating initiators (e.g., cobra venom factor and zymosan-activated serum) [80,81].

Although f-met-leu-phe produces only modest chemoattraction of monocytes and macrophages, its C-methyl ester derivative, f-met-leu-phe-M, has a 1000-fold greater specificity for mononuclear cells [82]. Microspheres of f-met-leu-phe-M might be useful as an adjuvant treatment in carefully selected cancer patients. Based on the considerations of tumor-host imbalance discussed above [74], the most appropriate use would be for treatment of microscopic tumor foci suspected to remain at the margins of surgically resectable tumors. Such a use is based on the rationale that intralesional and marginal macrophages show little activity in tumoricidal assays. This is thought to result from the effects of locally released suppressors (prostaglandin E_2 and other incompletely identified natural products) that impair local cellular resistance [83].

Magnetic Neutrophils

In certain clinical disorders, an indirect approach of targeting white cells by chemoattraction may not work due to the presence in patient sera of chemotactic factor inactivators [84] and neutrophil-directed inhibitors of chemotaxis [58]. These disorders include Hodgkin's disease, chronic lymphocytic leukemia, sarcoidosis, alcoholic cirrhosis, hemodialysis, Chron's disease, and severe bacterial infections (in particular, abdominal abscesses with neutrophil anergy). Although failure of chemotaxis is not observed in all patients or at all times, when such complications occur, they are life threatening. Hence, the author and co-workers have developed a means of making neutrophils ingest Fe_3O_4 so that they can be targeted directly to sites of severe infection [6].

Normal human blood was processed to enrich for granulocytes and eliminate erythrocytes [86]. The enriched fraction was adhered to specially treated culture plates that allowed subsequent cellular detachment with minimal effects on neutrophil function [6]. Nonadherent cells (primarily lymphocytes) were discarded. Magnetite particles, 10 to 15 nm in size, were opsonized with human IgG to facilitate neutophil binding and ingestion via Fc surface receptors. The adherent cells (granulocytes and monocytes) were allowed to ingest opsonized magnetite for 60 min, after which excess particles were washed away. Magnetized cells were detached by gentle agitation and suspended in saline for testing. The granulocytes in this suspension retained 80% of their native functional activity, as assessed by chemiluminescence assays for zymosan stimulation of O_2^- [6]. Magnetite ingestion was assessed in two ways: by cytological visualization using a Prussian blue iron stain [6,8] and by magnetic resonance relaxation methods [6]. Cytologically, the predominant cell type was neutrophilic, and about 60% of the magnetite iron was located intracellularly and 40% on the cell surface. By magnetic resonance assessment (see Carrier Localization, under Section III.E), each adherent cell carried between 7 and 20 pg of magnetite (range for three donor preparations) [6]. This was equivalent to 0.8 to 2.2% Fe_3O_4 (wet weight). Although we predicted these contents would be too low for magnetic capture in vivo (with a 0.55 T field), significant magnetic localization was observed, as described below.

Lung targeting was performed by injecting 0.5 to 1.0×10^6 adherent cells intravenously into mice that had been made neutropenic with methotrexate [6]. This pretreatment reduced the animals' own white blood cells to such low numbers that all the neutrophils quantified in lung sections were donor cells. For lung capture, the magnet was held next to the right chest wall for 20 min postinjection. Mice were sacrificed at 40 min and their lungs inflated to constant size with intratracheal formalin. Neutrophils and associated magnetite particles were quantified morphometrically, using a double histochemical stain developed to identify neutrophils and magnetite in the same tissue section [8]. The results are shown in Table 4.

Magnetic localization increased neutrophil numbers in target lung by a multiple of 2.6. Furthermore, these neutrophils remained responsive to intra-alveolar f-met-leu-phe. This was documented by three morphologic observations: neutrophil migration from initial intravascu-

TABLE 4 Neutrophil Localization in Target Lung at
40 Min

Magnetite in cells	Magnet over target lung[a]	Cells per square centimeter[b]
No	No	33.4 ± 2.3
Yes	No	32.0 ± 6.4
Yes	Yes	84.0 ± 7.2

[a]0.55 T field; 0.01 T/mm gradient over target lung.
[b]Each section was 5 μm thick; cells stained histo-
chemically for neutrophil esterase + magnetite iron,
as described in the text (n = 5).
Source: From Ref. 6.

lar sites into lung alveoli, septal edema caused by neutrophil O_2^-, and
neutrophil degranulation (assessed by the release of intracellular
magnetite) [6].

Why did such a low neutrophil content of Fe_3O_4 allow these cells
to become captured magnetically against microvascular flow forces?
Gamma camera [87] and histological images [6] of lungs at 2, 20, and
40 min after injection provide the answer. The in vitro processing
required for granulocyte isolation produced minimal alterations in neutrophil membranes. This caused the cells to become "sticky" and undergo transient bioadhesion to pulmonary vascular endothelium. Such
adhesion occurred for all categories of neutrophils (with or without
magnetite) and lasted for less than 20 min [6,87]. Hence, the neutrophils that remained in target lung at 40 min were actually captured by
two mechanisms: cellular adhesion, followed by magnetic retention.
These results show that functional neutrophils can be targeted directly
by magnetic means [6]. Of equal importance, they indicate that it
may be possible to target inert microspheres by bioadhesion alone [6,9].

Interleukin 2 Microspheres

Interleukin 2 (IL-2) is a 15,000 MW glycoprotein made by activated
T lymphocytes that increases cellular immune repsonses to certain tumors and infections [26]. IL-2 activates multiple cell types, including
T helper cells, cytotoxic T lymphocytes, natural killer (NK) cells,
and probably macrophages [26,73]. It is an appropriate molecule for
drug development because it is relatively stable, active in mice as well
as in man, and available in large quantities as a recombinant gene product. High doses of IL-2 have mediated the regression of established

pulmonary and hepatic metastases in several murine tumors [88] and disseminated human melanomas and renal cell carcinomas that were unresponsive to conventional therapy [26]. A marked lymphocytic infiltrate of Leu 4+, Leu 2+, and Dr(+) cells has been documented in one case of regressing human melanoma [26]. Despite these promising initial results, tumor treatment is fraught with difficulties. IL-2 is cleared from the plasma in 5 min [25]. Consequently, as much as 3 million units per kilogram must be administered for each round of therapy. Two or more rounds may be required for tumor control, at a cost of $30,000 to $100,000 per round. High-dose therapy produces severe side effects, including anemia and thrombocytopenia (requiring red cell and platelet transfusions), fever, hypotension, gastritis, azotemia, jaundice, skin eruptions, malaise, and confusion [89]. IL-2 also induces a capillary leak syndrome, which can lead to severe, occasionally fatal pulmonary edema and ascites [26,89].

Because of these almost unacceptable limitations on systemic administration, the author and co-workers have developed a controlled release, microsphere form of IL-2 that is adaptable for magnetic targeting to tumors and passive localization in the lung or bone marrow (with moderate selectivity for each target, based on microsphere size) [6]. In vitro bioassays of drug release were performed with the IL-2-responsive CTLL-2 cell line. By stabilizing the carrier matrix, release half-times of up to 42 min have been achieved, and longer times are anticipated.

A targetable, controlled release form of IL-2 would allow localization in tumors and infections in a similar fashion as occurs for lymphocyte-mediated delivery and would overcome the prohibitive cost of systemic administration. It has been suggested that IL-2's capacity to increase capillary permeability might provide the additional advantage of increasing monoclonal antibody access to tumors. However, for this to be practical, permeability changes would have to be restricted to the tumor rather than induced systemically, as occurs with free IL-2 (D. F. Ranney and P. Antich, work in progress). This is because antibodies gain access to tissues by passive diffusion (ultrafiltration) wherever there is increased microvascular permeability. If this occurred in the liver and lungs (established sites of IL-2 induced capillary leak), as well as in tumor, the tissue localization of subsequently administered antibody would be nonselective, and its tumor efficacy would be impaired. Hence, the preferred method of IL-2 delivery is one that targets it to tumor or bone marrow (the major source of IL-2-responsive precursor cells). Studies are in progress to test the in vivo effects of IL-2 entrapped in tumor-selective magnetic microspheres and bone-marrow-selective nonmagnetic nanospheres (D. F. Ranney, H. Huffaker, M. Tutt, V. Kumar, and M. Bennett, unpublished studies).

Biophysical Agents

Physical modulation of tumor growth has been approached in a number of ways, including resection, cautery, and cryotherapy; regional embolization (usually combined with chemotherapy as chemoembolization); brachytherapy (embolization with radioisotopic spheres); and hyperthermia. The procedures other than hyperthermia are reviewed extensively in the surgical and radiological literature and will not be covered here.

Hyperthermia is a potentially important adjuvant technique for treating cancer, especially superficial tumors. It is produced as a by-product of inflammation by white blood cells. This is amenable to magnetic amplification by white cell chemoattractants and neutrophils (see above). At present, clinical hyperthermia is produced by either contact heating or exposure to microwave, radiofrequency, or ultrasonic energy [90]. The rationale for hyperthermia is based on thermocouple measurements, which indicate that tumor tissue can be heated more efficiently than surrounding normal tissue [91]. This is thought to result from sluggish perfusion in the less viable, central cores of solid tumors. These regions are frequently hypooxygenated and hence, less susceptible to ionizing radiation. Consequently, hyperthermia synergizes with standard radiation therapy. In small primary tumors, metastatic nodules, and the perimeters of large tumors, perfusion may be greater than in normal tissue [90,91]. Such regions might benefit from accentuated heating by magnetic microsphere techniques. This is based on the capacity of magnetic susceptor materials to couple with oscillating external magnetic fields and generate heat [90]. Magnetic spheres have been injected by needle into the capsular regions of superficial tumors [90,92] and could also be captured magnetically in deep tumors following intra-arterial injection [6,9,30-32,46,47,64]. Both methods deposit spheres preferentially in the vascularized regions of tumors where heat dissipation is most rapid. It is hoped that selective augmentation of hyperthermia would result and compensate for differential heat loss.

To produce hysteresis heating under clinical conditions, susceptor materials must undergo magnetization reversal (open-type hysteresis loop) at the relatively low field strength-frequency products that are required to minimize eddy current heating and nerve-muscle activation (shock) [90]. The hysteresis component of heating is given by the following general equation [90]:

$$P = f \oint H \, dB$$

where
P = heat (over time and volume)
f = frequency of the applied field

$\oint$ = integral over the hysteresis loop
H = magnetic field strength
dB = derivative of the magnetic induction

A safe upper limit for the coercive field is 8 kA/m [90].
To date, the microspheres most extensively tested in hysteresis
heating are ones prepared by Corning Glass Works [90,92]. The initial
spheres [90] comprised a fine-grained magnetic phase of lithium ferrite,
which was microencapsulated and stabilized in a glass-ceramic matrix.
They had an overall dimension of 4.5 μm, a specific gravity of 3.5
g/cm^3, and a magnetization ranging from 181 × 10^7 to 226 × 10^7 T/kg·m^3,
depending on the composition and dispersal of lithium-ferrite. This
prototype material did not exhibit optimal heating characteristics at
low fields. Consequently, preliminary in vivo tests were carried out
at 10 kHz using a moderately high magnetic field of 43.8 kA/m [90].
The biological field frequency constraint was overcome by using a
mouse limb model in which the animals were anesthetized with ketamine
and tissue volumes were kept low. The oscillating field was generated
by a water-cooled, six-turn copper tubing (inductance of 4.3 H), powered by a 30 W, 10 kHz generator. Microspheres were injected around
the growing perimeters of subcutaneous Meth-A sarcomas at a tissue
dose of 0.75 g/cm^3 [90]. By X-ray analysis, spheres remained immo-
bilized at the site for at least 8 days. By thermocouple analysis, temperature increments of 12, 14, and 17.5°C were achieved in microsphere-
injected tumors after 5, 10, and 60 min of hysteresis, respectively.
This compared with 0, 0, and 4°C rises for uninjected tumors. Microsphere amplification of heating occurred only at the exact zone of ceramic implantation.

Limited testing of antitumor efficacy has been carried out with
modified glass-ceramic spheres containing Fe$_2$O$_3$. These were implanted
subcutaneously around weakly antigenic adenocarcinomas of the breast
(BW10232), which were grown in the inguinal regions of C57Bl/6J mice
[92]. A 10 kHz hysteresis field of 0.05 T was applied. This achieved
sufficient heating (43.5°C maximum temperature) to produce tumor
growth delay and complete remission in 50% and 12% of the animals,
respectively (n = 33). None of the control mice (which received spheres
alone or were exposed to the field alone) had a significant tumor response. These results indicate that it may be possible to achieve clinically relevant temperatures of 42.5°C in human tissues by hysteresis
methods. However, more extensive studies of efficacy and toxicity
will be required to properly evaluate the materials and field parameters.
Microspheres with more susceptible materials and larger or more con-
densed magnetic domains will be required to reduce total tissue doses.
It has not yet been reported whether transarterial magnetic targeting
can produce the required tumor concentrations of susceptor spheres
at acceptable systemic doses.

Diagnostic Agents

In special situations, it may be necessary to localize diagnostic agents selectively in nonreticuloendothelial organs. These include cases in which systemic toxicity is high (e.g., fluorodeoxyglucose), the dose required to obtain adequate sensitivity is high (e.g., enhancement of MR images and spectra), the target tissue requires MR relaxation "marking" with magnetic materials (e.g., to confirm tissue locations from which metabolic spectra were obtained), and agent access to tissue is impeded (e.g., neuropeptides and neurotransmitters). Ferromagnetic spheres can provide the highly selective targeting required in these instances.

G. Regulatory Considerations

Recent appreciation of the differences in targeting efficiencies among drug carriers should lead to more appropriate regulatory guidelines for each carrier. For example, the guidelines which require that 90% of an entrapped agent be recovered from its carrier in drug balance studies could be modified slightly for magnetic microspheres because the total dose of drug is only 10% of that for free drug. Such an appropriate change would eliminate the need for chemical and enzymatic digestion of spheres, as is presently required to recover 90% of the drug. (Only about 85% is spontaneously released from the albumin matrix as low molecular weight species.) Such digestion produces artificial metabolites that are not encountered in vivo but whose levels must be held within narrow limits from batch to batch to satisfy quality control requirements. Hence, in evaluating drug delivery, it is important to remember that the fractions of injected drug that are localized by various methods in nonreticuloendothelial target sites are as follows: magnetic microspheres, 25 to 50%; monoclonal antibodies, 2 to 7% (at low doses without prior sensitization); liposomes and standard microspheres, 0.1 to 1%; and standard drugs, 0.001 to 0.01%. For a more extensive review of microspheres and drug therapy, the reader is referred to the referenced text [93].

IV. MAGNETIC MODULATION OF DRUG RELEASE FROM IMPLANTED POLYMERS

Polymeric drug implants in the form of microspheres, rectangular slabs, and zero-order hemispheric castings have received recent attention as devices for controlled release over months to years. Potential agents include contraceptives, insulin and other peptide hormones, antiarrhythmics, nitrites, beta blockers, and antitumor drugs [94-98]. A long-standing limitation of simple implants was that their release rates generally decreased with time, and at best, remained constant until the supply of drug was exhausted. One way that has been devised to solve this problem is the addition of ferromagnetic beads to the polymer matrix and application of a slowly oscillating (5-15 Hz) magnetic field at the site of implantation. Depending on the type and physical form of polymer and drug, this method allows release rates to be incremented by a factor of up to 30. These systems for magnetic modulation were initially devised and most of the subsequent studies published by Langer et al. [99].

The most extensively studied matrix is ethylene vinyl acetate copolymer (EVAc), with others being polyvinyl alcohol (PVA) and polymeric hydroxyethyl methacrylate (polyHEMA) [94-100]. As obtained commercially, these materials must be washed extensively at 37°C in water, 95% ethanol, and absolute ethanol, to remove impurities that cause mild inflammation in vivo. Entrapped proteins diffuse relatively rapidly out of polyHEMA, less rapidly from PVA, and slowly from EVAc [94-100]. The agent most extensively tested is bovine serum albumin; however, comparable release kinetics have been reported for microparticulate insulin [96,97]. As is observed for most polymers, burst release occurs over the first few hours of incubation, after which the spontaneous release rate plateaus and then gradually declines [94].

Polymer matrices have been prepared by either casting in solvent (the usual method) or sintering. Solvent casting gives slower release rates. Typically, this is carried out by dissolving washed EVAc at a 10% concentration in dichloromethane [94,96,99]. Powdered drug is mixed into 10 ml of polymer solution, and the mixture is poured quickly into a leveled glass mold that has been cooled to dry-ice temperature. Immediately, 1.4 mm magnetic steel beads are dropped into the mixture using a loading device that deposits 263 beads at 3 mm spacing across a 7 × 7 × 0.5 cm slab [99]. To completely seal the beads, a top layer of polymer-drug is added 30 sec later. The slab is allowed to solidify for an additional 10 min and then is transferred to -20°C for drying over 48 hr. Casting and drying at low temperatures prevent migration of the drug powder and beads. (Magnetic beads are obtained from Ultraspheres, Inc. (Marie, Michigan), and consist of 79.17% iron, 17% chromium, 1% carbon, 1% manganese, 1% silicone, 0.75% molybdenum, 0.4% phosphorus, and 0.4% sulfur) [94]. The alternative method of sintering is performed by freezing finely powdered EVAc in liquid nitrogen, grinding and sizing the resulting particles to 300 μm or less, adding the drug, and compressing the mixture to 20,000 psi for 30 min in a Carver hydraulic press [96]. This produces individual disks 5 mm in diameter and 3 mm thick.

Spontaneous drug release is influenced by the following factors: (a) drug solubility (e.g., sodium insulin is released faster than zinc insulin), (b) the size of drug particles (e.g., increases in particle diameter from 75 to 425 μm doubles or triples the release rate), (c)

the proportion of drug to polymer (e.g., increases in the fractional
weight of insulin from 20% to 50% doubles or triples the release rate),
and (d) the porosity of the polymer matrix [94,96].

Modulation of drug release has been reported only for extracorporeal permanent magnets. Alternating fields have been applied by using
a single magnet attached to a carousel that revolves just beneath the
multiple specimen holder [100] and by attaching multiple magnets to a
reciprocating rocker arm, which approaches the multispecimen holder
from below [99]. In both cases, angular torque is placed on the magnetic beads. This somewhat complicates the analysis of bead movement
relative to that which would apply to a univectorial force. Electron
micrographs of magnetically triggered and control polymers indicate
that the principal mechanism of release modulation involves deformation
of the matrix adjacent to each bead. This results in "squeezing" of
entrapped drug powder through the tortuous channels created during
casting. These channels usually connect to all external surfaces of
the slab. An exception to this is the coated hemispheric casting, from
which drug is allowed to escape only through a single hole drilled at
the base of the hemisphere. Typically, magnetic triggering is carried
out for several hours followed by a similar interval of spontaneous
(basal) release. Modulation increases with both the strength and frequency of the field [95]. For example, the ratio of magnetic to basal
release of bovine serum albumin from EVAc increases from 1.4 to 3.0
as the field is increased from 0.09 to 0.18 T, and from 1 to 5.5 as the
frequency is increased from zero to 11 Hz [95].

Magnetic implants have several potential advantages over programmable pumps. They minimize the complexity and size of the device.
Drug is stored as a dry powder rather than a solution. Hence, it occupies a smaller volume and retains potency longer than it might in the
fluid reservoir of a mechanical pump. Magnetic implants are also relatively inexpensive, and hence, are suitable for large-scale animal studies. Their major problem is irreproducibility of drug release, both
from different pellets in the same magnetic tirggering interval and
from a single pellet in sequential triggering intervals. Standard deviations of 25 to 70% are commonly observed. An additional problem is
that the response to magnetic modulation decreases progressively with
time. The third difficulty is that a new device must be surgically implanted each time an old one expires, whereas with programmable
pumps, the reservoir can be refilled by percutaneous injection. It
might be possible to achieve improved reproducibility of magnetic modulation by using electromagnets to eliminate angular torque and employing precision methods to drill the exit holes in hemispheric implants.
Still, it is probable that magnetic polymers will find their major applications in experimental animals rather than humans.

V. MAGNETICALLY PROGRAMMABLE INFUSION PUMPS

Magnetic methods are in widespread use for external programming of cardiac pacemakers. The same technique has been successfully applied to an implantable infusion pump (P. Tarjan, personal communication). Although such pumps were developed to a prototype stage, the newer method of radiofrequency (rf) signaling has superseded the magnetic approach because of greater programming flexibility and bidirectional transmission capability. For at least one type of rf-programmable pump (Drug Administration System, Medtronic, Inc., Minneapolis), the receiver is initially switched to a programmable mode by a permanent magnet located in the extracorporeal programming head [101]. Reprogramming occurs only if the magnetic field and a recognizable rf pulse sequence are presented simultaneously. This particular pump has reached the stage of investigational testing in humans, and premarket approval is expected in the near future.

Experimental applications of programmable pumps have included continuous, time-pulsed or circadian infusion of antitumor agents into the systemic and portal veins [102,103]; control of pain in cancer patients by intrathecal or epidural infusion of morphine [104]; and treatment of motor spacticity in multiple sclerosis with intraspinal infusion of baclofen (a drug that binds γ-ammobutyric acid receptors) [105]. Programmable pumps have several advantages over polymeric implants. Drug output can be increased to compensate for biological tolerance to pain medications; catheter tips can be inserted into very small spaces or vessels where polymer slabs and even injectable microspheres will not fit; pump reservoirs require infrequent filling—only once every 2 to 6 weeks depending on drug stability [101-103]; and the pumps are designed to run for up to 2 years on their original batteries [101-103]. Potential disadvantages include the requirement for drug stability in solution at 37°C, relatively high expense, bulkiness of the central pump unit, failure rates of up to 12% [104], occasional plugging of the outflow catheter [101,104], and minor difficulty in accessing the injection port. Despite these problems, with continued improvements in design, programmable pumps appear to have important future applications in clinical drug delivery.

VI. SUMMARY AND PERSPECTIVE

For all the devices discussed in this chapter, magnetics can be viewed as serving a common function of opening the initial gate of a multibarrier or multistep drug delivery process. Indeed, the only indications for using magnetics are to achieve noninvasive effects that require force acting at a distance on relatively simple operations.

Magnetic drug targeting is a technologically involved but highly efficient means of localizing toxic or labile pharmaceuticals in single or multiple regional sites. For about 40 to 60% of the new peptide and recombinant protein biopharmaceuticals, it is the only way at present to localize 25 to 50% of the injected dose in nonreticuloendothelial target tissues and thereby achieve adequate drug levels, control bioavailability within the tissue, localize the effects of agents that must act as tissue-constrained hormones, and avoid toxic blood levels during targeting. Experimental animal testing has proceeded to the point where it is possible to (a) evaluate carrier localization and drug effects by noninvasive, high-resolution MR methods; (b) build the improved magnets required to obtain homogeneous carrier deposition across the 30 to 40 cm dimensions of human body cavities; (c) supplement transarterial magnetic targeting with intrameduallary drug administration to treat bony as well as soft tissue components of osteogenic sarcomas; and (d) institute the minor modifications in regulatory guidelines indicated for carriers that reduce total body drug doses by a factor of 10. Still, if clinical applications are approved, they will be limited to life-threatening diseases and specialized centers. The major impact of magnetic targeting would probably occur in the next 25 years. By that time, it is likely that drugs, prodrugs, and bioadhesion carriers with high selectivities and targeting efficiencies for specifically diseased tissues will have been developed. A side benefit of research on magnetic targeting is the recent elucidation that it actually works by two mechanisms: magnetic capture plus bioadhesion to microvascular endothelium. This implies that it should be possible to target drug carriers by bioadhesion alone. Such targeting may become feasible within the next 5 years for physiological modulation of tissues with normal endothelium; for bioadhesion targeting to be applicable to most pathological disorders, however, more needs to be learned about the endothelial changes that accompany specific clinical diseases.

Magnetic modulation of drug release from polymeric implants is an ingenious approach devised to compensate for the decay in drug release that occurs over time. This method simultaneously minimizes the cost, size, and complexity of implanted devices. Unfortunately, several factors have compromised the clinical utility of such implants: the irreproducibility of magnetic modulation, the decrement of magnetic modulation that occurs over time, and the necessity to surgically replace each implant as it expires. At present, the most promising applications involve large-scale animal studies for which programmable pumps are too bulky or expensive to be practical.

Externally programmable infusion pumps utilize magnetic intervention to only a limited degree, namely that of activating radiotelemetry circuits that allow bidirectional information transfer and accommodate complex programming routines. These pumps exhibit the flexibility required for complex clinical applications of the future. Drug targeting of a limited nature can be achieved by inserting their catheter tips into thecal, subarachnoid, or ventricular spaces. However, it is doubtful if intravascular (e.g., portal vein or intra-arterial) drug infusions will provide sufficient improvement in the fractional extraction of drug by proximal target organs to constitute true drug targeting by the standard pharmaceutical criterion of site-specific deposition which improves the therapeutic index by at least half an order of magnitude. Nevertheless, the availability of continuous, time-pulsed, and circadian infusions can improve host tolerance of antitumor agents and increase the efficacy of analgesics and other CNS medications. In tumor therapy, improved drug tolerance represents a form of biological response modification. With continued design improvement, advances in miniaturization, and decreased failure rates, these pumps hold great promise for controlled drug delivery in critical and chronic clinical diseases.

ACKNOWLEDGMENTS

I thank Dr. Peter Antich for valuable input on magnetic field configurations and hysteresis hyperthermia, Ms. Holly Huffaker for performing many of the studies included in this chapter, Mrs. Carla Peacock for typing the manuscript, and Mrs. Linda J. Bolding for preparing the photographs. The author's studies were supported by the National Institutes of Health (NIH CA15673), the departments of Pathology and Radiology of the University of Texas Health Science Center at Dallas, and grants from Eli Lilly and Company, the Upjohn Company, and the Dallas Foundation for Health, Education and Research.

REFERENCES

1. J. R. Graybill, P. C. Craven, R. L. Taylor, D. M. Williams, and W. E. Magee, J. Infect. Dis., 145:748 (1982).
2. G. Lopez-Berestein, R. Mehta, R. L. Hopfer, K. Mills, L. Kasi, K. Mehta, V. Fainstein, M. Luna, and E. M. Hersh, J. Infect. Dis., 147:939 (1983).
3. G. Lopez-Berestein, V. Fainstein, R. Hopfer, K. Mehta, M. P. Sullivan, M. Keating, M. G. Rosenblum, R. Mehta, M. Luna, E. M. Hersh, J. Reuben, R. L. Juliano, and G. P. Bodey, J. Infect. Dis., 151:704 (1985).
4. S. S. Davis, in Biological Approaches to the Controlled Delivery of Drugs, Vol. 507 (R. L. Juliano, ed.). New York Academy of Sciences, New York, 1987 (in press).
5. R. L. Taylor, D. M. Williams, P. C. Craven, J. R. Graybill, and D. J. Druz, Am. Rev. Respir. Dis., 125:610 (1982).

6. D. F. Ranney, in *Biological Approaches to the Controlled Delivery of Drugs*, Vol. 507 (R. L. Juliano, ed.). New York Academy of Sciences, New York, 1987 (in press).
7. K. J. Widder, A. E. Senyei, and D. F. Ranney, in *Advances in Pharmacology and Chemotherapy*, Vol. 16 (R. J. Schnitzer, S. Garattini, A. Goldin, G. Hawking, and I. J. Kopin, eds.). Academic Press, New York, 1979, pp. 213-271.
8. D. F. Ranney, *Science*, 227:182 (1985).
9. D. F. Ranney, *Biochem. Pharmacol.*, 35:1063 (1986).
10. H. E. Stockinger, *Am. Ind. Hyg. Assoc. J.*, 45:127 (1984).
11. M. J. Poznansky and R. L. Juliano, *Pharmacol. Rev.*, 36(4):277 (1984).
12. R. T. Borchardt, in *Biological Approaches to the Controlled Delivery of Drugs*, Vol. 507 (R. L. Juliano, ed.). New York Academy of Sciences, New York, 1987 (in press).
13. G. Majno, in *Handbook of Physiology*, Vol. 3 (P. Dow, ed.). American Physiological Society, Washington, DC, 1965, pp. 2293-2275.
14. M. Simionescu, N. Simionescue, and G. Palade, *J. Cell Biol.*, 67:863 (1975).
15. D. F. Ranney, J. C. Weinreb, J. M. Cohen, S. Srikanthan, L. King-Breeding, P. Kulkarni, and P. Antich, in *Contrast Agents in Mangetic Resonance Imaging* (V. M. Runge, C. Claussen, R. Felix, and A. E. James, Jr., eds.). Excerpta Medica, Princeton, NJ, 1986, pp. 81.
16. K. R. Maravilla, B. Mickey, R. M. Peshock, J. C. Weinreb, H. K. Riley, and J. Deiehl, in *Contrast Agents in Mangetic Resonance Imaging* (V. M. Runge, C. Claussen, R. Felix, and A. E. James, Jr., eds.). Excerpta Medica, Princeton, NJ, 1986, p. 106.
17. H. Eichstaedt and R. Felix, in *Contrast Agents in Mangetic Resonance Imaging* (V. M. Runge, C. Claussen, R. Felix, and A. E. James, Jr., eds.). Excerpta Medica, Princeton, NJ, 1986, p. 150.
18. R. K. Jain, *Biotechnol. Prog.*, 1:81 (1985).
19. M. V. Pimm and R. W. Baldwin, *Eur. J. Clin. Oncol.*, 20:515 (1984).
20. K. J. Mayberry-Carson, B. Tober-Meyer, J. K. Smith, D. W. Lambe, Jr., and J. W. Costerton, *Infect. Immunity*, 43:825 (1984).
21. A. L. Hubbard, in *Biological Approaches to the Controlled Delivery of Drugs*, Vol. 507 (R. L. Juliano, ed.). New York Academy of Sciences, New York, 1987 (in press).
22. G. Harris, in *Drug Carriers in Biology and Medicine* (G. Gregoriadis, ed.). Academic Press, New York, 1979, p. 167.
23. G. E. Hatch, D. E. Gardner, and D. B. Menzel, *J. Exp. Med.*, 147:182 (1978).

24. C. V. Dang, W. R. Bell, D. Kaiser, and A. Wong, *Science*, 227: 1487 (1985).
25. J. H. Donohue and S. A. Rosenberg, *J. Immunol.*, 130:2203 (1983).
26. M. T. Lotze, A. E. Chang, C. A. Seipp, C. Simpson, J. T. Vetto, and S. A. Rosenberg, *JAMA*, 256:3117 (1986).
27. L. J. Old, E. Stockert, E. A. Boyse, and J. H. Kim, *J. Exp. Med.*, 127:523 (1968).
28. J. Weinstein, in *Biological Approaches to the Controlled Delivery of Drugs*, Vol. 507 (R. L. Juliano, ed.). New York Academy of Sciences, New York, 1987 (in press).
29. U. S. Ryan, J. W. Ryan, C. Whitaker, and A. Chiu, *Tissue Cell*, 8:125 (1976).
30. K. J. Widder, A. E. Senyei, S. D. Reich, and D. F. Ranney, Magnetically responsive microspheres as a carrier for site-specific delivery of adriamycin, *Proc. Am. Assoc. Cancer Res.*, 19:17 (1978).
31. K. J. Widder, A. E. Senyei, S. D. Reich, and D. F. Ranney, Magnetically responsive microspheres: A carrier system for area-specific delivery of adriamycin, *Fed. Proc.*, *Fed. Am. Soc. Exp. Biol.*, 37:316 (1978).
32. K. J. Widder, A. E. Senyei, and D. G. Scarpelli, *Proc. Soc. Exp. Biol. Med.*, 158:141 (1978).
33. E. L. Neuwelt, P. A. Barnett, M. Glasberg, and E. P. Frenkel, *Cancer Res.*, 43:5278 (1983).
34. Y. Iwasawa, C. N. Gillis, and G. Aghajanian, *J. Pharmacol. Exp. Ther.*, 186:498 (1973).
35. J. W. Ryan, A. Chung, L. C. Martin, and U. S. Ryan, *Tissue Cell*, 10:555 (1978).
36. J. D. Lopes, M. dos Reis, and R. R. Bretani, *Science*, 229:275 (1985).
37. N. Bodor, in *Biological Approaches to the Controlled Delivery of Drugs*, Vol. 507 (R. L. Juliano, ed.). New York Academy of Sciences, New York, 1987 (in press).
38. I. Y. R. Adamson, *Environ. Health Perspect.*, 55:25 (1984).
39. H. Tillander, *Acta Radiol.*, 35:62 (1951).
40. H. Tillander, *Acta Radiol.*, 45:21 (1956).
41. E. H. Frei, J. Driller, H. N. Neufeld, I. Barr, L. Bleiden, and H. M. Askenzazy, *Med. Res. Eng.*, 5:11 (1966).
42. J. F. Alksne, A. Fingerhut, and R. Rand, *Surgery*, 60:212 (1966).
43. P. H. Meyers, F. Cronic, and C. M. Nice, *Am. J. Roentgenol. Ther. Nuclear Med. (N.S.)*, 90:1068 (1963).
44. T. Nakamura, K. Konno, T. Morone, N. Tsuya, and M. Hatano, *J. Appl. Phys.*, 42:1320 (1971).
45. U. Schroder, A. Stahl, and L. G. Salford, in *Microspheres and Drug Therapy: Pharmaceutical Immunological and Medical Aspects* (S. S. Davis, L. Illum, J. G. McVie, and E. Tomlinson, eds.). Elsevier, Amsterdam, 1984, p. 427.

46. J. M. Bartlett, R. C. Richardson, G. S. Elliott, W. E. Blevins, W. Janus, J. R. Hale, and R. L. Silver, in *Microspheres and Drug Therapy*: *Pharmaceutical Immunological and Medical Aspects* (S. S. Davis, L. Illum, J. G. McVie, and E. Tomlinson, eds.). Elsevier, Amsterdam, 1984, p. 413.

47. R. M. Morris, G. A. Poore, D. P. Howard, and J. A. Sefranka, in *Microspheres and Drug Therapy*: *Pharmaceutical Immunological and Medical Aspects* (S. S. Davis, L. Illum, J. G. McVie, and E. Tomlinson, eds.). Elsevier, Amsterdam, 1984, p. 439.

48. E. Tomlinson, in *Biological Approaches to the Controlled Delivery of Drugs*, Vol. 507 (R. L. Juliano, ed.). New York Academy of Sciences, New York, 1987 (in press).

49. L. Ghitescu, A. Fixman, M. Simionescu, and N. Simionescu, *J. Cell Biol.*, 102:1304 (1986).

50. E. M. Purcell, *Berkeley Physics Course*, Vol. 2. McGraw-Hill, New York, 1965, p. 369.

51. R. M. White, *Science*, 229:11 (1985).

52. A. T. Schlafke-Stelson and E. E. Watson, eds., *Proceedings of the Fourth International Radiopharmaceutical Dosimetry Symposium*, Oak Ridge, TN, 1986, pp. 1-700.

53. D. D. Stark and J. T. Ferrucci, Jr., *Diagn. Imaging*, 7:118 (1985).

54. V. M. Runge, J. A. Clanton, C. M. Lukehart, C. L. Partain, and A. E. James, Jr., *Am. J. Roentgenol.*, 141:1209 (1983).

55. H.-J. Weinmann, R. C. Brasch, W.-R. Press, and G. E. Wesby, *Am. J. Roentgenol.*, 142:619 (1984).

56. R. B. Lauffer and T. J. Brady, *Magn. Resonance Imaging*, 3:11 (1985).

57. R. L. Nunnally, E. E. Babcock, S. D. Horner, and R. M. Peshock, *Magn. Resonance Imaging*, 3:399 (1985).

58. M. Chopp, J. A. Helpern, J. R. Ewing, and K. M. Welch, *Magn. Resonance Imaging*, 2:329 (1984).

59. C. R. Malloy, A. D. Sherry, and F. M. H. Jeffrey, *FEBS Lett.*, 212:58 (1987).

60. R. E. London, in *Progress in NMR Spectroscopy* (J. W. Emsley, J. Fenney, and L. A. Suitcliffe, eds.). Pergamon Press, Elmsford, NY, 1987 (in press).

61. J. Alexander, N. Dianiak, H. J. Berger, L. Goldman, D. Johnstone, L. Reduto, T. Duffey, P. Schwartz, A. Gottschalk, and B. L. Zaret, *New Engl. J. Med.*, 300:278 (1979).

62. K. J. Widder, A. E. Senyei, and D. F. Ranney, *Cancer Res.*, 40:3512 (1980).

63. Z. A. Tokes, K. L. Ross, and K. E. Rogers, in, *Microspheres and Drug Therapy*: *Pharmaceutical Immunological and Medical Aspects* (S. S. Davis, L. Illum, J. G. McVie, and E. Tomlinson, eds.). Elsevier, Amsterdam, 1984, p. 139.

64. K. J. Widder, R. M. Morris, G. Poore, D. P. Howard, Jr., and A. E. Senyei, *Proc. Natl. Acad. Sci., U.S.A.*, 78:579 (1981).
65. B. A. Rhodes, I. Zolle, J. W. Buchanan, and H. N. Wagner, Jr., *Radiology*, 92:1453 (1969).
66. I. Zolle, B. A. Rhodes, and H. N. Wagner, Jr., *Int. J. Appl. Radiat. Isot.*, 21:155 (1970).
67. V. M. Petriev, T. R. Bochkova, D. G. Kachirov, and S. V. Seryi, *Med. Radiol.*, 21:39 (1976).
68. S. Higashi, Y. Yamamuro, Y. Katnatani, Y. Ikada, S.-H. Hyon, and K. Jamshidi, in *Advances in Drug Delivery Systems* (A. M. Anderson and S. W. Kim, eds.). Elsevier-North Holland, Amsterdam, 1985, p. 167.
69. J. Cohen, *J. Antimicrob. Chemother.*, 13:409 (1984).
70. A. M. Stamm and W. E. Dismukes, *Chest*, 83:911 (1983).
71. J. Schwarz, in *Pathology Annual*, Vol. 8 (S. C. Sommers, ed.). Appleton-Century-Crofts, New York, 1973, p. 81.
72. G. Medoff, F. Valeriote, and J. Dieckman, *J. Natl. Cancer Inst.*, 67:131 (1981).
73. R. B. Herberman, *Cancer Treat. Rep.*, 69:1161 (1985).
74. G. Poste, in *Biological Approaches to the Controlled Delivery of Drugs*, Vol. 507 (R. L. Juliano, ed.). New York Academy of Sciences, New York, 1987 (in press).
75. E. A. Carswell, L. J. Old, R. L. Kassel, S. Green, N. Fiore, and B. Williamson, *Proc. Natl. Acad. Sci. U.S.A.*, 72:3666 (1975).
76. L. Helson, C. Helson, and S. Green, *Exp. Cell Biol.*, 47:53 (1979).
77. K. Haranaka, N. Satomi, and A. Sakurai, *Int. J. Cancer*, 34:263 (1984).
78. K. J. Tracey, B. Beutler, S. F. Lowry, J. Merryweather, S. Wolpe, I. W. Milsark, R. J. Hariri, T. J. Rahey, III, A. Zentella, J. D. Albert, G. T. Shires, and A. Cerami, *Science*, 234:470 (1986).
79. R. D. Diamond, R. Krzesicki, B. Epstein, and W. Jas, *Am. J. Pathol.*, 91:313 (1978).
80. G. O. Till, K. Johnson, R. Kunkel, and P. A. Ward, *J. Clin. Invest.*, 69:1126 (1978).
81. A. C. Helfin and K. L. Brigham, *J. Clin. Invest.*, 69:1126 (1978).
82. P. P. K. Ho, A. L. Young, and G. L. Southard, *Arthritis Rheum.*, 21:133 (1978).
83. O. J. Plescia, A. H. Smith, and K. Grinwich, *Proc. Natl. Acad. Sci. U.S.A.*, 72:1848 (1975).
84. P. A. Ward, *Am. J. Pathol.*, 77:520 (1974).
85. E. G. Maderazo, P. A. Ward, C. L. Woronick, and R. Quintilliani, *J. Lab. Clin. Med.*, 89:190 (1977).
86. K. M. Lohr and R. Snyderman, *J. Immunol.*, 129:1594 (1982).
87. G. S. Worthen, C. Haslett, L. A. Smedly, A. J. Rees, R. S.

Gumbay, J. E. Henson, and P. M. Henson, *Fed. Proc., Fed. Am. Soc. Exp. Biol. Med.*, 45:7 (1986).
88. S. A. Rosenberg, J. J. Mule, P. J. Spiess, C. M. Reichert, and S. L. Schwartz, *J. Exp. Med.*, 161:1169 (1985).
89. C. G. Moertel, *JAMA*, 256:3141 (1986).
90. N. F. Borelli, A. A. Luderer, and J. N. Panzarino, *Phys. Med. Biol.*, 29:487 (1984).
91. M. von Ardenne and W. Kruger, in *Thermal Characteristics of Tumors: Applications in Detection and Treatment*, Vol. 335 (R. K. Jain and P. M. Gullino, eds.). New York Academy of Sciences, New York, 1980, p. 356.
92. A. A. Luderer, N. F. Borelli, J. N. Panzarino, G. R. Mansfield, D. M. Hess, J. L. Brown, and E. H. Barnett, *Radiat. Res.*, 94: 190 (1983).
93. S. S. Davis, L. Illum, J. G. McVie, and E. Tomlinson, eds., *Microspheres and Drug Therapy: Pharmaceutical Immunological and Medical Aspects.* Elsevier, Amsterdam, 1984, pp. 1-448.
94. R. Langer, L. Brown, and E. Edelman, in *Methods in Enzymology: Drug and Enzyme Targeting*, Part A, Vol. 112 (K. J. Widder and R. Green, eds.). Academic Press, New York, 1985, p. 399.
95. R. Langer, R. Siegel, L. Brown, K. Leong, J. Kost, and E. Edelman, in *Macromolecules as Drugs and as Carriers for Biologically Active Materials*, Vol. 446 (D. A. Tirrell, L. G. Donaruma, and A. B. Turek, eds.). 1985, p. 1.
96. L. Brown, L. Siemer, C. Munoz, and R. Langer, *Diabetes*, 35: 684 (1986).
97. L. Brown, C. Munoz, L. Siemer, E. Edelman, and R. Langer, *Diabetes*, 35:692 (1986).
98. J. Murray, L. Brown, and R. Langer, *Cancer Drug Delivery*, 1:119 (1984).
99. D. A. T. Hsieh, R. Langer, and J. Folkman, *Proc. Natl. Acad. Sci. U.S.A.*, 78:1863 (1981).
100. E. R. Edelman, J. Kost, H. Bobeck, and R. Langer, in *Journal of Biomaterials Research*, Vol. 19 (A. N. Cranin, ed.). Wiley, New York, 1985, p. 67.
101. N. J. Vogelzang, M. Ruane, and T. R. De Meester, *J. Clin. Oncol.*, 3:407 (1985).
102. N. J. Vogelzang, *J. Clin, Oncol.*, 2:1289 (1984).
103. W. J. M. Hrushesky, *Science*, 228:73 (1985).
104. R. D. Penn, J. A. Paice, W. Gottschalk, and A. D. Ivankovich, *J. Neurosurg.*, 61:302 (1984).
105. R. D. Penn, in *Neurologic Clinics*, Vol. 3 (L. I. Kranzler, R. D. Penn, and G. J. Dohrmann, eds.). Saunders, Philadelphia, 1985, p. 439.

12

Externally Modulated Drug Delivery Devices

JOSEPH KOST / Ben-Gurion University of the Negev, Beer-Sheva, Israel

I. INTRODUCTION

Polymer controlled drug delivery systems have attracted increasing interest over recent years. In these systems, the drug is incorporated into a polymeric material. The role of drug release is determined by the properties of the polymer-drug system and is only weakly dependent on environmental factor such as pH and interpatient variations. Already, devices are commercially available for the sustained administration of drugs such as pilocarpine, scopolamine, nitroglycerin, estradiol, clonidine, progesterone, and levonorgesterol [1].

Controlled drug release preparations can (a) maintain the drug concentration in the desired therapeutic range by means of a single dose, (b) localize delivery of the drug to a particular body compartment, which lowers the systematic drug level, (c) reduce the need for follow-up care, (d) preserve medications that are rapidly destroyed by the body, and (e) improve patient comfort and/or compliance. However, one problem central to the entire field of controlled release is that all the systems so far developed display release rates that either are constant or decay with time.

Augmented delivery on demand could be beneficial in a number of situations. These include delivery of insulin for patients with diabetes mellitus, antiarrhythmics for patients with heart rhythm disorders, and nitrates for patients with angina pectoris. Other possible applications include selective β-adrenergic blockade, birth control and general hormone replacement, immunization, cancer chemotherapy, and long-term immunosuppression [2,3].

The systems in which external or feedback control has been studied are still largely experimental. Examples of various control techniques include pumps that can be activated to provide different flow rates [4], polymers responding to pH stimuli [5], nonerodible polymers containing enzymes that cause the polymer to swell and regulate the rate of delivery in response to external stimuli [6,7], pH-sensitive erodible polymers containing enzymes in hydrogels that degrade more rapidly in response to external stimuli [8], and lectin drug systems that release additional drug due to the affinity of an external molecule for the lectin [9,10].

This chapter describes externally modulated drug delivery systems. In these systems release rate of substances from polymeric matrices can be repeatedly modulated at a desired rate, by external control.

II. MAGNETICALLY MODULATED SYSTEMS

Polymeric systems that are capable of delivering drugs at an increased rate on demand have recently been developed [11-14]. The systems consist of drug powder dispersed within a polymeric matrix—generally, ethylene vinyl acetate copolymer (EVAc)—together with some magnetic beads. The particles used are either magnetic steel beads composed principally of iron (79%), chromium (17%), carbon (1%), manganese (1%), silicon (1%), molybdenum (0.75%), and phosphorus (0.04%), or small samarium cobalt magnets. One method of formulating these systems is to add approximately 50% of the drug-polymer mixture to a glass mold, which has been cooled to -80°C using dry ice. The magnetic particles are added followed by the remaining drug-polymer mixture [12] (Fig. 1). For the in vitro experiments, the magnetic tablets are placed in glass vials.

Release rates are controlled by an oscillating external magnetic field, which is generated by a device that rotates permanent magnets beneath the vials. By placing small plastic cages containing animals on the table top, it can also be used for in vivo studies (Fig. 2). Polymer matrices containing drug and magnets can release up to 30 times more drug when exposed to the magnetic field, and release rates return to normal when the magnetic field is discontinued.

The magnetically controlled implant does not cause inflammation in vivo. This was confirmed by the lack of edema, cellular infiltrate, or neovascularization as judged by gross and histological examination in rabbits [13].

A. System Parameters

Recently, factors that are critical in controlling the release rates of these systems have been studied. They are characterized by two main

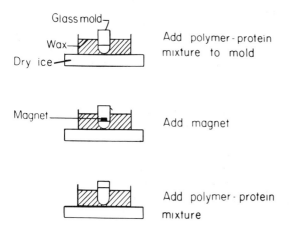

Fig. 1 Procedure for preparation of magnetically controlled release polymers.

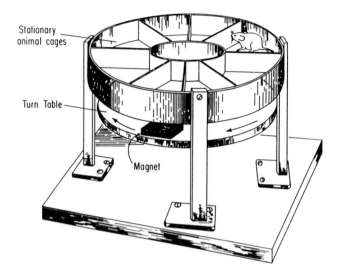

Stationary animal cages

Turn Table

Magnet

Fig. 2 Schematic diagram of the device used to generate an oscillating magnetic field.

groups: magnetic field characteristics and the mechanical properties of the polymeric matrix.

Studies were conducted wherein the amplitude of the magnetic field was varied by increasing the distance between the external and embedded magnets or by changing the embedded magnet's strength [12]. It was found that the extent of release enhancement increases as the field amplitude rises. For example, at a field frequency of 11 Hz, a mean rate release enhancement of 12.4 times was obtained for matrices containing 1100 G magnets, as opposed to 1.5 times for matrices containing less than 100 G magnets. When the frequency of the applied field was increased from 5.0 Hz to 11.0 Hz the rate of release rose in a linear fashion (Fig. 3).

The magnet orientation has been studied using samples containing a single 1100 G magnet [12]. In half the cases, the magnet was placed perpendicular to the applied field and in the other half it was oriented parallel to the field. The mean release rate enhancement was 2.1 times in the parallel cases and 12.4 times in the perpendicular cases. The difference between the two is presumably due to the rotational torque. When placed in parallel, the magnet rotates in an attempt to align its pole vector with the field; therefore, the displacement is smaller.

The mechanical properties of the polymeric matrix also affect the extent of magnetic enhancement [14]. For example, the modulus of elasticity of the polymeric matrix can easily be altered by changing

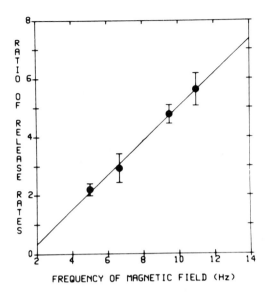

Fig. 3 The average ratio of the rates of bovine serum albumin release from EVAc matrices during field-applied and field-absent periods plotted versus magnetic field frequency. (From Ref. 12.)

the vinyl acetate content of the polymer (Table 1). Figure 4 shows that the release rate enhancement induced by the magnetic field increases as the modulus of elasticity of the EVAc decreases.

B. Mechanism

The release of macromolecules from EVAc systems not containing magnetic beads has been studied extensively [14-18]. It was found that

TABLE 1 Modulus of Elasticity of EVAc Copolymers

Vinyl acetate content (%)	Modulus of elasticity (psi)
16	4480 ± 46
30	970 ± 5
40	430 ± 12
50	110 ± 4

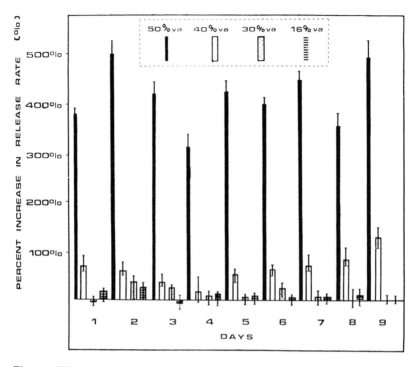

Fig. 4 The percentage increase in bovine serum albumin release during exposure to the oscillating magnetic field for the different vinyl acetate (va) contents of the EVAc copolymer matrices. (From Ref. 14.)

although molecules with molecular weights greater than 300 cannot permeate the polymer, the direct incorporation of macromolecules in the polymer-macromolecule casting procedure caused a tortuous and complex series of pores to form within the matrix (Fig. 5). Factors affecting permeation of water into the polymer and drug out of these pores determine the release rates [18].

Video recordings of the polymer matrix surface, with magnetic beads, show that the beads actually move within the matrix in response to the external magnetic field and move adjacent material containing polymer and drug with it, "squeezing" out the dissolved drug through the pores. McCarthy et al. [19] proposed a model for the enhanced release. They suggested that the major effect stems from the alternate compression and expansion deformation of the pores, causing the fluid within to undergo a pulsatile flow, which alone (no net convection) is able to greatly improve diffusive mass transfer. The mechanism by which the magnetic field is able to increase release rates is currently under investigation.

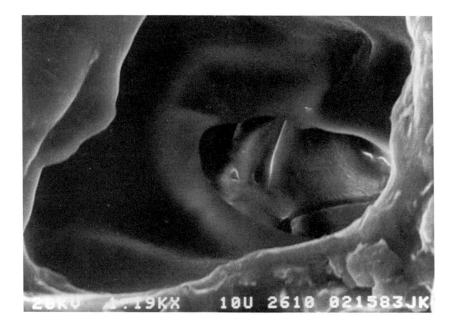

Fig. 5 Interconnecting pores shown on a scanning electron micrograph of an EVAc copolymer matrix containing bovine serum albumin (BSA) after long exposure to the release media.

C. In Vivo Experiments

In vivo experiments have been conducted using implants composed of EVAc-embedded magnets and bovine zinc insulin, placed subcutaneously in diabetic rats for 2 months [20]. After implantation, the blood glucose level decreased due to diffusion of insulin from the polymer. When the diabetic rats were exposed to an oscillaitng magnetic field, the blood glucose levels were further lowered from 50 to 200 mg/dl below this basal level, depending on the magnetic field conditions.

These results were confirmed by radioimmunoassay (RIA). This phenomenon was not observed in the following cases: (a) control rats receiving EVAc implants with insulin without a magnet, (b) control rats receiving implants with a magnet but without insulin, (c) diabetic rats not containing any implant, and (d) healthy rats not containing any implant. All these animals were exposed to the same manipulations as the experimental group of animals.

III. ULTRASONICALLY MODULATED SYSTEMS

Recent studies [21] suggest the feasibility of ultrasonically controlled polymeric delivery systems in which release rates of substances can be repeatedly modulated at will from a position external to the delivery system. Both bioerodible and nonerodible polymers were used as the drug carrier matrices. The bioerodibles were poly[bis(p-carboxy-phenoxy)alkene anhydride], synthesized by following the method described by Conix [22]. The nonerodible polymer was ethylene vinyl acetate copolymer (EVAc: Dupont Chemical Co. Elvax, 40P).

Drug-incorporated polyanhydride matrices were formulated by either compression or injection molding. A mixture of finely ground and sieved polymer (90-150 mm) and 10% of p-nitroaniline, as a model drug, was pressed into circular disks in a Carver test cylinder outfit, at 30 kpsi and 5°C above the glass transition temperature for 10 min. Injection molding was performed in the ASCI Mini Max Injection Molder at temperatures of 10°C above the melting temperature of the polymer [23].

Bovine zinc insulin (Eli Lilly) or bovine serum albumin (Sigma) was mixed with 10% w/v of EVAc in methylene chloride. The suspension was quickly poured into a glass mold, which had been cooled on dry ice. When the solution was solidified (10 min), the sample was removed from the mold and placed consecutively in a freezer under vacuum at -20°C for 48 hr and then for an additional 48 hr at 20°C [24].

The ultrasonic source was a RAI Research Corporation ultrasonic cleaner model 250, which operated at a frequency of 75 kHz. Drug-incorporated polymeric matrix was placed in a jacketed vial filled with 0.1 M phosphate buffer pH 7.4 at 37°C. The vial in turn was immersed in the ultrasonic bath filled with water (Fig. 6). The sample was then exposed to alternating periods of triggering and nontriggering. After each period, the buffer in the vial was replaced and the amount of drug released and polymer degraded was determined by ultraviolet spectroscopy.

A pronounced enhancement of polymer degradation and drug release rates was observed when the samples were exposed to ultrasound (Fig. 7). Enhancement of release rates while exposed to ultrasound was also observed in nonerodible polymers (Fig. 8). This suggests that the ultrasound also promotes the diffusional release of the drug, which explains the higher increase in the rate of drug release compared to the rate of drug degradation.

A. System Parameters

Experiments have also been conducted in which the drug concentration was continuously monitored by circulating the buffer to a ultraviolet Fig. 6

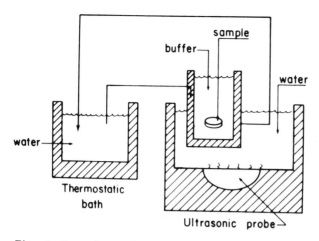

Fig. 6 Experimental setup for the ultrasonic triggering of drug-incorporated polymeric matrices. (From Ref. 21.)

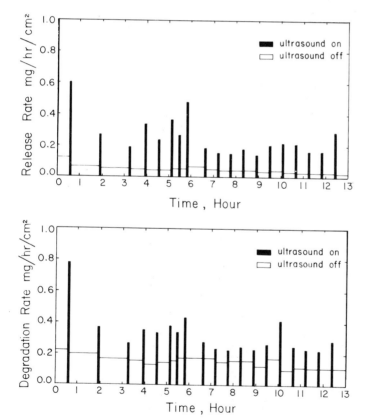

Fig. 7 The effect of ultrasound on degradation and release rates of p-nitroaniline from poly[bis(p-carboxyphenoxy)-methane] as a function of time. (From Ref. 21.)

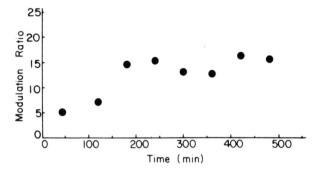

Fig. 8 Modulation ratio (ratio of the release rates at a given period of ultrasound exposure to the average of the release rates immediately preceeding and following this exposure) versus time for insulin release from EVAc copolymer exposed to alternating triggering periods of 30 min. (From Ref. 21.)

spectrometer in a closed-loop manner [21]. The release rates are represented by the slope of the curve in Fig. 9. As can be seen, the release rates, at different periods, are constant with time. The response time is less than 2 min upon turning on the ultrasound and almost instantaneous when turning it off.

It has also been demonstrated that the extent of enhancement can be regulated [21]. This can be seen in Fig. 10. By varying the intensity of the ultrasound, the degree of enhancement for both the polymer degradation and the drug release can be altered.

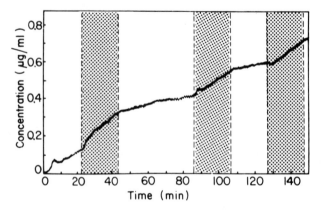

Fig. 9 Release rates of p-nitroaniline from poly[bis(p-carboxyphenoxy)hexane] with on-line detection. The shaded areas are the periods in which the device was exposed to ultrasound. (From Ref. 21.)

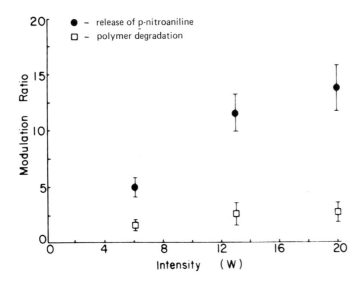

Fig. 10 The effect of ultrasound intensity on modulation ratio for the release of p-nitroaniline from poly[bis(p-carboxyphenoxy)methane]. (From Ref. 21.)

B. Mechanism

Experimental evidence indicates that cavitation induced by the ultrasonic waves may be responsible for augmented polymer degradation and drug release [21]. Figure 11 shows that in experiments conducted in a degassed buffer, where cavitation was minimized, the observed enhancement in degradation and release rates was much smaller.

In accompanying experiments, additional factors, such as temperature and mixing, were also examined [21]. Exposure of the samples to ultrasound increases the temperature inside the polymer. Figure 12a shows the temperature increase of the device while exposed to ultrasound. Figure 12b presents the effect of such temperature increase on release rates. These results suggest that the enhanced release due to the ultrasound is not due to an increase in temperature. Figure 13 shows the effects of mixing on polymer degradation and drug release. Release experiments were performed under vigorous shaking to examine the effect of ultrasound on the diffusion boundary layer. As can be seen, the effect of the ultrasound on the augmented release is independent of the degree of mixing. The increase in release rates is minimal under conditions of vigorous shaking. This suggests that even if the ultrasound eliminates or diminishes the diffusion boundary layer, this effect cannot account for the 10- to 30-fold increase in release.

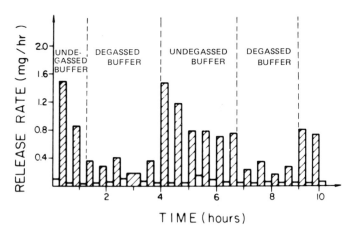

T I M E (hours)

Fig. 11 Release rates of bovine serum albumin from EVAc copolymer versus time. The sample was exposed to ultrasound alternatively in degassed and ungassed buffers. (From Ref. 21.)

The mechanism by which ultrasound enhances the degradation and release rates is still unclear. One explanation might be the higher penetration of water into the polymer. This exposes more anhydride linkages for hydrolysis. In polymer solutions exposed to ultrasound, main chain rupture is thought to be induced by shock waves created during the cavitation, which are assumed to cause a rapid compression with subsequent expansion of the liquid [25]. Apart of the action of shock waves, the collapse of cavitation bubbles may create pronounced perturbation in the surrounding liquid, possibly inducing other increase effects as well.

C. In Vivo Experiments

Recent studies have demonstrated the feasibility of in vivo ultrasound-mediated drug release enhancement [26]. Implants composed of polyanhydride copolymer (80% polycarboxyphenoxy-propylene, 20% sebacic acid) loaded with 10% p-aminohippuric acid (PAH) were implanted subcutaneously in the upper back of catheterized rats. The p-aminohippuric acid was totally eliminated from the body in the urine. The concentration of the PAH in urine was assayed by high-performance liquid chromatography. When the rats were exposed to the ultrasound, a significant increase in the PAH concentration of urine was evaluated. The enhancement release was observed during exposure and up to 20 min after exposure was terminated. Subsequently PAH concentration returns to the basal rate prior to the ultrasound application. No skin damage was observed at the application area.

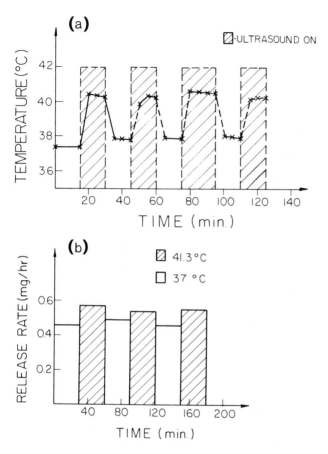

Fig. 12 (a) Temperature profiles of samples exposed and unexposed to ultrasound. (b) The effect of temperature on the release rates of bovine serum albumin from EVAc copolymers. (From Ref. 21.)

IV. CONCLUSION

Drug delivery techniques appear to have gone through two evolutionary stages: first, uncontrolled delivery of a bolus and, more recently, the introduction of zero-order or constant release rate systems. However, metabolite concentrations are normally closely regulated by the body in response to changes in the concentrations of other metabolites (i.e., insulin release is dependent on glucose concentration and both undergo fairly wide but short-term concentration changes). A third generation of drug delivery systems is needed to truly approach this physiological ideal.

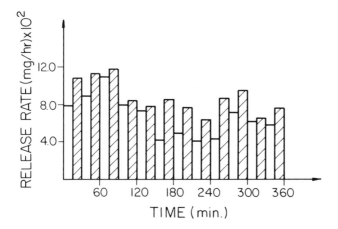

Fig. 13   The effect of vigorous shaking on release rates of bovine serum albumin from EVAc copolymers; shaded areas are release rates during the shaken periods. (From Ref. 21.)

The externally modulated drug delivery devices reviewed in this chapter have some of the properties necessary for achieving this goal. Such devices could be used in a closed-loop controlled delivery system in which the amount of release drug can be regulated by a minicomputer, perhaps contained in a watchlike device, according to the physiological level that is required. Using diabetes as an example, by implanting a glucose detector and minicomputer, release rates from the magnetically triggered device could be adjusted automatically such that the release of insulin would be in response to the patient's physiological needs. Alternatively, even without such a sensor, the triggering device could be programmed to be activated near mealtime, or the patient could activate the device manually at desired times.

One of the goals of future research in externally controlled release systems is to achieve a better understanding of the factors controlling release kinetics. The factors already studied provide the ability to control release rates externally. For example, the rates can be increased by changing the frequency or intensity of the externally applied magnetic or ultrasonic field. However, actual clinical implementation require still further in vitro and in vivo studies.

The development of a demand-responsive drug delivery system offers alternatives to much more cumbersome and inefficient means of therapeutics. The use of a polymer-based system minimizes the complexity and size of the potential implant. Because the drug is stored as a dry powder and not in solution, it occupies a much smaller volume than it would take up in the reservoir of a mechanical pump. Combined with the fact that the polymer matrix requires no moving parts, the magnetic polymer system can contain more than 100 times more drug per unit volume than a standard Infusaid or Siemens pump [27-29]. The concept of modulated controlled release offers a new way of thinking about drug delivery. Such processes will stimulate additional research on polymer-based systems for improved therapy and pharmacological studies examining optimal drug delivery patterns.

REFERENCES

1. J. Kost and R. Langer, *Pharm. Int.*, 7:3, 60 (1986).
2. R. Langer and N. Peppas, *J. Macromol. Sci. Rev., Macromol. Chem. Phys.*, C23:61 (1983).
3. J. Kost and R. Langer, *Trends Biotechnol.*, 2:47 (1984).
4. M. Sefton, Implantable pumps. In *Medical Application of Controlled Release* (R. Langer and D. Wise, eds.). CRC Press, Boca Raton, FL, 1984, p. 129.
5. F. Alhaique, M. Marchetti, F. Riccieri, and E. Santucci, *J. Pharmcol.*, 33:413 (1981).
6. J. Kost, T. Horbett, B. Ratner, and M. Singh, *J. Biomed. Mater. Res.*, 19:1133 (1985).
7. K. Ishihara, M. Kobayashi, N. Ishimanu, and I. Shinohara, *Polym. J.*, 16:8, 625 (1984).
8. J. Heller and P. Trescony, *J. Pharm. Sci.*, 68:919 (1979).
9. M. Brownlee and A. Cerami, *Science*, 206:1190 (1979).
10. S. Kim, S. Jeong, S. Sato, J. McRea, and J. Feijen, in *Recent Advances in Drug Delivery Systems* (J. Anderson and S. Kim, eds.). Plenum Press, New York, 1984, p. 123.
11. D. Hsieh and R. Langer, in *Controlled Release of Bioactive Materials* (Z. Mansdorff and T. J. Roseman, eds.). Dekker, New York, 1983, pp. 121-131.
12. E. Edelman, J. Kost, H. Bobeck, and R. Langer, *J. Biomed. Mater. Res.*, 19:67-83 (1985).
13. D. Hsieh, R. Langer, and J. Folkman, *Proc. Natl. Acad. Sci. U.S.A.*, 78:1863-1867 (1981).
14. J. Kost, R. Noecker, E. Kunica, and R. Langer, *J. Biomed. Mater. Res.*, 19:935-940 (1986).
15. W. Rhine, D. Hsieh, and R. Langer, *J. Pharm. Sci.*, 69(3):265-270 (1980).
16. T. Hsu and R. Langer, *J. Biomed. Mater. Res.*, 19:445-460 (1985).
17. R. Bawa, R. Siegel, B. Marasca, M. Karel, and R. Langer, *J. Controlled Release*, 1:259-267 (1985).
18. R. Siegel and R. Langer, *Pharm. Res.*, 1:2-10 (1984).
19. M. McCarthy, D. Soong, and E. Edelman, *J. Controlled Release*, 1:143-147 (1984).

20. J. Kost, E. Edelman, L. Brown, and R. Langer, *Transactions of the Second World Congress on Biomaterials*, April 1984, p. 34.
21. J. Kost, K. W. Leong, and R. Langer, in *Polymers in Medicine: Biomedical and Pharmaceutical Applications*, Vol. II (E. Chiellini, ed.). Plenum Press, New York, 1986, p. 387.
22. A. Conix, *Macromol. Synth.*, 2:95 (1966).
23. K. W. Leong, B. C. Brott, and R. Langer, *J. Biomed. Mater. Res.*, 19:941 (1985).
24. W. Rhine, D. Hsieh, and R. Langer, *J. Pharm. Sci.*, 69(3):265 (1980).
25. W. Schnabel, *Polymer Degradation.* Hanser International, Munchen, 1981.
26. J. Kost, K. W. Leong, and R. Langer, *J. Die Makromolekulare Chemie* (in press).
27. L. Brown, C. Munoz, L. Siemer, E. Edelman, and R. Langer, *Diabetes*, 35:692 (1986).
28. H. Buchwald, J. Barbosa, R. L. Varco, T. D. Rodhe, W. Rupp, R. Schwartz, F. Goldenberg, T. Rublein, and P. Blackshear, *Lancet*, 1:1233-1235 (1981).
29. K. Irsigler, K. H. Kritz, G. Hagmuller, M. Franetzki, K. Prestele, H. Thurow, and K. Geison, *Diabetes*, 19:1-9 (1981).

13

Transdermal Drug Delivery Devices

SHARAD K. GOVIL / Schering-Plough Corporation, Miami, Florida

I. INTRODUCTION

Typically, all the conventional dosage forms, with the lone exception of continuous intravenous infusion, follow second-order kinetics with respect to the release of drug(s) from the dosage form. This means that the dosage form releases drug initially at a faster rate, thus leading to a quick rise in the blood level of the drug, and then falls exponentially until a further dose is administered. This results in a peaks-and-valleys pattern of drug concentration in blood and tissues. Thus, for most of the time the concentration of drug is either above the required therapeutic level or below it. Equality of the rate of absorption and the rates of metabolic elimination would result in the equilibrium distribution of the drug in tissue and blood but is, however, missing in case of conventional dosage forms. This factor, as well as some other factors such as repetitive dosing and unpredictable absorption, led to the concept of the drug delivery systems or the therapeutic systems. As explained by Zaffaroni, "A dosage form that releases one or more drugs continuously in a predetermined pattern for a fixed period of time, either systematically or to a specified target organ, is a therapeutic system or a drug delivery system" [1]. Essentially the advent of drug delivery systems brings rate-controlled delivery with fewer side effects, increased efficacy, and constant delivery.

The development of drug delivery systems is also the result of certain trends in thinking of the past decade or two: namely, that drug absorption and efficacy can be enhanced by redesigning the delivery processes rather than the drug molecules or the chemical entities. When the aim is to deliver drugs through skin in a predetermined and controlled fashion, the result is transdermal drug delivery.

Transdermal delivery systems provide the following advantages over conventional therapy.

1. Gastrointestinal absorption problems are avoided.
2. First-pass effect is avoided, thus minimizing drug input.
3. This approach is useful when oral administration is to be avoided or is contraindicated.
4. Drugs with narrow therapeutic range can be delivered.
5. Better control of blood levels for potent drugs is possible.
6. Patient compliance can be increased.
7. Drugs with short half-lives are utilized.
8. Therapy can be quickly terminated by simple removal of the system from the skin surface.

However, transdermal drug delivery is neither practical nor affordable when required to deliver large doses of drug(s), when the drug or the formulation is skin sensitizing or irritating, when the drug is extensively metabolized in skin, or when molecular size is great enough to prevent the molecules from diffusing through the skin.

II. FACTORS IN TRANSDERMAL MEDICATION

The design, development, and success of transdermal delivery systems can be traced to four factors, which are interrelated. These are (a) drug formulation, (b) biopharmaceutics of the drug, (c) characteristics of skin, and (d) adhesion of the system to skin. Figure 1 describes these interrelationships graphically, as also outlined by Cleary [2]. Each of these factors in turn is then influenced by several other factors, which are briefly outlined here.

The *formulation* characteristics that determine the efficacy of the device are as follows:

> Boundary layers
> Thickness
> Temperature
> Geometry of system
> Polymers
> Vehicles
> Porosity of membranes
> Tortuosity, etc.

The design of the delivery device depends on the following *skin* parameters:

> Species (caucasian/black)
> Condition of skin (healthy/diseased, pretreated, secretion, hair
>   density, etc.)
> Site-to-site permeability

The adhesion parameters that determine delivery device design are essentially the adhesive formulation and the skin. The *adhesive formulation* is affected by the following:

> Size and shape
> Cohesiveness
> Curing
> Arrangement of other layers
> Flexible/nonflexible and breathable/nonbreathable backing material
> Type and characteristics of the polymer, etc.

The *biopharmaceutical* parameters affecting the design of delivery devices are as follows:

> Half-life of the drug
> Pharmacological blood levels
> Therapeutic window

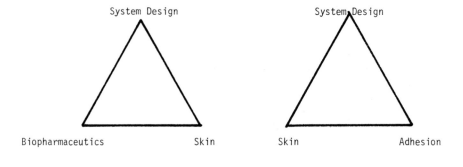

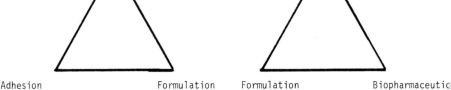

Fig. 1 Factors and interrelationships in transdermal delivery system design. (Courtesy of Key Pharmaceuticals, Inc., Miami, Florida.)

Amount of drug required to permeate the skin
Hydration state of the skin

III. TYPE OF TRANSDERMAL DEVICES

There are five types of transdermal drug delivery device currently available in the market (see Fig. 2). To be more precise, there are two concepts in the design of transdermal delivery, namely, the reservoir type and the matrix type. The others are extensions of these two concepts. These concepts are discussed in Sections A to F.

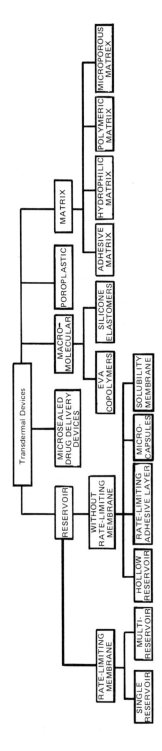

Fig. 2 Classification of transdermal delivery devices.

389

A. Reservoir-type Devices

Reservoir-Type Devices with Rate-Limiting Membrane

In the reservoir type of devices the drug is stored in a reservoir from which it diffuses through a rate-limiting membrane to the site of absorption. In concept, this type of system is good when the stratum corneum is not the principal rate-limiting barrier for the diffusion of drug(s) and rate control from the device is desired. One of the advantages of such a system is the near-constant release rate of drug from device. However, rupturing of the rate-limiting membrane may also result in a quicker than desired release of drug from the device. The reservoir type of transdermal device is exemplified by the Transderm-Scop (Ciba Pharmaceuticals), Transderm-Nitro (Ciba Pharmaceuticals), Catapres-TTS (Boehringer-Ingelheim), and Estraderm (Ciba Pharmaceuticals) systems. All four devices have basic similarities in design. They all contain backing membrane, reservoir of drug, rate-limiting membrane, adhesive, and a peel-off release liner.

While all four transdermal devices are quite similar in basic design, there are several processing differences. Figure 3 depicts a typical reservoir type of device with rate-controlling membrane. Transderm-Scop (scopolamine) and Catapress-TTS (clonidine) patches are known as multilaminates. Here the adhesive polymers are dissolved in a vehicle and drug is added while another solution of the drug is prepared separately. The drug layer and the adhesive layers are then coated as a thin continuous film onto a moving web passing through drying ovens. Once the layers have dried, the drug layer, the adhesive layer, the rate-controlling membrane, and the backing layer, along with the release liner, are laminated together. Then individual units are punched out. In the Transderm-Nitro and Estraderm systems the drug reservoir is filled as liquid (Estraderm) or ointment (Transderm-Nitro) between the impermeable backing and the rate-limiting membrane. The delivery rate of the drug from such systems can be varied by varying the polymer ratios, permeability coefficient of the rate-controlling membrane, thickness of the adhesive, and so on. The release rate of drug from such membrane-controlled transdermal delivery devices can be expressed as follows:

$$\frac{dQ}{dt} = \frac{C_r}{1/p_{rm} + 1/P_a} \tag{1}$$

where P_{rm} is the permeability coefficient of the rate-controlling membrane, P_a the permeability coefficient of the adhesive, and C_r the concentration of drug in the reservoir [3]. A system for the transdermal administration of scopolamine, Transderm-Scop, is represented in Fig. 4 [4]. The individual layers and possible components are as follows:

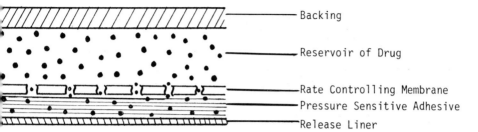

Fig. 3 Scheme for reservoir-type transdermal delivery devices with rate-controlling membrane.

Backing: polyethylene terephthalate, metallized polypropylene, metallized PVC, or metallized polyethylene
Reservoir: scopolamine in mineral oil (10-100 cp.), polyisobutylene.
Microporous membrane: polypropylene or PVC or cellulose acetate nitrate or polyacrylonitrile of 0.1 to 0.85 porosity and 1 to 10 tortuosity and 0.01 to 0.001 cm thickness
Adhesive: polyisobutylene (high molecular weight, low molecular weight) and mineral oil
Release liner: siliconized PVC/polypropylene/polyethylene terephthalate

Figure 5 depicts the construction of a transdermal nitroglycerin therapeutic system (Transderm-Nitro) with a rate-limiting membrane. The device [5] has the following components:

Backing: metallized plastic
Reservoir: nitroglycerin on lactose in colloidal SiO_2 and silicone medical fluid

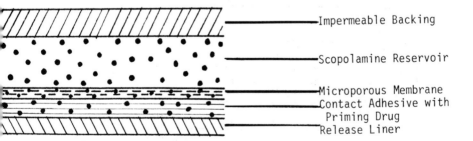

Fig. 4 Design of a transdermal scopolamine therapeutic system.

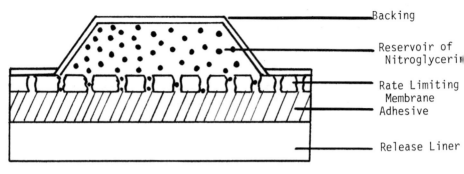

Fig. 5 Transdermal therapeutic nitroglycerin system with rate-limiting membrane.

   Membrane: Ethylene vinyl acetate (EVAc) copolymer
   Adhesive: pressure-sensitive silicone adhesive

   Boehringer-Ingelheim's transdermal clonidine system (Catapress-TTS), diagrammatically depicted in Fig. 6, consists of the following components [6]:

   Backing: pigmented polyester film
   Reservoir: clonidine in mineral oil, polyisobutylene, and colloidal
      SiO_2
   Membrane: microporous polypropylene membrane
   Adhesive: clonidine in mineral oil, polyisobutylene, and colloidal
      SiO_2

   Figure 7 describes schematically a transdermal estradiol system (Estraderm). The device has the following components [7]:

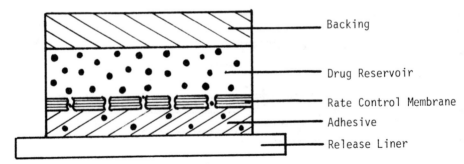

Fig. 6 Clonidine transdermal therapeutic system with rate-limiting membrane.

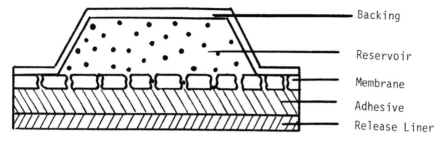

Fig. 7 Transdermal estradiol system with rate-limiting membrane.

Backing: aluminized polyethylene terephthalate
Reservoir: estradiol in ethanol and hydroxypropylcellulose
Membrane: EVA copolymer
Adhesive: high molecular weight and low molecular weight poly-
isobutylene in light mineral oil
Release liner: siliconized polyethylene terephthalate

Hercon Device

Another type of reservoir system with rate-limiting membrane was
designed and patented by the Hercon Division [8] for the transdermal
delivery of pharmaceutical agents. The Hercon NTG System was recently approved by the U.S. Food and Drug Administration (FDA).
The system as depicted in Fig. 8 consists of three polymer layers.
The central layer is the reservoir of drug. One of the outer sides
of the reservoir is the impermeable or barrier membrane, while the
other layer is the rate-controlling layer, and it is this layer that con-

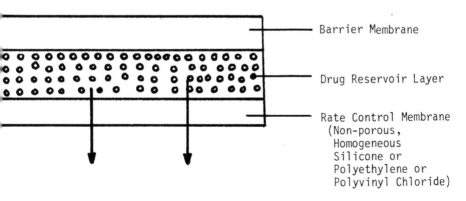

Fig. 8 The Hercon NTG System, a transdermal controlled release device. (Adapted from Ref. 8.)

tacts the skin. A peripheral adhesive ring (not shown) on the barrier layer secures the system on the skin. The advantages of this system include its flexibility, the possibility of varying rate control by varying the polymers in the reservoir and the control layers, and the accommodation of both the solids or liquid reservoir.

Multireservoir Rate-Limiting Devices [9]

U.S. Patent 4,379,454 (Campbell and Chandrasekharan) describes multireservoir, rate-limiting membrane-type devices. A characteristic feature of these systems is that an enhancer is stored in a compartment, separate from the drug reservoir. The system as shown in Fig. 9 has a conventional impermeable backing of materials described earlier, followed by the reservoir of a vehicle or an enhancer, a rate-limiting membrane, and a drug reservoir in the adhesive. This reservoir may also contain stabilizer, diluent, and other inert materials such as a gelling agent. The rate-limiting membrane here is present to control the permeation rate of the vehicle/enhancer and should preferably be impermeable to the drug. The drug is dispersed in any pressure-sensitive adhesive. In one structural modification of this system, the drug reservoir is accommodated between the rate-limiting membrane and the adhesive layer as a separate compartment (Fig. 10). Multireservoir-type devices are distinctly advantageous where intimate contact between the vehicle/enhancer and the drug is not desired.

Another modification of such systems is depicted in Fig. 11, where both the enhancer and the drug are dispersed in an adhesive polymer or a polymeric matrix followed by an adhesive overlay. Here the enhancer or vehicle is microencapsulated inside a diffusion-controlling membrane, and these microcapsules together with the drug are dispersed in an adhesive polymeric matrix that adheres well to the skin. The membrane may be made of microporous materials described in connection with earlier devices. The release rate of enhancer from the microcapsules governs the release rate of drug from the formulation.

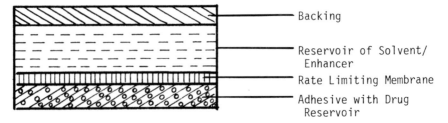

Fig. 9 Scheme for multireservoir-type transdermal devices. (Adapted from Ref. 8.)

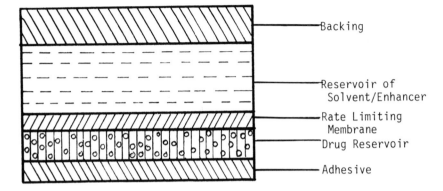

Fig. 10 Scheme for modified multireservoir-type transdermal devices.
(Adapted from Ref. 9.)

A similar type of system containing a peripheral ring of adhesive
(Fig. 12) may also be preapred. This may be preferred when the drug
and the enhancer have lower than desired permeation rates through
the adhesive layer.

Reservoir-Type Devices Without Rate-Limiting Membrane

Devices with Rate-Limiting Adhesive Layer

In the previously described reservoir systems with rate-limiting
membranes, the drug reservoir was sandwiched between an impermeable
backing and a microporous rate-controlling membrane. The adhesive
diffusion control reservoir types of device differ in that a dispersion
of drug in the adhesive polymer (reservoir) is spread as a thin layer
on the impermeable backing. Layers of rate-limiting adhesive polymers
without any drug are then spread on top of the reservoir layer.

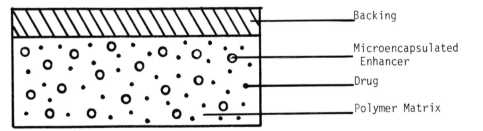

Fig. 11 Scheme for a transdermal device containing microencapsulated
enhancer.

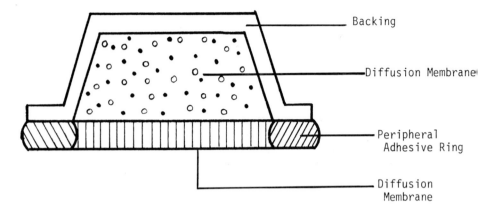

Fig. 12 Scheme for a transdermal device with microencapsulated enhancer and peripheral adhesive ring. (Adapted from Ref. 9.)

This concept has been utilized by Pharma-Schwartz (Monheim, Germany) in the development of their transdermal nitroglycerin delivery system, Deponit [10]. The release rate from such a system (see, e.g., Fig. 13) may be described as follows:

$$\frac{dM}{dt} = \frac{KDC}{h} \tag{2}$$

where
  K = partition coefficient of glyceryl trinitrate (GTN) between reservoir and adhesive layer
  D = diffusion coefficient of adhesive
  H = thickness of adhesive
  C = concentration of nitroglycerin in reservoir

Microencapsulated Drug Reservoir-Type Devices [11]

When the drug is dispersed as microcapsules all throughout the contact adhesive, the rate-controlling step in the delivery is the diffusion of the drug through the walls of the microcapsules. The permeaction rate of drug across the microcapsule is a function of the porosity, thickness, and diffusion coefficients of the membrane and also of the solubility of the drug in the membrane.

Obviously, the most important component in such a system is the *microencapsulation agent*. Several hydrophilic or hydrophobic polymers are available for this purpose. Hydrophilic polyether gels, crosslinked polyvinyl alcohols/partially hydrolyzed acetate, acrylates, and methacrylates are some examples of hydrophilic polymers, while hydro-

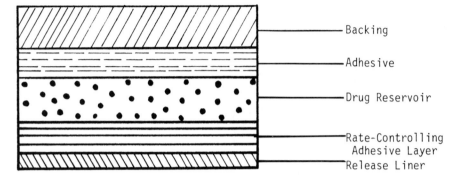

Backing

Adhesive

Drug Reservoir

Rate-Controlling
Adhesive Layer
Release Liner

Fig. 13 Diagrammatic view of a transdermal device with adhesive diffusion control. (Adapted form Ref. 10.)

phobic polymers may be exemplified by silicones (organopolysilocone rubbers), soft nylon, and plasticized or unplasticized polyvinyl chloride.

The microencapsulates are then dispersed into pressure-sensitive adhesives and a thin layer of the dispersion is cast on the backing material, as indicated in Fig. 14. The thickness of the adhesive layer varies with the amount of drug required for loading.

Reservoir Devices with Solubility Membranes [11-13]

This type of system as depicted in Fig. 15 has drug dispersed in a polymer matrix as reservoir which is sandwiched between an impermeable backing and a solubility membrane. The nonreservoir side of the solubility membrane is coated with a pressure-sensitive adhesive. The system is characterized by two rate-controlling steps: (a) the polymeric matrix material, which is capable of dissolving the drug and thus controls the rate of the passage of drug to the solubility membrane, and (b) dissolution of the drug in the solubility membrane. This solubility

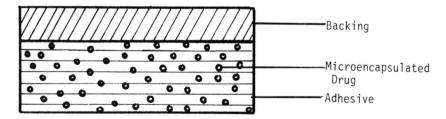

Backing

Microencapsulated
Drug

Adhesive

Fig. 14 Microencapsulated drug reservoirs in a transdermal device. (Adapted from Ref. 11.)

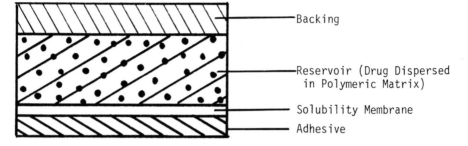

Fig. 15 Scheme for transdermal devices with solubility membranes.

membrane may be formed of any of the microencapsulation agents described previously [11]. The solubility profile of the drug is different in the two rate-controlling steps, and thus precise delivery of the drug to the adhesive can be attained by varying the ratio or the composition of the polymeric matrix and the solubility membrane.

Transdermal Devices with Hollow Reservoirs [13]

Figure 16 illustrates a reservoir type of transdermal delivery system, in which the reservoir is in the form of a hollow cylinder having an impermeable backing and a rate-limiting membrane that controls the release of drug into the adhesive layer. The reservoir may be prepared by one of the following procedures: (a) by moulding into a hol-

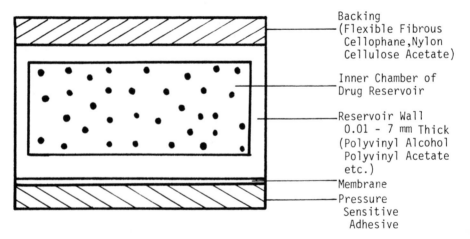

Fig. 16 Scheme for hollow cylindrical reservoir-type transdermal devices.

low container with the drug entrapped, or (b) by forming an envelope of polymeric materials that is permeable to passage of drug with the drug encased. The microencapsulating agents described earlier are suitable for the preparation of the reservoir. The delivery rate of the drug is governed by the thickness and diffusivity of the lower reservoir wall/membrane.

Normally the reservoir of a transdermal delivery device may contain beside the drug some pharmaceutical carriers (saline, sterile water, dextrose, lactose, mineral oil, light vegetable oils, triglycerides of lower fatty acids, glycols, polyvinyl pyrrolidone, Klucel, etc.).

B. Matrix-Type Transdermal Devices

The drug in a matrix-type system is uniformly dispersed throughout a hydrophilic or lipophilic polymer matrix, which is then cured into a polymeric disk of predetermined thickness and surface area. The matrix is then glued to aluminum foil, which is sealed to drug-impermeable backing through an absorbent pad [10]. Most such systems do not have an adhesive overlay but instead possess a peripheral adhesive ring. Figure 17 illustrates a typical matrix type of transdermal delivery device. Several structural modifications are possible.

As described by Hymes and Rolf [14], the polymeric matrix is an "open cell molecular sponge" saturated with a dispersion or solution of drug in a solvent. The solvent molecules are organized by the polymer network such that the dispersed and/or dissolved drug is held in the microspaces of the network. Such an orientation and organization of drug and solvent molecules inside the polymeric network is affected to a great degree by the ionization of the polymer cross-linking and configuration of the polymer. The matrix should have the following characteristics.

There should be zero chemical interaction of the matrix polymers with the drug.

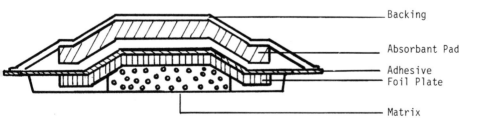

Backing

Absorbant Pad

Adhesive
Foil Plate

Matrix

Fig. 17 A typical matrix-type transdermal device.

The matrix should not impart excessive resistance to the diffusion
of the entrapped drug; that is, the molecular weight, the glass
transition temperature, the functional groups, and their orientation must be appropriate for the release of a particular drug.
The matrix should be stable and be able to hold the drug in stable
condition.
The matrix should be nonirritating to skin and also should adhere
well to the skin to provide an appropriate bridging between
the skin and the drug.
Structural integrity should be maintained at high temperatures
and humidities.

Commonly employed agents for matrix formulation are polyvinyl pyrrolidone, ethylene vinyl acetate copolymers, polyesters, microporous
polypropylenes, polyvinyl chloride, and polysaccharides.

Polymeric Matrix-Type Transdermal Devices

The polymeric matrix type of transdermal delivery devices are exemplified by Nitro-Dur (Key Pharmaceuticals, Miami, Florida), as shown in
Fig. 18. The release from matrix-type devices shows a square root of
time dependence:

$$\left[\frac{dM}{dt} = \frac{LC_m D_m}{2t} \right]^{1/2} \tag{3}$$

where L is the loading dose in the matrix, C_m is the concentration
of the drug in the matrix, and D_m the diffusion coefficient of the drug
in the polymer. At steady state the release may be expressed as follows:

$$\frac{M}{t^{1/2}} = [(2L - C_m) C_m D_m]^{1/2} \tag{4}$$

According to Cleary and Keith [15] the critical components in the design of Nitro-Dur fall into four categories: (a) aluminum foil package,
(b) absorbent pad, (c) adhesion components, and (d) polymer-GTN
matrix. Because of the complicated deisgn of the entire system (Fig.
18), in the case of Nitro-Dur the selection of proper components is as
critical as that of the active unit.

The *aluminum foil package* has an aluminum foil release liner (cover
strip) and an aluminum foil baseplate. The GTN matrix is completely
surrounded by these two components during its shelf life. At the time
of application, the aluminum foil cover strip is peeled off, exposing

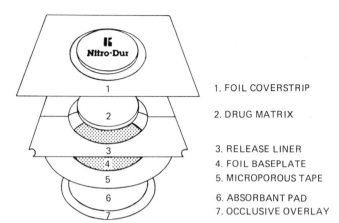

1. FOIL COVERSTRIP

2. DRUG MATRIX

3. RELEASE LINER
4. FOIL BASEPLATE
5. MICROPOROUS TAPE

6. ABSORBANT PAD
7. OCCLUSIVE OVERLAY

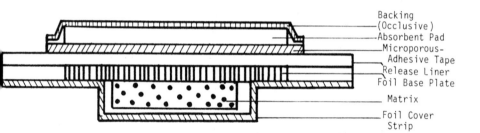

Backing
(Occlusive)
Absorbent Pad
Microporous-
Adhesive Tape
Release Liner
Foil Base Plate
Matrix
Foil Cover
Strip

Fig. 18 The Nitro-Dur matrix device. (Exploded diagram courtesy of Key Pharmaceuticals, Inc., Miami, Florida; cross-sectional view adapted from Kydonieus and Berner.)

the matrix. The aluminum foil baseplate and the cover strip serve to eliminate the possibility that GTN and other potentially volatile components will evaporate. The foil baseplate stays behind the matrix for the duration of the application and thus serves as a barrier for GTN and other liquid components of the matrix.

Transepidermal water loss as well as active sweating may result in buildup of moisture droplets at the interface of the patch and the skin, which may result in some change in the adhesion. The Nitro-Dur system has a *microporous adhesive tape* just above and around the baseplate, and a *nonocclusive absorbent pad* just underneath the backing. The microporous adhesive tape allows for the permeation of excessive moisture and maintenance of good adhesion during wear.

The *pressure-sensitive adhesive* is behind the release liner at the periphery of the matrix to provide adhesion of the unit to the skin. Besides having appropriate peel strength, creep, tack, and adhesive properties, the adhesive on the tape must allow for ease in removing the release liner and should also adhere properly to the baseplate. Any of the acrylics and silicone-type or latex-type adhesives may be used. The adhesive is on the periphery of the matrix; hence diffusivity of the drug through the adhesive is not a concern.

The *polymeric matrix* of Nitro-Dur consists of polyvinyl alcohol (PVA) and polyvinyl pyrrolidone (PVP) forming the lattice structure, while the GTN and other liquid components occupy the interstices. The release of GTN from the matrix is dependent on the extent of polymer cross-linking. Ethylene glycol dimethacrylate (EGDMA), Glycidyl methacrylate (GMA), gamma rays, and dialdehydes (glutaraldehyde) are some of the agents useful for cross-linking.

A lactose triturate of GTN is mixed with the PVA and PVP mixture while in a liquid state. A matrix of GTN partitioned between lactose, polymers, and other fluid phases is formed upon cooling.

U.S. patents describe a polymeric matrix for the transdermal delivery of clonidine. The matrix consists of 6 to 20% polyvinyl alcohol, 2 to 10% polyvinyl pyrrolidone, and about 2 to 60% of a polar plasticizer, in addition to clonidine. The polar plasticizer may be glycerol, polyethylene glycol, polypropylene glycol, or mixtures of these in different ratios. Besides PVA and PVP, the other components of matrix may be 1 to 9% agar or agarose, gum arabic, acacia, tragacanth, polyacrylic acid, polymethacrylic acid, polyvinyloxazolidone, polyvinylmorpholinone, and polyvinylpiperidone. Normally, partially hydrolyzed (90%) PVA of the 50,000 to 150,000 molecular weight range is used; PVP should be in the 15,000 to 80,000 molecular weight range. Matrices without the polar plasticizers are usually less flexible and have poor diffusional properties.

The matrix may be formed by adding PVA and PVP to the water and polar plasticizer mixture with agitation and heating the mixture to approximately 95°C for extension of the polymers.

The drug is then added with mixing. The mixture is then cast and cooled to facilitate gelation. Dispersing agents such as sodium dodecyl sulfate, Tween 20, or other detergents may also be added (0.1-10%).

Microporous Matrix-Type Devices [16]

The patented microporous rate-controlling matrix of Zaffaroni [16] was designed for, but not limited to, antibiotics, hypnotics, sedatives, cardiovascular agents, and so on. The device (Fig. 19) consists of a backing material and a drug-containing microporous matrix, which rests on a pressure-sensitive adhesive layer. The drug passes through

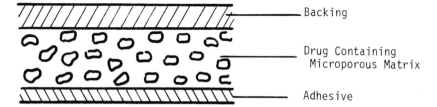

Backing

Drug Containing
Microporous Matrix

Adhesive

Fig. 19 Microporous matrix for transdermal delivery.

the rate-controlling microporous material, which continuously monitors the flow of the drug to the skin by monitoring the viscous or diffusive transfer mechanisms. The matrix is impregnated with a diffusive medium in which the drug can dissolve and which also determines the drug release rate. The drug permeation is also governed by the pressure-induced viscous flow of drug molecules through the pores of the microporous matrix. By varying composition, pore size, effective thickness of the microporous rate-controlling material, viscosity of formulation, and impregnating solvent, the delivery rate can be controlled and varied.

The *microporous materials* may be isotropic (uniform structure throughout the matrix), or anisotropic (heterogeneous structure). The materials usually employed for this purpose include polyamides (polyhexamethylene adipamide, nylon, etc.), polyvinyl chloride, poly-sulfones, acrylonitriles, polycarbonates, polyvinylidene fluoride, acrylic resins, polyurethanes, polyvinyl acetate, cellulose esters, epoxy resins, and cross-linked PVP.

The drug is usually added to the matrix material in a liquid form and is uniformly distributed and then converted to a microporous structure. Normally the polymer film is cast and then immersed in a non-solvent medium that is compatible with the solvent but does not dissolve the polymer. The original solution then forms a polymer-rich phase and a polymer-poor phase. Both phases are physically continuous but have interspersed pores. In antoher method, the preformed microporous material is impregnated with drug by immersion in a solution of the drug.

The *impregnation fluids* normally employed include water, 2 to 6 carbons containing alcohols, 1-2 butanediol, cyclohexanol, amylacetate, benzyl propionate, etheral oils, and so on. Plasticizers may also be included in the diffusive medium and include octyldiphenyl phosphate, long-chain fatty amides, higher alcohols, and high-boiling esters.

The pressure-sensitive adhesives used for this purpose are acrylates, natural or synthetic rubbers, such as silicones, polyisobutylenes, and similar materials. Various nonocclusive or occlusive backings are used and include cellophane, polypropylene, polyethylene, aluminum foil, paper, polyesters, and many other substances.

Hydrophilic Matrix Devices (Lec-Tec Matrix)

Hymes and Rolf [14] have described a new type of transdermal matrix system employing hydrophilic gel membranes. The device consists of a semi-solid state polymeric matrix acting as a reservoir as well as a hydrophilic bridge to the skin, which facilitates drug permeation into and through the skin by wetting the skin.

The hydrophilic matrix consists of polysaccharides such as algin, xanthan, and guar, or synthetic hydrophilic polymers such as polyvinyl sulfonates, PVA, PVP, polyacrylate, and polyacrylamides. The matrix also contains hydrogen-bonding liquids such as water, glycerol, propylene glycol, and polyethylene glycol. The formulation may also include an aqueous emulsion of adhesive to improve the tack of the patch. A gel is formed at room temperature; however, heating may also be used to facilitate gelling. The hydrogen-bonding rearrangement results in a properly cross-linked gel that is stable and swells in high-humidity conditions. According to Hymes and Rolf, the hydrogen bond network resulting from hydration of hydrogel structure is, on a molecular level, fluxional. The system is self-adhering and can be removed and reapplied. The transdermal delivery rate from such a system is a function of the reservoir (matrix) formulation, the hydrophilic bridges formed between the system and the skin, and the drug concentration within the aqueous phase of the skin.

Adhesive Matrix Devices

The final matrix type of system is characterized by an adhesive matrix, which also acts as a reservoir of drug and represents a new concept in transdermal delivery. This type of system is exemplified by Nitro-Dur II (Key Pharmaceuticals) as shown in Fig. 20. Here the nitroglycerin is dispersed in an acrylic adhesive. This acts as an adhesive matrix, which is coated onto a Saranex type of backing material with a clear polypropylene type of release liner.

C. Microsealed Delivery Devices [10]

The microsealed transdermal device is the result of the hybridization of the reservoir and matrix types of system and is represented by Nitro Disc (G. D. Searle Pharmaceuticals, Chicago). In this system (Fig. 21) an aqueous suspension of drug is prepared in a water-soluble polymer. The suspension is then dispersed into a lipid-soluble polymer with high-speed-shear force, to form microscopic spherical reservoirs with the drug entrapped. Immediately, the system is cross-linked by the addition of polymeric cross-linking agents, and a matrix is formed. This matrix is then attached to an aluminum foil plate at the back, to prevent evaporation of the GTN. The aluminum foil plate is then attached to an adhesive polyurethane (flexible) foam pad which forms the

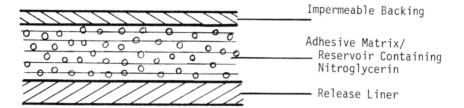

Impermeable Backing

Adhesive Matrix/
Reservoir Containing
Nitroglycerin

Release Liner

Fig. 20 Diagrammatic representation of the Nitro-Dur II.

backing. This system has a peripheral adhesive ring. The release rate of the drug from the microsealed delivery device, may be expressed [10] as follows:

$$\frac{dM}{dt} = \frac{D_p D_s X' K_p}{D_p h_d + D_s h_p X' K_p} \left[\beta S_p - \frac{D_L S_L (1 - \beta)}{h_L} \left(\frac{1}{K_L} + \frac{1}{K_m} \right) \right] \quad (5)$$

where K_L, K_m, K_p are the partition coefficients for the interfacial partitioning of the drug from liquid to matrix, from polymer membrane to skin, and from matrix to polymer membrane, respectively. The D_L, D_p, and D_s are diffusion coefficients in liquid, polymer membrane, and skin, respectively. The h_L, h_p, and h_d are the thickness of liquid, polymer membrane, and the hydrodynamic boundaries around the polymer membrane. while β is the ratio of drug concentration in the inner edge of the interface and the solubility in the matrix. In addition, $X' = d'/\beta'$, where d' is the ratio of drug concentration in the bulk of the elution solution to the drug solubility in the elution solution and β' is the ratio of the drug concentration at the outer edge of the polymer membrane to the drug solubility in polymer membrane.

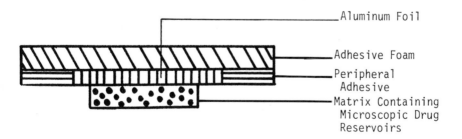

Aluminum Foil

Adhesive Foam

Peripheral
Adhesive

Matrix Containing
Microscopic Drug
Reservoirs

Fig. 21 Scheme for a microreservoir transdermal delivery device.

D. Poroplastic- or Moleculon-Type Devices

The Poroplastic devices which are being developed at Moleculon (Cambridge, Massachusetts) utilize Poroplastic films. The Poroplastic films consist of ultramicroporous cellulose triacetate membranes which are not sensitizing to skin and are fairly stable at even higher than normal temperatures and at biological pH [17].

The film as described in the proprietary literature [18] is made utilizing the concept of the water coagulation of cellulose triacetate solution in organic acids at low temperatures. The coagulation is performed under controlled conditions and the extent of water content may be varied to a great degree. The percent weight of water in a Poroplastic film is used to give an identification number for different grades of Poroplastic films. According to Obermayer [17], the water may be exchanged subsequently for another vehicle by a diffusional exchange process, and hence a Poroplastic membrane is also known as "solid composed mostly of liquid." The liquid in the film is held by capillary action; therefore Poroplastics are also compared to molecular sponges but with a much smaller pore size. The Poroplastics are available in different molecular weight cutoff ranges, which are directly related to the percentage of water present in the film. The greater the amount of water in the film, the greater is the pore diameter; for example, for films with 70% water the apparent pore diameter is 0.0014 μm, for 85% water the pore diameter is 0.0025 μm, and for 92% water content the pore diameter is 0.006 μm.

The internal diffusivities are very high in Poroplastic films because of the presence of liquid(s), and this results in higher permeability of drugs through such films. However, the rate-control feature can be added to such systems by reducing the percentage of liquid, by changing the type of liquid (to reduce the solubility of drug), by adding a rate-limiting membrane external to the film, or by changing the structure (such as tortuosity) or collapsing pores to some extent.

The cellulose triacetate film is chemically inert and functions just to hold the vehicle and the drug; hence the permeation rate is basically governed by the formulation and the vehicle characteristics. Some of the model vehicles for a Poroplastic film include polyethylene glycols (low molecular weight), propylene glycol, water, alcohols, aliphatic esters, mineral oils, silicone fluids, and glycerol.

The design features of the three types of Poroplastic transdermal device are summarized in Table 1 and shown in Fig. 22.

E. Transdermal Delivery of Macromolecules

Typical requirements for transdermal delivery of drugs include low molecular weight ($\leq$ 500-1000, preferably < 500), low melting characteristics ($\leq$ 150-200°F), aqueous solutions neither too acidic nor too

TABLE 1 Design Features of Poroplastic Patches

Simple monolith	Zero order	Reservoir
1. Drug solution in membrane.	1. Drug crystals are present in membrane.	1. Concentrated solution of drug behind the Poroplastic film acts as a distinct reservoir.
2. Drug content depletes with time and permeability decreases.	2. As drug permeates, more crystals dissolve to maintain saturated solution.	2. As drug permeates out of the film, more drug enters the film from the reservoir.

basic (between 5 and 9 pH units, preferably in the pH range of 6.0-8.0), and preferably unit oil/water partition coefficients. Typical macromolecules do not possess these characteristics and hence are not ideal candidates for transdermal delivery. Only recently have any attempts been made to characterize diffusional properties of some low molecular weight peptides. While there are no FDA-approved transdermal devices for the delivery of peptides, advances have been made lately in the fabrication of systems for the rate-controlled delivery of macromolecules (for hormones, enzymes, interferon, bioactive peptides, etc.) [19]. The devices under consideration may be divided into two categories: (a) devices based on *ethylene vinyl acetate copolymers* (EVAc) and (b) devices based on *silicone elastomers*. Both systems utilize one common concept: that is, because of the large molecular size of drug the matrix must have channels to facilitate the release of macromolecules. These devices are used as implants, but since the release is diffusion controlled and the technology can be modified somewhat to suit transdermal delivery, the technology alone is discussed here in brief.

EVAc Copolymer-Type Macromolecule Delivery Devices

The general procedure [20] for designing EVAc copolymer-type macromolecule delivery systems essentially follows the flowchart shown in Fig. 23. When the polymer solution is mixed with presieved macro-

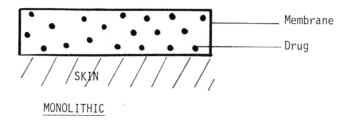

MONOLITHIC

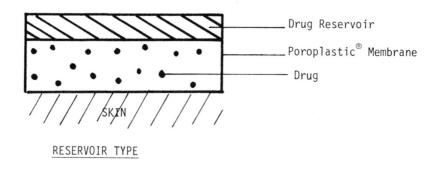

RESERVOIR TYPE

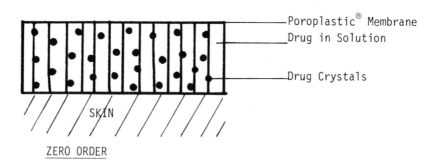

ZERO ORDER

Fig. 22 Different types of Poroplastic transdermal device. (Adapted from Ref. 17.)

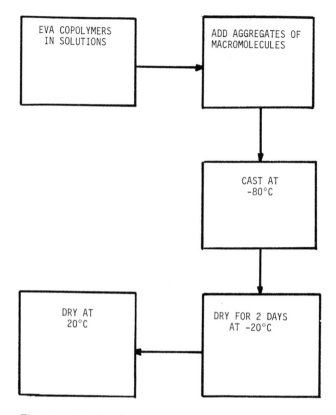

Fig. 23 Fabrication procedure for casting macromolecule delivery systems containing EVAc copolymers. (Adapted from Ref. 20.)

molecular aggregates and molded at -80°C, a gel is produced which is then dried at -20°C to remove the solvent. Apparently, the release kinetics are affected in a desired manner when the casting is done this way at low temperatures [21]. Presieved aggregates are incorporated so that heterogeneity is minimum, and extremely low temperatures are used in drying to achieve physical stability of the matrix. The release kinetics are affected appreciably by loading, size distribution of aggregates, and the coating [20].

Alternately, aqueous dispersions may be used so as to incorporate small amounts of biologically active substances in EVAc [22]. In this method the aqueous solution of drug is mixed with the polymer solution and the temperature is reduced to allow the water to freeze. Low temperature drying is used to evaporate the organic solvent while water is removed by lyophilizaiton. This procedure creates channels which facilitate the release of the drug. The diffusion-controlled EVAc matrix type of device for the delivery of macromolecules may be *hemisphere shaped* [23] or of the magnetically *modulated release type* [24]. A solvent casting method is used in both cases (Fig. 23) but for a few modifications. For hemispherical devices (Fig. 24) the matrix is prepared in a hemispherical mold. After drying first at -20°C and then at +20°C, it is dipped in the EVAc solution. The coating is repeated and the device is dried again at the two temperatures (-20 and +20°C). During the coating, a stick is inserted in the flat surface so that the final device has a cavity in the center of the flat surface. This device, with proper geometric parameters, gives a fairly good zero-order release.

Magnetically modulated devices modulate the release rate, whenever needed, by the application of magnetic field. The basic principle of construction is similar to that described in Fig. 23. The EVAc-macromolecule solution/dispersion is cast into a slab at -80°C and the magnetic beads are embedded, and then another layer of the solution is cast on top of the first layer. The entire device is dried at -20°C and at 20°C.

Silicone Elastomer-Type Macromolecular Delivery Devices [19,25]

This type of device is made by using different medical-grade silicone elastomers in certain ratios. The macromolecular powder is added to the mixture very slowly, with constant mixing, and then a calculated amount of polymerizing agent is also added. The mixture is kept under vacuum and then extruded into a Tygon or Silastic tubing and allowed to cure overnight at room temperature. When the cross-linking is complete, the tubing is cut into small pieces of preset dimensions. One end of the tubing is coated with impermeable Silastic coating, while the other end is left open to allow the drug release.

IV. PRESSURE-SENSITIVE ADHESIVES

Pressure-sensitive adhesives are very similar to contact adhesives, the major difference being the requirement of pressure to effect the bond. Pressure-sensitive materials usually consist of a rubbery elastomer and a modifying tackifier. The substrate may be coated by a solvent system or a hot melt. Usually, these systems are highly thixotropic and have good "quick tack." The temperature capability is often limited, and some of these systems are subject to oxidative degradation.

The pressure-sensitive adhesives currently used in transdermal delivery devices may be classified into three categories: butyl rubbers and polyisobutylenes, acrylics, and silicones.

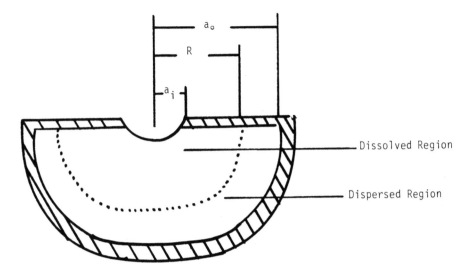

Dissolved Region

Dispersed Region

Fig. 24   Scheme of a hemisphere shaped delivery device: a_o - outer radius, a_i = inner radius, and R = distance of interface between dissolved and dispersed regions. (Adapted from Ref. 23.)

A. Butyl Rubber and Polyisobutylenes

Elastomeric polymers [26] are used widely in pressure-sensitive adhesives both as primary elastomers and as tackifiers and modifiers. Butyl rubber is a copolymer of isobutylene with trace levels of isoprene while polyisobutylene is a homopolymer. Butyl rubber is fairly inert and stable because the C—H backbone is fairly large (contains 40,000-60,000 units) with only few double bonds and other reactive sites. Since it is a hydrocarbon the polymer has low solubility in water, but it is is soluble in hydrocarbon solvents. The side groups attached to the polymer chain are small and regularly spaced and the structure is compact and unstrained. Because of these properties, the permeability of the polymer to gas, air, and moisture is very low.

The polyisobutylenes are very similar to butyl rubbers but differ in terminal unsaturation and have a wide molecular weight range. The low molecular weight ones are tough, strong, and elastic rubbers. These polymers (butyl rubbers and polyisobutylenes) depend on crosslinking rather than crystallinity for their strength. This makes the internal structure completely amorphous and gives them flexibility, tack, internal mobility, and similar desirable properties. They have a low glass transition temperature (-60°C), indicating maintenance of these physical properties at subambient temperatures. These polymers have little or no polarity and hence show poor attraction toward other surfaces, even though the tack is good. Therefore, resins and other polarity-imparting substances are added to give better surface properties.

Butyl rubbers are made by copolymerizing isobutylene with less than 3% of isoprene. The presence of isoprenic double bonds permits cross-linking. Butyl rubbers are mainly differentiated on the basis of the number of isoprene units per 100 monomer units in the chain, as well as molecular weight. Stabilizers of several types (zinc dibutyl dithiocarbamate, BHT, etc.) are FDA approved. Metallic stearates are added to all butyl rubbers during preparation to prevent coagulation of polymer particles [18,27]. Butyl rubbers are also available in several halogenated grades, in low molecular weight, semiliquid form, and in various partially cross-linked grades. The halogenation tends to increase the reactivity of the double bonds and supplies extra reactive sites for cross-linking.

The low molecular weight polyisobutylenes are permanently tacky, clear to white-yellow semiliquids containing no stabilizers [29]. They have wide acceptability by the FDA and show some flow at elevated temperatures (150-180°C). They are primarily used as tackifiers. Such polymers provide tackiness, softness, and flexibility and assist in improving adhesion by wetting other surfaces. Low molecular weight polyisobutylenes are especially useful in increasing adhesion to polyolefin plastic surfaces.

The high molecular weight polyisobutylenes are tough, rubberlike solids, containing traces of BHT stabilizer [30]. They have good acceptance by the FDA and impart flow resistance and strength. They are also used in hot melts, where they enhance flexibility and impact resistance, particularly at low temperatures.

The adhesive strength of isobutylenes may be increased by (a) adding high molecular weight polyisobutylene (PIB) with butyl rubber and curing the butyl rubber portion (since the PIB does not cure, hence the cohesive strength is governed by the butyl rubber portion); (b) partial curing of butyl rubber; and (c) blending either PIB or butyl with chlorobutyl portion and curing only the chlorobutyl portion with a curative such as zinc oxide.

The *tack* of pressure-sensitive adhesives may be increased with Vistanex LM, depolymerization of butyl rubber, or addition of *tackifiers*, resins such as phenolformaldehyde resin (SP-1068), modified resins, resin esters, and hydrocarbons (Escorez 112, Escorez 1304, Escorez 1315) [31].

B. Acrylic Adhesives

The pressure-sensitive acrylic adhesives derive their pressure sensitivity from acrylic esters, which result in polymers of low glass transition temperatures (T_g) and can be copolymerized with acrylic acid and many other functional monomers. Generally, suitable monomers include alkyl acrylate and methacrylates with 4 to 17 carbon atoms and these are excellent pressure-sensitive adhesives. 2-Ethylhexyl acrylate, butyl acrylate, and acrylic acid are commonly used monomers. The polymer properties can be varied by copolymerization with other monomers. Normally the glass transition temperature is used to predict the pressure-sensitive adhesive application of a polymer and the effect of a comonomer on the copolymer properties. Pressure-sensitive properties, such as peel adhesion, may be correlated with T_g [32]. A polymer that is too soft and fails cohesively when peeled can be improved by copolymerization using a monomer that increases T_g. Similarly, a hard polymer that fails in peel because of stick-slip manner may be improved by incorporation of a low-T_g monomer. The homopolymer must have a low T_g to give good tack. 2-Ethylhexyl acrylate ($T_g = -54°C$) and n-butyl acrylate ($T_g = -54°C$) have good tack and make good pressure-sensitive adhesives. Homopolymers with high T_g are generally not tacky enough. Polymer flexibility and tackiness can be increased by increasing the side chain length until the chains start forming crystalline regions, which results in stiffening. For a straight-chain polymer, n-octyl acrylates afford maximum softness ($T_g = -80°C$) in the acrylate series, and n-decyl or n-dodecyl in the methacrylate series [33,34]. Branching of side chains results in stiffening of polymers having lengths in the propyl and hexyl range. For long-chain polymers, increased branching results in reduction of crystalline regions, and softening occurs. It has also been shown [35] that peel adhesion of copolymers of methacrylate with alkyl or aryl acrylates, in a molar ratio of 9:1, increases with the increasing length of comonomer side chain. For long-chain polymers, increased branching results in the reduction of crystalline regions and softening occurs.

Molecular weight has a profound effect on the mechanical properties of acrylic polymers [36]. Low molecular weight polymer normally exhibit good tack but poor shear resistance. Such polymers need crosslinking to be acceptable adhesives. High molecular weight polymers exhibit resistance to creep. This is not observed normally in low molecular weight polymers unless they have high secondary bonding. Nevertheless, there is a better correlation of adhesive properties with intrinsic viscosity than with average molecular weight. It is the rate of polymerization that determines the molecular weight range. Both the tack and resistance to peel increase with increasing molecular weight. The maximum tack and resistance to peel are observed at not too high molecular weight, and it is the same region where transition from cohesive to adhesive failure takes place. Increases in molecular weight beyond this point result in reduction and leveling of these properties. Good pressure-sensitive adhesives are in this range and show only small variations in tack with increasing molecular weight beyond the transition range. Shear resistance also increases with increasing weight. According to published reports [37], in the region of slow peel rates the peel strength increases with increasing molecular weights, since the peel strength is increased by viscous flow of the adhesive.

Cross-Linking

The main purpose of cross-linkers is to improve the shear resistance of pressure-sensitive adhesive especially at high temperatures. The improvement in shear resistance is fairly dramatic even at a low density of cross-linking. With cross-linking, the free movement of polymer molecules is considerably reduced and a decrease in tack is noticed. The viscoelastic properties of the polymers are affected such that the elastic component is increased, while there is a reduction in the viscous component. The peel adhesion also frequently decreases with cross-linking. The change from a cohesive failure to an adhesive failure during peeling is shifted toward lower peel rates and higher temperature with the increased cross-linking density. An adhesive that has been cross-linked may not demonstrate this transition at all, but there may be a total adhesive failure [36].

The introduction of divinyl monomers during polymerization is well established for cross-linking. Divinyl benzene, ethylene glycol dimethacrylate, and many other monomers are used similarly for cross-linking while maintaining a low cross-linking density. Different vinyl monomers carrying functional groups can be easily copolymerized with acrylic monomers, providing sites for cross-linking. To maintain flexibility and a high stress relaxation rate, the long and flexible chains must be cross-linked. There are two basic approaches to cross-linking:

1. Functional groups are introduced along the polymer chain and an additive consisting of several functional groups capable of reacting with the pendant functional groups is introduced later.
2. Several functional groups capable of interaction are introduced into the polymer chain, providing sites for intermolecular cross-linking.

Functional groups that are frequently used for cross-linking [38, 39] include carboxyl, amide, hydroxyl, allylic double bond, and amine. Salts of multivalent metals are also added for cross-linking.

C. Silicone Adhesives

Silicone pressure-sensitive adhesives exhibit the flexible characteristics of silicone rubber and the temperature resistance of the silicone resins. Moreover, they are nonreacting and are functional between extremely low and high temperatures, giving them versatility. Such adhesives are based on two components, a gum and a resin. The resin functions as a tackifier and for optimizing the physical properties of the pressure-sensitive adhesive. A broad range of tack and peel adhesion properties is achieved with the variation of the gum/resin ratio. The chemical reaction required proceeds via condensation reaction of SiOH gorups in the polymers. The inter- and intramolecular condensation is responsible for physical properties of the adhesive. Adhesives containing a high amount of gum are very tacky at room temperature, while those with higher amounts of reson are tacky only at elevated temperatures. There are two different types of silicone gum: methyl and phenyl [40].

The methyl-based silicone pressure-sensitive adhesives exhibit a wide range of viscosities (100-90,000 cp) and, typically contain approximately 50% solids. Normally the peel adhesion of a tacky adhesive increases with the addition of a dry-type adhesive. A dry type of methyl-based adhesive having peel strength of 1110 g/cm may be blended with a tacky adhesive to raise its peel strength from 400 g/cm to about 800 g/cm (about 30% dry type and 70% tacky type). These methyl types of adhesive are universal. The phenyl-based adhesives are available in two viscosity ranges: 6,000 to 25,000 cp and 50,000 to 100,000 cp. Phenyl adhesives have good tack and peel strength, and high viscosity [40].

Silicone adhesives normally exhibit 0 to 1500 g/cm^2 tack on Polyken Probe Tack Testers. Methyl adhesives with low tack at room temperature exhibit good adhesive properties at about 90°C and high pressure, hence are good for making laminates.

Curing of silicone adhesives may be achieved by addition of 2,4-dichlorobenzoyl peroxide or benzoyl peroxide at high temperatures. This results in an adhesive with high-temperature shear properties while nearly maintaining the peel strength.

V. TACKIFIERS

The adhesive properties of pressure-sensitive adhesives depend primarily on the viscoelastic properties of the adhesive mass. In such adhesive formulations, the elastomer adds the elastic component while a tackifier provides the viscous properties. The principal properties of adhesives are tack, resistance to peel, and resistance to shear, and these are controlled by the characteristics of the elastomer-tackifier mixture. Schlademan [41] has described *tack* as a measure of viscous flow under conditions of fast strain rates and low stress magnitudes, while *shear adhesion* (creep) is a measure of viscous flow at low strain rates and medium stress levels. *Peel adhesion* is a measure of resistance to flow at intermediate strain rates and medium to high stress

levels and is also a measure of the cohesive strength of the adhesive.
A good adhesive has a proper balance of these properties.

The tackifiers used in pressure sensitive adhesives are divided
into two types: rosin types and hydrocarbon resins. The rosin group
consists of rosin, modified rosins, their esters, and so on. The hydrocarbon resin group consists of polyterpenes, synthetic hydrocarbons,
phenolic resins, and similar compounds.

VI. RELEASE COATINGS

Release liners are an intergral component of transdermal delivery devices. They provide protection from undesirable contact of the product
with other surfaces. Several factors contribute toward the properties
of the release coatings used in the release liners.

The release coating should not be wetted by the adhesive; that
is, contact between the release liner and the adhesive should be poor.
A smooth but tough plastic film may be used as a release liner without
any release coating. Better anchorage of adhesive to backing may
also be imparted by prime coatings to provide better release of the
release liner. One of the most important considerations is that the
surface of release liner be nonporous so as to prevent the soft-adhesive
flow into the pores which would otherwise result in the need for increased
unwinding force. The release coating, according to Satas [42], should
meet the following requirements:

1. The coating should provide an adequate release. The release
   level should be low enough to permit an easy unwind. The
   release should be slow at low peel angle and fast at 90° peel.
2. The release should be reproducible, also meaning that the
   release should not depend on the amount of release agent.
3. The release agent should be firmly anchored to the surface
   of the release liner or the release backing and should not be
   susceptible to being transferred to the adhesive.

The release coating is normally applied as a dilute solution or a
dispersion over the release backing ($2-3$ g/m^2).

Solvent-borne silicone release coatings are applied to a variety of
substrates such as supercalendered two-side-sized kraft, glassine,
kraft-glassine, foil, and polyethylene/polypropylene film [43].

Water-borne silicone systems have historically been applied for
non-pressure-sensitive applications and hence will not be discussed
here.

The most recent development in silicone release technology consists of the solventless silicone coatings, which are applied at 100%
solids level. These were designed specifically for pressure-sensitive

release and consist of a vinyl functional polymethyl hydrogen siloxane cross-linker and a noble metal catalyst. They can give thin films (0.03-0.04 mil thick). Solventless silicone coatings are applied to two-side sized, supercalendered kraft substrates [43].

REFERENCES

1. A. Zaffaroni, New approaches to drug administration, Abstract of papers presented at 31st International Congress of Pharmaceutical Sciences, Washington, DC, 1971, p. 19.
2. G. W. Cleary, *Transdermal Concepts and Perspectives*. Drug Information, Clinical & Technical Affairs, Key Pharmaceuticals, Inc., 18425 N.W. 2nd Ave., Miami, FL.
3. Y. W. Chien, in *Transdermal Delivery of Drugs*, Vol. I (A. F. Kydonieus and B. Berner, eds.). CRC Press, Boca Ration, FL, 1987, p. 86.
4. J. Urguhart, S. D. Chandrasekharan, and J. E. Shaw, Bandage for transdermally administering scopolamine to prevent nausea, U.S. Patent 4,041,894 (June 28, 1977).
5. *Physician's Desk Reference*, 40th ed. (E. R. Barnhart, ed.). Medical Economics Co., Oradell, NJ, 1986, p. 819.
6. S. K. Chandrasekharan, S. Darda, A. S. Michaels, and G. W. Cleary, Therapeutic system for administering clonidine transdermally, U.S. Patent 4,201,211 (May 6, 1980).
7. P. S. Campbell and S. K. Chandrasekharan, Dosage for coadministering drug and percutaneous absorption enhancer, U.S. Patent 4,379,454 (April 12, 1983).
8. A. F. Kydonieus, in *Transdermal Delivery of Drugs*, Vol. I (A. F. Kydonieus and B. Berner, eds.). CRC Press, Boca Ration, FL, 1987, p. 145.
9. P. S. Campbell and S. K. Chandrasekharan, Dosage for coadministering drug and percutaneous absorption enhancer, U.S. Patent 4,379,454 (April 12, 1983).
10. Y. W. Chien, in *Transdermal Delivery of Drugs*, Vol. I (A. F. Kydonieus and B. Berner, eds.). CRC Press, Boca Ration, FL, 1987, p. 86.
11. A. Zaffaroni, Bandage for the controlled metering of topical drugs to skin, U.S. Patent 3,731,683 (May 8, 1973).
12. A. Zaffaroni, Bandage for administering drugs, U.S. Patent 3,598,123 (Aug. 10, 1971).
13. A. Zaffaroni, Therapeutic adhesive patch, U.S. Patent 3,699,963 (October 1972).
14. A. C. Hymes and D. Rolf, in *Transdermal Delivery of Drugs*, Vol. I (A. F. Kydonieus and B. Berner, eds.). CRC Press, Boca Ration, FL, 1987, p. 157.

15. G. Cleary and A. Keith, in *Transdermal Delivery of Drugs*, Vol. I (A. F. Kydonieus and B. Berner, eds.). CRC Press, Boca Ration, FL, 1987, p. 117.

16. A. Zaffaroni, Bandage for the administration of drug by controlled metering through microporous materials, U.S. Patent 3,797,494 (March 19, 1974.

17. A. S. Obermayer, in *Transdermal Delivery of Drugs*, Vol. I (A. F. Kydonieus and B. Berner, eds.). CRC Press, Boca Ration, FL, 1987, p. 161.

18. Moleculon Research Corporation, internal document on Poroplastic toxicology, *References on Toxicity of Cellulose Triacetate Membranes*. Moleculon, Cambridge, MA.

19. D. S. T. Hsieh, in *Transdermal Delivery of Drugs*, Vol. I (A. F. Kydonieus and B. Berner, eds.). CRC Press, Boca Ration, FL, 1987, p. 161.

20. W. D. Rhine, D. S. T. Hsieh, and R. Langer, *J. Pharm. Sci.*, 69:265 (1980).

21. R. Langer and J. Folkman, *Nature*, 263:797 (1976).

22. D. S. T. Hsieh and R. Langer, Methods of making Prolonged release body, U.S. Patent 4,357,312.

23. D. S. T. Hsieh, W. D. Rhine, and R. Langer, *J. Pharm. Sci.*, 72:17 (1983).

24. D. S. T. Hsieh, R. Langer, and J. Folkman, Magnetic modulation of release of macromolecules from polymer, *Proc. Natl. Acad. Sci. U.S.A.*, 78:1863 (1981).

25. D. S. T. Hsieh, C. C. Chang, and D. S. Desai, *Pharm. Technol.*, 9(6):39 (1985).

26. D. J. Buckley, *Rubber Chem. Technol.*, 32(5):1475 (December 1959).

27. *Introduction to Rubber Technology* (W. L. Dunkel, R. F. Neu, R. L. Zapp, and R. L. Morton, eds.). Van Nostrand, New York, 1959, p. 309.

28. R. M. Thomas and W. J. Sparks, in *Synthetic Rubber* (G. S. Whitby, ed.). Wiley, New York, 1954.

29. An introduction to Vistanex LM low molecular weight polyisobutylene. Brochure SC-79-131, Exxon Chemical Co. U.S.A., Houston, 1979.

30. Vistanex polyisobutylene, properties and applications. Brochure SYN-76-1434, Exxon Chemical Co., U.S.A., Houston, 1974.

31. J. J. Higgins, F. C. Jagisch and N. E. Strucker, in *Handbook of Pressure Sensitive Adhesive Technology* (D. Satas, ed.). Van Nostrand Reinhold, New York, 1982, p. 283.

32. D. W. Aubrey, in *Development in Adhesives*, Vol. 1 (W. C. Wake, ed.). Applied Science Publishers, Barking, England, 1977, p. 127.

33. C. E. Rehberg and C. H. Fischer, *J. Am. Chem. Soc.*, 40:1203 (1944).
34. C. E. Rehberg and C. H. Fisher, *J. Am. Chem. Soc.*, 40:1429 (1948).
35. T. J. Mao and S. L. Reegen, in *Proceedings of the Symposium on Adhesion and Cohesion* (P. Weiss, ed.). Elsevier, Amsterdam, 1962, p. 202.
36. D. Satas, in *Handbook of Pressure Sensitive Adhesive Technology* (D. Satas, ed.). Van Nostrand Reinhold, New York, 1982, p. 307.
37. D. W. Aubrey, G. N. Welding, and T. J. Wong, *J. Appl. Polym. Sci.*, 13:2193 (1969).
38. T. J. Miranda, *J. Paint Technol.*, 38:469 (1966).
39. *Offic. Dig.*, June 1961, p. 679.
40. D. F. Merrill, in *Handbook of Pressure Sensitive Adhesive Technology* (D. Satas, ed.). Van Nostrand Reinhold, New York, 1982, p. 344.
41. J. A. Schlademan, in *Handbook of Pressure Sensitive Adhesive Technology* (D. Satas, ed.). Van Nostrand Reinhold, New York, 1982, p. 353.
42. D. Satas, in *Handbook of Pressure Sensitive Adhesive Technology* (D. Satas, ed.). Van Nostrand Reinhold, New York, 1982, p. 370.
43. M. D. Fey and J. E. Wilson, in *Handbook of Pressure Sensitive Adhesive Technology* (D. Satas, ed.). Van Nostrand Reinhold, New York, 1982, p. 384.

14

Iontopheretic Devices

PRAVEEN TYLE* / American Cyanamid Company, Princeton,
New Jersey

BRUCE KARI / Children's Hospital, St. Paul, Minnesota

---

*_Current affiliation_: Sandoz Pharmaceutical Corporation, Lincoln, Nebraska

I. INTRODUCTION

In conventional transdermal drug delivery, the delivery of the drug
to the site of action at therapeutic levels is sometimes hindered because
many drugs are ionized and, as such, are unable to penetrate the skin
surface adequately. The stratum corneum is the main barrier limiting
the passive transepidermal (skin pores) routes constitute the major
penetration pathways for the ionized molecules [1-5]; however, the
surface area occupied by these pathways is relatively small (Fig. 1).
The only skin appendages applicable are hair follicles, sebaceous
glands, and the eccrine sweat glands [1]. Penetration of ionic drugs
by the transfollicular and transappendageal routes can be facilitated
by the application of electricity.

Iontophoresis (or ion transfer) is defined as the migration of ions
when an electrical current is passed through a solution containing ionized species. A schematic representation of this phenomenon is shown
in Fig. 2. Drugs in the ionic form, contained in a reservoir, can be
"phoresed" out with a small current and driven into the body through
the skin [6-12]. The potential affects ions already present in tissues
but, more importantly, it also affects ionized drugs at the skin surface
and can drive them into the body through the skin pores [1]. Electrical
potential by itself does not change skin permeability [4,13]. Positive
ions can be introduced into the tissues from the positive pole, while
those of negative charge can be introduced from the negative pole.

Various reports exist in the literature showing a relative increase
in the absorption rate and total amount of drug absorbed when iontophoresis is used compared to the conventional methods of transdermal
drug delivery. This noninvasive drug delivery means minimizes
trauma, risk of infection, and damage to the wound and is an
important alternative to the needle.

II. THERAPEUTIC APPLICATIONS

As early as 1908, LeDuc [14] showed that chemicals could be carried
across an avascular membrane using electric potential as an electro-
motive force. Strohl et al. [15] found considerable activity in the
blood after electrophoretic introduction of radioactive sodium iodide
into the skin of rats, guinea pigs, and rabbits, whereas the penetration by "simple diffusion" (meaning application without electric current)
was negligible. Their results are shown in Fig. 3. It is suggested
that iontophoresis could markedly facilitate the transdermal transport

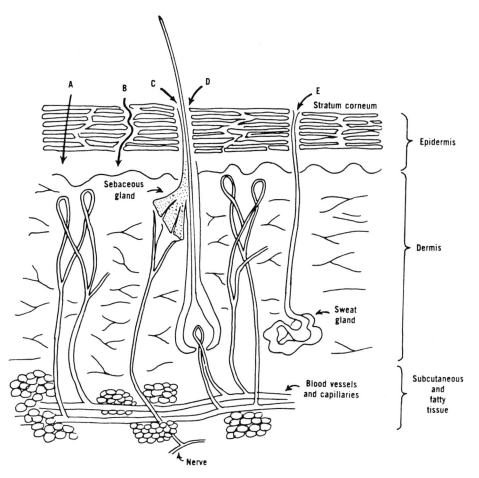

Fig. 1 Schematic presentation of probably routes of penetration.
Sites of percutaneous penetration: A = transcellular, B = diffusion
through channels between cells, C = through sebaceous ducts, D =
transfollicular, and E = through sweat ducts. (From Ref. 78.)

of ionized drug molecules [10-16]. In other words, percutaneous absorption can be regulated by the strength of the current.

A schematic representation of the complete circuit involved in the
process of iontophoresis is shown in Fig. 4. Drug contained in a gauze
pad is applied under an electrode of the same charge as the drug,
and a return electrode (over a gauze pad soaked in saline) opposite
in charge to the drug is placed at a distal location on the body surface.
The current below the level of the patient's pain threshold is then allowed to flow for an appropriate length of time. Shelley et al. [6] tested

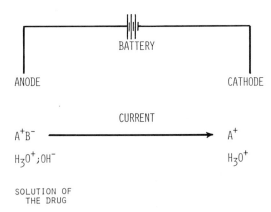

Fig. 2 Movement of active drug ions A^+ from anode to cathode under the influence of current.

nine antihistaminic compounds and concluded that they could be administered transdermally by iontophoresis to achieve local antihistaminic action. Also, the effect of iontophoresis was that of acceleration of absorption. They also concluded that since the acceleration was roughly equivalent for similar compounds, it is possible to correlate the effectiveness of compounds introduced by iontophoresis with their effectiveness when applied in topical preparations.

Iontophoresis at some unusual sites has also been reported. Iontophoresis of sulfa drugs, for pyocyaneous infection, was 3 to 12 times greater in the cornea and 3 to 15 times greater in the aqueous humor of the eye than that resulting from diffusion alone [16]. The results are shown in Fig. 5. The results of Rapperport et al. [10] show that the amount of penicillin deposited through burn eschar and into the avascular tissue was 200-fold greater with iontophoresis compared with simple diffusion.

Harris [17] concluded that iontophoresis is a clinically effective, painless, and safe mode of delivering ionized anti-inflammatory drugs to inflamed tissues. Delacerda [18] also showed that the effect of iontophoresis of anti-inflammatory drug in shoulder girdle myofascial syndrome is more effective than treatment with muscle relaxant and analgesic medicament or treatment with hydrocollator/ultrasound modalities.

Table 1 summarizes the various disease conditions in which iontophoretic drug delivery has been used. It should be realized that much of the work done prior to 1960 was based on clinical impressions rather than on a quantitative estimation of the amount of material introduced. Few controlled trials have been undertaken, and even when these approach the "double-blind" technique, comparison with results obtained by other methods has not been made.

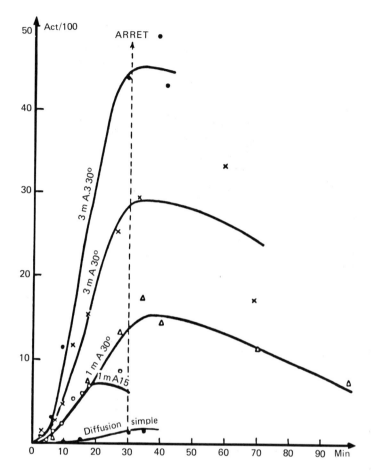

Fig. 3 Development of activity in the blood of rats as a function of intensity of current and length of application after electrophoretic introduction of radioactive sodium iodide into the skin. (From Ref. 15.)

Table 2 shows the effect of duration of iontophoresis, at a fixed current, on the rate of sweat production [23,24]. The drug used was 0.5% pilocarpine in the diagnosis of cystic fibrosis. The optimum sweating rate was attained when the quantity of electrical charge delivered reached a value at about 47 mC/cm^2 of skin. This deposits approximately 0.1 mg of pilocarpine per square centimeter, which is the recommended dosage for the diagnosis of cystic fibrosis. This technique is reported as reliable and more advantageous than other methods of

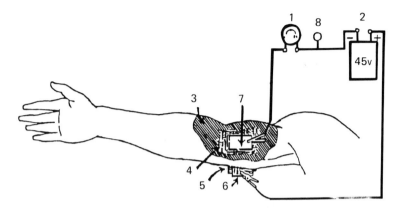

Fig. 4 Schematic representation of an iontophoresis circuit: 1 = milliammeter, 2 = battery, 3 = scar, 4 = gauze with drug, 5 = gauze with saline, 6 = electrode (positive), 7 = electrode (negative), and 8 = potentiometer. (From Ref. 10.)

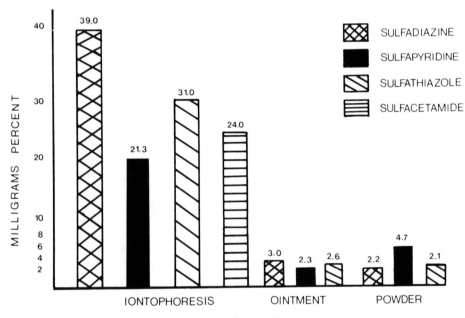

Fig. 5 Comparative concentrations of sulfa drugs in the aqueous humor of the eye after application by various methods. (From Ref. 16.)

TABLE 1 Drugs Used in Various Disease Conditions for Therapy by Iontophoresis

Drug	Condition/disease	Reference
1. Methylene blue and potassium iodide	Skin disorders (e.g., Demodex infection)	Jenkinson and Walton [7][a]
2. Pencillin	Burns	Rapperport et al. [10][b]
3. Histamine	Disease conditions of soft tissues, bursae, and tendons	Kling and Sashin [11][a]
4. Sodium iodide	Electrolytes	Strohl et al. [15][b]
5. Sulfa drugs	Pyocyaneus infection	von Sallmann [16][b]
6. Dexamethasone, sodium phosphate, and xylocaine	Musculoskeletal inflammatory conditions	Harris [17][a] Delacerda [18][a]
7. Copper	Contraception	Riar et al. [19][b]
8. Insulin	Diabetes	Kari [21][b] Stephen et al. [22][b] Siddiqui et al. [99][b]
9. Pilocarpine	Cystic fibrosis	Webster [23][b]
10. Ragweed pollen extract	Hay fever	Abramson [31][a]
11. Thyrotropin releasing hormone	Hormone deficiency	Burnette and Marrero [34][c]
12. Phosphorus		O'Malley and Oester [35][b]
13. Citrate	Rheumatoid arthritis	Coyer [51][a]
14. Dexamethasone sodium phosphate and lidocaine hydrochloride	Primary tendinitis	Bertolucci [52][d]

TABLE 1 (*continued*)

Drug	Conditions/disease	Reference
15. Vidarabine monophosphate (Ara-AMP)	Keratitis (herpes virus)	Kwon et al. [54][b] Hill et al. [56][b]
16. Lignocaine hydrochloride or lidocaine	Topical analgesia/local anesthetic	Comeau et al. [9,28][d] Russo et al. [12][d] Echols et al. [27][a] Siddiqui et al. [38][c] Petelenz et al. [55][d] Schleuning et al. [59][a] Gangarosa [60,61][a] Arvidsson et al. [62][a]
17. Acetyl β-methylcholine chloride	Arteriosclerosis	Cohn and Benson [57][a]
18. Acetyl β-methylcholine	Arthritis	Martin and Eaton [58][a]
19. Idoxuridine	Herpes simples, keratitis	Gangarosa et al. [60,63][d
20. Sodium fluoride	Dentin	Gangarosa [60][a]
21. Methylprednisolone succinate	Postherpetic neuralgia	Gangarosa et al. [64][a]
22. Lidocaine, epinephrine, and corticosteroid	Temporomandibular joint-myo-fascial pain dysfunction syndrome	Gangarosa and Mahon [65][a]
23. Sodium salicylate	Planter warts	Gordon and Weinstein [66][a]
24. Calcium	Myopathy	Kahn [67][a]
25. Acetic acid	Calcium deposits	Kahn [68][a]

26.	Zinc	Nasal disorders	Weir [69][a]
27.	Esterified glucocorticoids	Peyronie's disease	Rothfeld and Murray [70][a]
28.	Vasopressin	Lateral septal neuron activity	Marchand and Hagino [71][c]
29.	Alkaloids	Chronic pain	Csillik et al. [73][a]
30.	Optidase	Arthrosis	Ulrich [74][a]
31.	Natrium salicylicum butazolindin	Acute thrombophlebitis	Kostadinov et al. [75][a]
32.	Penicillin	Pneumonia and abscesses of lungs	Sokolov et al. [76][b]
33.	Papaverine and nicotinic acid	Cervical osteochondrosis with neurological symptoms	Ostrokhovich and Strelkova [77][b]
34.	Grasses	Allergy	Shilkret [80][a]
35.	Metoprolol	Beta-blocker (angina pectoris)	Okabe et al. [82][b]
36.	Zinc oxide	Ischemic ulcer	Cornwall [84][a]
37.	Triamcinolone	Aphthous stomatitis	Lekas [85][b]
38.	Hyaluronidase	Hemorrhages, scleroderma, and lymphedema	Boone [53][a], Popkin [86][a], Schwartz [87][a]
39.	Meladine	Vitiligo	Moawad [88][b]
40.	Iodine	Scar	Tannenbaum [89][a]
41.	Poldine methyl sulfate	Plantar and palmar hyperhydrosis	Hill [90][a], Gric et al. [91][b]
42.	Water	Hyperhidrosis	Tapper [43][a], Levit [92][b], Midtgaard [94][a]

TABLE 1 (continued)

Drug	Conditions/disease	Reference
43. Glycopyrronium bromide and water	Hyperhidrosis	Abell and Morgan [95][a]
44. 6-Hydroxydopamine	Ocular infection	Caudill et al. [81][b] Gordan et al. [96][b]
45. Gentamicin sulfate	Antibiotic (ocular infections)	Barza et al. [98][b]
46. Inotropic catecholamine	Cardiac failure	Sanderson et al. [100][b]

[a]Based on clinical impressions (qualitative).
[b]Based on controlled comparative study (quantitative, but not double blind).
[c]Based on in vitro experiments.
[d]Based on double-blind study (well-controlled study).
Source: Partly form Ref. 83.

TABLE 2 Effect of the Duration of Iontophoresis, at a Fixed Current, on the Subsequent Rate of Production of Sweat[a]

Iontophoresis duration (min)	Volume of sweat (μl)	Rate of sweat production (g/m^2/min)	Quantity of electricity delivered to skin (mC/cm^2)	Pilocarpine deposited at skin surface (mg/cm^2)
1	26	3.0	15.7	0.03
2	30	3.5	31.4	0.07
2.5	50	5.8	39.3	0.09
3	60	7.0	47.1	0.10
5	61	7.1	78.5	0.17
7	66	7.7	109.9	0.24

[a]Experimental conditions: iontophoresis, using 0.5% pilocarpine, at a fixed current of 1.5 mA, applied to a circular area of skin (5.73 cm^2) on the flexor surface of the forearm. The same area of skin was stimulated for each experiment to ensure identical sweat gland contribution; 15-min collection under heated cup, immediately following iontophoresis.
Source: Ref. 23.

collecting sweat because it is rapid, with minimal discomfort, and accurate, and the chance of producing hyperpyrexia in critically ill infants or children is eliminated [22].

Riar et al. [19] found that copper iontophoresis is a promising method for male contraception. Copper was deposited in the form of a depot from which it is released into the lumen and thereafter acts as a spermicidal agent. One deposition was sufficient for 9 months. Copper was deposited by iontophoresis into vasa deferentia of animals, using a 1 mA current for 30 to 90 sec in rats and 3 mA current for 60 sec in rabbits. Gangarosa et al. [20] measured electrical conductivities in vitro of several local anesthetics, vasoconstrictors, corticosteroids, anticancer drugs, and antiviral agents and found them suitable for iontophoretic delivery. This provides a useful method for selection of drugs for potential testing by iontophoresis.

Recently, macromolecules have been delivered iontophoretically for systemic action. The results from recent studies conducted using insulin are discussed in detail in Section V. Iontophoretic delivery of local anesthetic agents has been the subject of several reports (see Table 1). These agents are discussed here briefly.

A. Local Anesthetic Agents

A typical local anesthetic drug is a weakly basic tertiary amine that is soluble in lipids but poorly soluble and unstable in water [25]. Conversely, salts of these bases are readily soluble in water and stable in solution. The usual local anesthetic solution contains a salt (commonly the hydrochloride) of the base. In this aqueous solution, the positively charged quaternary amine species is in equilibrium with the uncharged base according to [25] the following relation:

$$R \equiv NH^+(\text{cation}) \rightleftharpoons R \equiv N(\text{base}) + H^+$$

Since the pK_a of most local anesthetics lies between 7.5 and 9.0, the solution at tissue pH (isoelectric range, 3-4; pH of skin surface is 3.78 [26]) contains more cations than base, as derived from the Henderson-Hasselbalch equation. Because of their pK_a, hydrochloride salts of local anesthetics conduct iontophoretically best at pH 5. This pH keeps almost all local anesthetic molecules in the positively charged form. Increasing the pH tends to lower the conductivity by converting positively charged molecules to un-ionized molecules. However, iontophoresis of local anesthetics can be performed successfully even when the pH is close to the pK_a; since there will be adequate numbers of local anesthetic ions to carry the current [20].

Lidocaine ($pK_a = 7.86$) is one of the most widely used local anesthetic agents. The marketed solutions of lidocaine hydrochloride are mostly ionized [27]. Anesthetizing a person can be painful if done by the conventional intradermal injection method and time-consuming if done by using topical ointments. On the other hand, iontophoresis of a compound of this nature may be virtually painless, as well as bringing in a more uniform concentration throughout the skin area of interest. By this method, the drug, lidocaine hydrocloride, can be applied to the skin by means of a sponge that has been soaked in its solution. The positive electrode can then be placed over it and current passed. The negative electrode contacts the skin at some distant point to complete the circuit. To ensure good electrical contact, the negative electrode is coated with electroencephalograph electrode paste. Complete coating is important here as well, to prevent minor direct current burns resulting from metal-to-skin contact. A sponge rubber cuff that prevents any possibility fo metal-to-skin contact can also be used. Drug penetration should occur at least through the stratum corneum, a result that cannot be obtained presently from the topical application of conventional solutions or ointments of either the ionized or the unionized forms fo lidocaine. Various reports showing the effectiveness of lidocaine hydrochloride by iontophoresis exist (see Table 1). Russo et al. [12] found that when lignocaine was administered topically by iontophoresis to volunteers, it produced a local anesthesia of significantly longer duration than did administration by swabbing, thus avoiding the use of needles. Comeau and co-workers [9,28] showed the relationship between the duration of anesthesia with different concentrations of lidocaine, and the duration of iontophoresis. Problems of physical retention of drug and controlled release can also be solved.

III. MECHANISM OF ACTION AND THEORY

Skin consists of 15 to 20% lipids (triglycerides, free fatty acids, cholesterol, and phospholipids), 40% proteins (mostly keratin), and approximately 40% water [29,37]. The isoelectric point of skin is between 3 and 4, which is another way of saying that pores have a positive charge below pH 3 and a negative charge above pH 4 [26,29,37]. Because of this original negative charge in the superficial skin layers, it is relatively "easy" to introduce basic drugs (e.g., methylene blue) through the skin [1]. Electroosmosis, the transport of the liquid water as a whole, can interfere with the mechanism of iontophoresis. This causes migration of undissociated molecules in solution [4]. Because the skin has a negative charge, iontophoresis will effect the movement of water into the body from the positive pole electroosmotically toward the outer surface of the skin at the negative pole. This leads to shrinkage of the skin pores at the positive pole and causes swelling at the negative pole after intensive iontophoresis [29]. This process is helpful in case of cation transfer from the positive pole, as it acts in the same direction, facilitating absorption of the cationic drugs. Electroosmosis is highest in solutions with a low conductivity; iontophoresis, on the other hand, is greatest in fluids with a high electrolyte concentration [4]. Gangarosa et al. [30] postulated that increased penetration of the drug idoxuridine after anodal iontophoresis may result from the water movement associated with the sodium ion transfer. They adopted the term "iontohydrokinesis" to describe water transport during iontophoresis, with no specific mechanism implied by the term.

In addition to ionic conduction and electroosmosis, phenomena such as solute-solvent and solute-solute coupling may account for observed enhancement of drug absorption when an electric field is present. Although a number of equations have been used to describe the observed rate of iontophoretic drug delivery, an exact relationship has not been defined, primarily because of the differences in the experimental conditions used by various authors. Moreover, many ionized parenterally administered drugs are supplied with admixtures of buffer salts, usually for the purpose of rendering them isotonic. These additional ions act as charged carriers or active competitors for the drug itself.

The iontophoretic procedure involves a number of variables that must be controlled in the interest of patient safety and optimal stimulation. Faraday's law has been used by some authors to provide dependable information concerning the rate of deposition of the drug at the skin surface. Faraday's law, in essence, states that the amount of material deposited at either electrode is proportional to the quantity of electricity passed through the system. However, due to the complexity of the factors involved during the process of iontophoresis, theoretical predictions based on Faraday's law and their correlations with experimental data are virtually impossible. Abramson [31] used Coulomb's law for predicting an electrophoretic treatment unit, independent of the area of the electrode.

Abramson and Gorin [1] defined an equation relating the iontophoretic dosage to the various components contributing to it. These included contributions due to electrical mobility, electroosmosis, and simple diffusion. Another equation, defining the iontophoretic current I passing through an electrode tip having a resistance R_E, and surrounding tissues release energy P in the form of heat as given [32] by the following relation:

$$P = I^2 (R_E + R_e) \tag{1}$$

where R_e is the resistance of the tissues. This relationship is not very practical and can be used only in in vitro experiments.

Masada et al. [33] used the following equation for describing their in vitro studies using a four-compartment diffusion cell electrode system:

$$E = \frac{Y}{Y_0} = (FZ \ \Delta V) \left\{ RT \ \left[\exp - \left(\frac{FZ \ \Delta V}{RT - 1} \right) \right] \right\}^{-1}$$ (2)

where

E = flux enhancement ratio
Y = flux with an electric field
Y_0 = flux with no electric field
ΔV = potential drop
Z = molecular charge
F = Faraday's constant
R = universal gas constant
T = absolute temperature

The authors found that at a low voltage (0-0.25 V) the data obtained by iontophoretic transport of benzoic acid, sodium benzoate, and tetraethylammonium bromide were in agreement with the theoretical flux enhancement. These experiments were done using a cellulose acetate membrane and hairless mouse skin. At high voltages, however, they observed a faster experimental flux enhancement than the theoretical predictions. Burnette and Marerro [34] studied the iontophoretic transport of thyrotropin releasing hormone (TRH), a tripeptide, using hairless mouse skin. They found that the steady state transport results were in agreement with their predictions based on the Nernst-Planck flux equations.

IV. EXPERIMENTAL VARIABLES

The technique of iontophoresis depends on several randomized physicochemical variables: electrolyte concentration, pH, vehicle type and composition, ionic strength, solubility of the drug, viscosity of the vehicle, drug concentration, duration and strength of the current, resistance of the skin, and size of the electrodes. The roles of these parameters in the iontophoretic delivery of drugs and in optimization of the technique are of utmost interest to the medical device and pharmaceutical industry. It might be mentioned here that a review of the literature indicated that various investigators had attempted to ascertain what effects these various physicochemical factors had on iontophoresis. However, their results were based mostly on clinical observations rather than on scientific experiments.

A. pH

Changes in the pH of the fluid at the driving electrode produced only minor changes in the uptake of radioactive phosphorus by various tis-

sues in rats [35]. Release of histamine from aqueous media during
iontophoresis also showed a similar behavior [36]. Harpuder has, however, shown a significant dependence on pH during electrophoretic
therapy [37]. The change in flux for lignocaine hydrochloride during
iontophoresis was related to the degree of ionization [38]. The results
obtained with the iontophoresis of sulfa drugs [16] were also shown
to be paralleled by the degree of ionization.

B. Ionic Strength

Only a few papers in the literature relate to the concern of ionic
strength during iontophoresis. A report on a decrease in the uptake
of phosphorus by tissue has been published [35].

C. Size and Charge of Electrodes

Electrode material used should be harmless to the body and sufficiently
flexible to be applied closely to the body surface. Tin/steel plates
are known to be the best for this purpose [8]. The electrode pad/
sponge chosen should be about 1 to 2 cm thick. One should avoid direct contact of electrode with the body. The charge of the electrode
under which the drug will be kept depends on the charge of the active
drug species. In the case of lidocaine hydrochloride, the positive
electrode is used, so that the positive lidocaine ions will migrate toward
the negative electrode. The distribution of active drug species within
the skin depends on the size and position of electrodes. They are
usually selected according to individual needs. The literature indicates that greater amounts of drugs are introduced by larger electrodes.
Results negating this observation also have been published [31,35].

D. Nature of Electrodes

Disposable electrodes capable of conforming to irregular skin surfaces
comprising a flexible material having one surface coated with a skin
adhesive adapted to be applied directly to the skin of the patient and
the nonconductive planar body having a tab to which an electrical connection can be made are highly desirable [38].

E. Duration and Intensity of Current

From Faraday's law we know that in an electrolytic solution the transported quantity of electricity depends on the strength of the current
and the duration of its passage [5]. The same number of ions will
be transported at different strengths of current if the time for current
flow is inversely related to their strengths. The rate at which the
ions are introduced into the body with various current strengths can

play an important role. When the current is stronger, more ions penetrate at one time, and their accumulation produces the desired local
effect and may even build up a reserve of ions that will later be diffused more deeply into the tissues, perhaps resulting in prolonged
drug effect. The strength of current used depends also on the sensitivity of the patient [40]. Using benzoate as a model ion, it is reported [41] that increases in the applied current produced a linear
increase in benzoate flux. However, upon current termination, benzoate flux does not return to the control values, suggesting compromised
barrier integrity of a variable nature. The authors speculated that
the diffusional path followed specifically by ionized species undergoes
sporadic current-related changes.

Iontophoretic technique is based on a direct current source. It
is designed to increase the current slowly and to remain at a predetermined level as long as the treatment requires, following which the current is slowly decreased to zero. The time for iontophoresis ideally
is 1 min for the increasing phase and 30 sec for the decreasing phase.
The intensity of the current used is between 40 μA and 10 mA regulated with a 25,000 ohm potentiometer [10]. Currents ranging from
5 to 10 mA have been found to be painless [10]. The intensity of the
current should not exceed 0.5 to 1 mA/in.^{3} for large electrodes [11,40].
This current can be distributed in the case of stimulation treatment of
a number of areas, by branching wires connected with the desired
pole. The relationship between the duration of the iontophoresis and
the time until the effect is perceived has not been widely investigated.

F. Resistance

The electrical resistance of the skin area where the iontophoretic application is desired can vary widely. The electrical resistance of the
human epidermis has been measured with a minute electrode [42]. When
the electrode was placed over the skin, the resistance was much lower
on sweat pores, especially when they discharged sweat [42]. When
the electrode was gradually inserted into the epidermis, no marked
change in resistance was found in the outermost layer, followed by
a thin layer where a slight fall in resistance began to occur.

G. Concentration

Increased uptake by the skin after iontophoresis with an increase in
drug concentration has been the subject of many reports [35,36]. Increased uptake of radioactive phosphorus by various tissues after iontophoresis with an increase in the concentration of ^{32}P is demonstrated
by O'Malley and Oester [35]. Bellantone et al. [41] also showed a
linear increase in benzoate ion steady state flux with greater donor
compartment concentrations in their in vitro system.

V. ADMINISTRATION OF INSULIN

While iontophoresis has proved to be a safe and useful technique for assuring penetration of charged molecules into surface tissues for localized effects [56], it has received little attention as a technique for delivering charged macromolecules for a systemic effect. However, the number of protein drug molecules needed for a physiological effect is often very low. Given this fact it might be possible to use iontophoresis as a method for administration of some proteins/peptides for systemic effect. Besides being effective at low concentrations, such drugs would also have to be ionizable and to have some solubility in skin tissues. One drug that has these characteristics is insulin. Besides being ionizable, insulin has traditionally been administered by subcutaneous injection into the skin tissues. The injected insulin then leaks into the capillaries for a systemic effect. Thus, iontophoresis could replace injection as a method for loading the skin tissues with insulin. Iontophoresis from a reservoir could also provide for a longer term supply of the drug.

There have been at least two reports describing iontophoretic administration of insulin in experimental animals. First, Stephen et al. [22] were successful in delivering a highly ionized and monomeric form of insulin by iontophoresis in pigs. However, their attempts in human volunteers failed because regular soluble insulin is only weakly charged and much of it is present in a polymeric form. In a second report, iontophoresis was used to administer regular soluble insulin to alloxan-diabetic rabbits [21]. The results from this study are described in detail below.

A. Materials and Methods

Alloxanization of Animals

New Zealand white rabbits weighing 3 to 4 kg were obtained from a local supplier. Animals were made diabetic by intravenous injection of 125 mg/kg of alloxan (Sigma Chemical Co., St. Louis) as a 10% solution in normal saline. Blood glucose levels were assayed 2 days after alloxan treatment to determine which animals had become diabetic and the degree of hyperglycemia. Animals with blood glucose levels greater than 200 mg/dl were included in the study. After alloxanization animals, were allowed free access to food and water.

Preparation of Animals for Iontophoresis

Hair was removed from backs of animals with electric clippers. Hair stubble was removed from iontophoresis sites by shaving with a razor 2 to 24 hr before iontophoresis. Care was taken to assure that no abrasions occurred due to shaving; however, shaving most likely did disrupt the stratum corneum. In some cases hair stubble was removed with a commercial depilatory compound (Nair). In these cases, animals were not used for 24 hr after use of the depilatory so that the skin could recover. After recovery, the skin was prepared by using a scapel held perpendicular to the skin and scraping with 20 to 40 gentle strokes to remove or disrupt the stratum corneum. Finally, tincture of benzoin was applied around the iontophoresis site to help secure the insulin reservoir in place and to help reduce leakage.

Iontophoretic Procedure

Iontophoresis of insulin was done with direct current generated by a 9 V power source (Fig. 6; Motion Control, Salt Lake City). Since this unit was originally designed for iontophoretic administration of dexamethasone sodium phosphate with lidocaine hydrochloride, it was necessary to modify the unit to deliver insulin such that the drug-containing reservoir became the negative pole. This reservoir consisted of a plastic chamber with a permeable membrane across the bottom, which consisted of a polyvinyl acetate copolymer. The chamber had a circle of adhesive plastic around its perimeter for the purpose of holding it on the skin. The top of the chamber was fitted with a rubber septum for introduction of insulin and a small circular metal snap to serve as the electrode. The positive pole was a dispersive Karaya electrode (Lec Tec, Minnetonka, Minnesota). This electrode consisted of a Karaya pad, which was in contact with the skin, and an aluminum foil back to serve as a dispersive electrode. The major components of the Karaya pad were Karaya, glycerin, and water. The Karaya pad also provided adhesive properties to maintain skin contact and allowed uniform passage of current densities to the skin. The positive electrode was placed within a few centimeters of the negative electrode; however, its exact position was not important.

Currents of less than 1.0 mA were used on a surface area of 6.2 cm^2. Currents exceeding 2.0 mA caused electrical burns and therefore were not used. The drug reservoir was filled with 3 ml of regular pork zinc insulin (Squibb Novo, Princeton, New Jersey), pH 7.0. This volume was required to completely fill the drug reservoir. When less than 300 units of insulin was used for iontophoresis, U-100 regular pork insulin was diluted with sterile diluting fluid for regular pork insulin (Eli Lilly and Company, Indianapolis). This solution contained glycerin (16 mg/ml) and m-cresol (2.5 mg/ml) and was adjusted to pH 7.0 with either NaOH or HCl.

Measurement of Blood Glucose and Serum Insulin

Blood samples were taken from ear veins and glucose levels measured immediately with Ames Dextrostix and an Ames Dextrometer (Ames Co., Elkhart, Indiana). Blood glucose levels (BGL) are reported as milli-

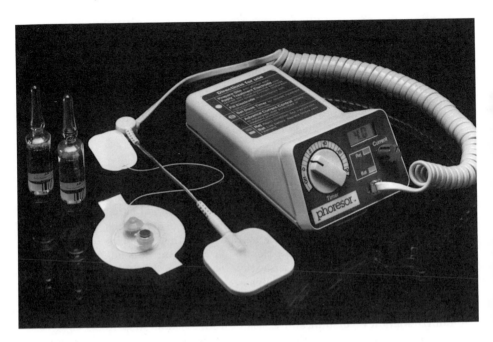

Fig. 6 The control unit and the electrode system of the Phoresor by Motion Control.

grams per deciliter. For BGL above 200 mg/dl, BGL were first estimated with Visidex II reagent strips (Ames). Based on these estimated values, whole blood samples were diluted with normal saline solution to obtain BGL less than 200 mg/dl. Diluted blood samples were also assayed with a Dextrometer.

Serum insulin concentrations (SIC) were measured quantitatively with an ^{125}I radioimmunoassay kit obtained from Diagnostic Products Corporation (Los Angeles) and are reported as microunits per milliliter. Serum samples for insulin measurements were collected using capillary serum separators obtained from Monoject Scientific (St. Louis). Serum samples were stored for approximately 12 hr at 4°C before insulin assays were done.

B. Results

Effects of Skin Preparation on Iontophoresis

The effect of skin preparation on iontophoresis of insulin was determined by comparing results obtained when hair stubble was removed with a depilatory only versus the use of a depilatory plus scraping.

In both cases, a reservoir containing 300 units of regular pork insulin (100 U/cm^3) was placed on the prepared site and a current of 0.8 mA was applied for 3 hr. When only a depilatory was used, SIC only increased from a mean ±SD of 3±4 μU/ml to 8±1 μU/ml and BGL decreased slightly going from a mean ±SD of 430±14 to 365±9 mg/dl after applying current for 3 hr. Furthermore, BGL and SIC were followed for an additional 4 hr after the current was turned off and no further changes were noted. However, when the skin was gently scraped to remove the stratum corneum 24 hr after using a depilatory, the mean ±SD SIC increased from 3±3 to 172 ±11 μU/ml and BGL decreased from a mean ±SD of 390 ±9 mg/dl to 194 ±6 mg/dl after 3 hr. These data suggested that the stratum corneum was a significant barrier to iontophoresis of insulin. Therefore, in the experiments reported here, the stratum corneum was always removed.

Response of Blood Glucose and Serum Insulin Levels to Iontophoresis of Insulin

Experiments were initiated by examining the response of BGL and SIC to iontophoresis of insulin in alloxan-diabetic rabbits. As shown in Fig. 7, some animals were used more than once. When an individual animal was reused, a different area of the back was chosen as the iontophoresis site. This raised the possibility of variation in the delivery of insulin due to differences in skin thickness at different sites on the back. However, in these experiments, if all other conditions were held constant no significant difference was noted in the effect obtained when different sites on the back of the same animal were used.

Two types of control experiment were run. In one control, an electrode not containing insulin was used with a current of 0.8 mA for 4 hr. Before iontophoresis, the mean ±SD BGL was 580 ±24 mg/dl and at the end of 4 hr of iontophoresis BGL was 749 ±80 mg/dl. Furthermore, the mean SIC (±SD) did not increase, being 14 ±2 μU/ml before iontophoresis and 12 ±11 μU/ml after iontophoresis. In another control experiment, an insulin-filled reservoir was placed on the back of a rabbit, but no current was applied. In these cases, BGL also remained well above normal and little serum insulin was detected. However, when an insulin-filled reservoir was used and a current of 0.4 mA applied, there was a significant decrease in BGL and a corresponding increase in SIC (Fig. 8). Moreover, in these experiments after turning the current off, BGL continued to decrease for 2 hr and SIC continued to increase for 1 hr.

Effects of Current Level on Iontophoresis of Insulin

Preliminary experiments demonstrated that similar results could be obtained using various current levels. To more closely examined the

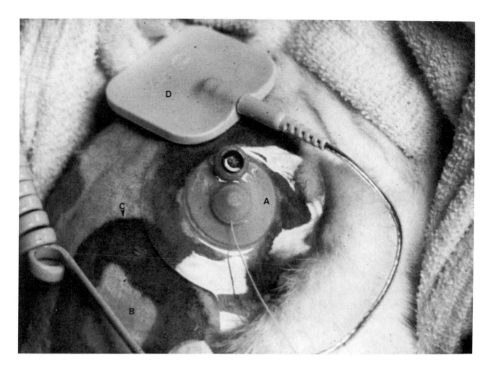

Fig. 7 The back of an alloxan-diabetic rabbit was prepared for cathodal iontophoresis as described. A drug reservoir was filled with 3 ml of insulin solution and placed on the iontophoresis site. The reservoir was connected to the negative pole of the power source. A positive electrode was placed on the back at an indifferent site. Key: A = insulin reservoir, B = previous iontophoresis site, C = tincture of benzoin, and D = positive electrode, which measured approximately 4.5 cm on a side.

effect of current levels, iontophoresis of insulin was done at 0.2, 0.4, and 0.8 mA for 2 hr and BGL and SIC were compared (Table 3). At all levels of current examined, both a decrease in BGL and an increase in SIC were detected after applying current. However, increasing the current from 0.2 to 0.4 mA increased the maximum SIC by approximately threefold (0.5 < P < 0.1, Table 3), while increasing the current to 0.8 mA did not produce higher SIC when compared with 0.4 mA (Table 3).

Serum insulin concentrations were increased by increasing the current from 0.2 to 0.4 mA. However, examination of BGL showed that this parameter was unaffected by increasing the current levels (Table 3). Furthermore, BGL did not start to rise again until approx-

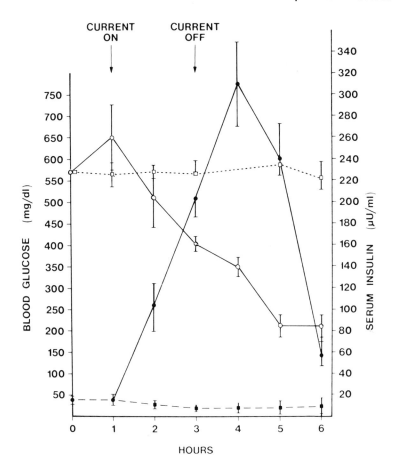

Fig. 8   Alloxan-diabetic rabbits were given insulin by iontophoresis using a current of 0.4 mA for 2 hr and reservoirs containing 300 units of regular pork insulin. In control experiments, animals were prepared in the same manner and a drug reservoir placed on the iontophoresis site; however, no current was applied. Key: open squares = control BGL, solid squares = control SIC, open circles = BGL in experimental animals, solid circles = SIC in experimental animals. All experimental values represent the mean ±SEM of four different experiments using four different animals.

imately 3 hr after turning the current off again, regardless of the current level. This suggested that the amount of insulin available at 0.2 mA was sufficient to have the desired physiological response and that the additional insulin available at higher current levels may have been wasted.

TABLE 3 Effect of Current Level on Iontophoresis of Insulin[a]

Animal identification number	Current (mA)	Initial BGL (mg/dl)[b]	Minimum BGL (mg/dl)[c]	Initial SIC (μU/ml)[b]	Maximum SIC (μU/ml)[c]
64	0.2	550	123	16	92
73	0.2	212	29	17	94
74	0.2	533	47	9	220
		432 ± 190[d]	66 ± 30	14 ± 4	135 ± 73
59	0.4	624	195	8	380
64	0.4	861	183	23	490
71	0.4	713	145	4	230
74	0.4	440	71	14	159
		659 ± 176[d]	104 ± 75	12 ± 8	315 ± 148
52	0.8	314	26	2	225
54	0.8	577	129	7	150
76	0.8	506	31	15	350
		466 ± 136[d]	62 ± 58	8 ± 7	243 ± 101

[a]Alloxan-diabetic rabbits were given insulin by iontophoresis using reservoirs containing 300 units of regular pork insulin and the indicated currents for 2 hr.
[b]Values obtained just before initiating iontophoresis.
[c]Lowest and highest values obtained during the course of the experiment.
[d]The values in these rows are the mean ± SD for the listed BGL and SIC.

Effect of Reservoir Insulin Concentration on
Iontophoresis of Insulin

Since increasing current levels from 0.2 to 0.4 mA appeared to affect
the maximum SIC, it was of interest to determine what effect the concentration of insulin available for iontophoresis would have. Therefore,
drug reservoirs were loaded with 10, 50, 100, and 500 U/ml of regular
pork insulin all in a total volume of 3 ml. In all cases, except for the
experiments using 100 U/ml, iontophoresis was done for 3 hr at 0.8
mA. For the experiments done with a concentration of 100 U/ml, 0.8
mA was used for 2 hr. Furthermore, since similar results were obtained with either 0.4 or 0.8 mA, 0.8 mA was used to make sure that
the effects observed were due to the insulin reservoir concentration
and not to current levels. Serum insulin concentrations always increased when current was applied regardless of the amount of insulin
in the reservoir. However, when reservoirs contained insulin concentrations of 10 or 50 U/ml, increases in SIC were much less when compared to higher reservoir insulin concentrations (Table 4). Thus,
increasing the reservoir concentration to 100 and 500 U/ml of insulin
increased the maximum SIC (Table 4). At 100 U/ml the maximum SIC
was fourfold that at 50 U/ml ($0.05 < P < 0.1$) and at 500 U/ml it was
10-fold greater ($P < 0.05$).

While SIC increased when the reservoir contained insulin concentrations below 100 U/ml, the initial decrease in BGL was similar at all
reservoir insulin concentrations (Table 4). However, when reservoirs
contained 100 or 500 U/ml of insulin, BGL continued to decrease or
only slightly increased after the current was off for 3 hr; but, when
10 or 50 U/ml of insulin was used, BGL increased 65 ±20 and 67 ±20
mg/ml, respectively, after the current was off for only 2 hr. This
suggested that at higher reservoir insulin concentrations, the subcutaneous tissues may have accumulated more insulin.

C. Discussion

The major purpose of these studies was to determine the feasibility
of using iontophoresis to deliver insulin in alloxan-diabetic rabbits
for a systemic effect. Currents of less than 1.0 mA used for 2 to 4
hr were sufficient to deliver insulin such that there were measurable
serum insulin concentrations and significant decreases in blood glucose
levels. The amount of insulin delivered could be controlled to some
extent by controlling the amount of insulin available for iontophoresis
or the level of current used. Moreover, in most cases, serum insulin
concentrations continued to increase and blood glucose levels continued
to decrease after the current was turned off, suggesting that the skin
and subcutaneous tissues were being loaded with insulin, which was
being removed by capillary washout. Furthermore, the temporal and

TABLE 4 Effect of Reservoir Insulin Concentration on Iontophoresis of Insulin[a]

Animal identification number	Reservoir insulin concentration (U/ml)	Initial BGL (mg/dl)[b]	Minimum BGL (mg/dl)[c]	Initial SIC (µU/ml)[b]	Maximum SIC (µU/ml)[c]
58	10	412	218	19	139
63	10	630	185	17	73
63	10	642	214	6	120
		516 ± 130	206 ± 18	14 ± 7	111 ± 34[d]
72	50	413	130	31	65
75	50	431	129	8	50
76	50	410	49	4	ND
		418 ± 11	103 ± 47	14 ± 15	57 ± 11[d]
52	100	314	26	2	225
54	100	577	129	7	150
76	100	506	31	15	350
		466 ± 136	62 ± 58	8 ± 7	243 ± 101[d]
75	500	455	61	7	340
80	500	374	24	14	700
81	500	622	189	4	700
		484 ± 126	91 ± 87	8 ± 4	580 ± 280[d]

[a] Alloxan-diabetic rabbits were given insulin by iontophoresis using a current of 0.8 mA and the indicated insulin reservoir concentrations.

[b] Values obtained just before initiating iontophoresis.

[c] Lowest and highest values obtained during the course of the experiment.

[d] The values in these rows are the mean ±SD for the listed BGL and SIC; ND = not done for technical reasons.

kinetic dynamics of insulin administration by the iontophoretic methods employed appeared to be very similar to what might be expected with subcutaneous insulin injections. However, it may be that the temporal and kinetic parameters of insulin administration by iontophoresis could be altered in other ways. For example, the amount and rate of insulin delivered at a given current level might be increased by the use of a more highly charged form of insulin, such as sulfated insulin. This could also reduce the total amount of insulin needed in a reservoir to obtain an effect. Moreover, it could be possible to deliver constant low amounts of insulin by the use of very low levels of current coupled with bursts of higher current levels to deliver a bolus of insulin as needed. This could theoretically provide for more rigorous glycemic control. Finally, the control of pH changes during iontophoresis might also improve insulin delivery by maintaining insulin as the most abundant charged molecule carrying the current.

Using regular soluble insulin, Stephen et al. [22] were unable to deliver significant amounts of insulin in human subjects by iontophoresis. They suggested that this was because regular soluble insulin is only weakly charged and much of it is present in a polymeric form. These factors no doubt affected the delivery of insulin. However, they did not disrupt or remove the stratum corneum, which is generally considered to be the portion of the skin that is the most significant barrier to transdermal drug delivery [83]. As our study shows, the stratum corneum proved to be a significant barrier to insulin iontophoresis; thus, had the previous investigators removed or disrupted the stratum corneum, they might have been able to deliver more insulin. While this difference existed between this study and that reported by Stephen et al. [22], both studies suggested the theoretical feasibility of iontophoresis as a noninvasive method for insulin administration. However, many factors remain to be investigated; and thus, the clinical feasibility of iontophoresis as a method for insulin delivery remains hopeful.

VI. DISADVANTAGES

Iontophoretic burns are often produced by low voltages and are caused without the sensation of pain. Tapper [43] has tried to pinpoint the cause and source of these burns, which usually can be prevented by a thick pad/gauge. Tapper [44] has described a method for constructing an iontophoretic electrode that will offer burn proteciton. He suggests the use of a feltlike material, preferably moistened, and having a thickness in excess of 3 mm, covering at least the area of the negative electrode in contact with the skin. Compliance with a current-time limitation according to the method essentially avoids iontophoretic burns. Formation of undesirable vesicles and bullae in the skin being treated can be avoided by periodically interrupting a unidirectional treatment current with a relatively short pulse of current in the opposite direciton [45]. Electric shocks are caused by a high current density at the skin surface. Cardiac arrest may be caused by an excessive electrical current passing through the heart. This situation can easily be avoided by conditioning the body to the current in a stepwise fashion. This would require an operator first to secure the patient to the device and then slowly advance the output control from zero to permit patient accommodation to the signal. After a given treatment period, the operator would slowly turn the output control down to zero and release the patient from contact with the output [43]. The literature contains reference to the use of brass, copper, zinc, gold, conductive plastic, and steel for avoiding this problem. The resistance contributed by the electrode in infinitesimally low compared with that of the skin and is not, per se, a factor potentially predisposing toward burns [23].

The limitations of iontophoresis depend on the properties of the drug species. The drug solution must be of a sufficiently ionized concentration to carry a measurable current (in excess of 10^{-10} A) in biological systems [32]. The skin itself imposes a barrier to the delivery of some medications: introduction of ionized solutes with molecular weight exceeding 8000 to 12,000 results in a very uncertain rate of delivery [97].

VII. EQUIPMENT AND DEVICES

The design and construction of equipment for iontophoresis is not unduly complex. The development of prototype devices that could deliver small amounts of therapeutically active materials is under way at various research laboratories. Some of these devices are also available on the market today. The limitations of an iontophoretic device are governed by three major factors: safety, convenience, and predictability. Many devices in the past were powered by household current, which caused the patient shock hazard in the event of the device malfunction [22]. These devices were modified to function with a constant voltage so that the current can be varied, depending on the resistance of the skin area being treated. This decreased the possibility of electric shocks. At present there is a need for devices with high patient compliance and acceptability.

Many types of device for the delivery of drugs, enzymes, dyes, and other ions have been employed. These vary in complexity from the simple battery and rheostat types to modern electronic circuit devices [79]. The optimal features of these devices for control of the amount of the drug delivered should include regulation of parameters such as current density, voltage, and time. Currently three types of iontophoresis unit are commercially available: line-operated units, simple battery-operated units, and rechargeable power sources [93]. Line-operated devices are widely used for pilocarpine iontophoresis for the diagnosis of cystic fibrosis. One of the battery-operated devices currently on the market is the Phoresor, manufactured by Motion Control (Fig. 6). The device is designed to deliver drugs such as lidocaine and dexamethasone. The Phoresor delivers a constant current and automatically adjusts to any change in resistance in the external circuit during the iontophoretic procedure. The features incorporated in this device and some other devices are listed in Table 5 [23,24,83]. This device features control for a slow increase in current to avoid any discomfort caused by changes in skin resistance. LecTec Corporation uses a wafer-thin membrane to push positively charged ions of a drug through the stratum corneum of the skin [46]. Nucleopore Corporation (Pleasanton, California) markets effective polycarbonate membranes as a microporous barrier to be used in iontophoretic devices. Based on patient safety, Webster [23] outlined some recommendations for the desired safety features in an iontophoretic device. Jochem et al. [47] have described a high-voltage electrometer for iontophoresing dyes or enzymes through extremely fine micropipettes. This device incorporates a controlled current source, direct current monitoring, balance bridge, electrode resistance, and capacitance compensation test circuits. A device for iontophoretic application of fluoride on teeth is discussed by Ishikawa et al. [48].

Another iontophoresis-based device, the Drionic, was recently released by the Food and Drug Administration for the market and has gained wide acceptance among consumers and medical professionals in its very short life [43,49]. The device is currently sold by prescription for about $100; it takes 30 min to soak the Drionic pad and another 20 min for the application. The device has been designed for self-use at home, primarily for antiperspirant action. Clinical studies showing the safety and effectiveness of the device have been reported [43]. The device is presently being developed for drug delivery purposes [43].

The FDA has classified iontophoretic devices for specialized uses (for the diagnosis of cystic fibrosis, fluoride uptake acceleration in dentistry, and anesthesia of the intact tympanic membrane) into class II (performance standards) and for all other uses into class III [50]. (Also see Chapter 2.)

In summary, iontophoresis is a very effective and viable technique for drug delivery. However, its therapeutic applications are not based soundly on clinical experiments but remain based considerably on clinical impressions. Therefore, future controlled clinical experiments are necessary to quantitate the contribution of this technique, relative to transcellular diffusion.

TABLE 5 Circuit Characteristics of Commercial Iontopheresis Systems

				Model or manufacturer				
Characteristic	Farrall model IPS-6D	Orion model 417	Medtherm	Sherwood	Wescor model 3600	Phoresor model PM600	Drionic	Metronic model 6850, 6820
Power source	Battery	Battery	AC line-operated	AC line-operated	Electronic charge displacement	Battery	Battery	Battery
Automatic current rate-of-change limitation	No	Yes, 20 sec rise	No	Yes, <10 sec rise	Yes, 30 sec rise decay	Yes, 20 sec rise	Yes, 2.5 sec rise	Yes, approx. 2 sec rise
Current control	Manual (limit at 4 mA)	Automatic (1.0 or 1.5 mA)	Manual	Automatic	Automatic (0.25 mA/cm²)	Manual	Automatic variable resistor	Automatic (limit 2 mA)
Circuit resistance sensor	Voltage limited, no shutdown	No	No	No	Audio signal automatic shutdown, >18 kilohm	No	Voltage-limited capacitor	Relative light intensity
Open-circuit sensor	Ammeter indication, no shutdown	Ammeter indication, no shutdown	Ammeter indication, no shutdown	Ammeter indication, no shutdown	Audio signal automatic shutdown	Audio signal automatic shutdown	Delay capacitor discharge	Light indicator

Source: Modified from Ref. 23 and 83.

REFERENCES

1. H. A. Abramson and M. H. Gorin, *J. Phys. Chem.*, 44:1094-1102 (1940).
2. S. Rothman, ed., *Physiology and Biochemistry of the Skin*. University of Chicago Press, Chicago, 1954, p. 38.
3. S. Rothman, *Hand. Normal. Pathol. Physiol.*, 4(107):143-149 (1929).
4. H. Schaefer, in *Skin Permeability* (H. Schaefer, A. Zesch, and G. Stuttgen, eds.). Springer-Verlag, Boston, 1982, pp. 640-641.
5. D. Abramowitsch and B. Neoussikine, eds., *Treatment by Ion Transfer*. Grune & Stratton, New York, 1946, p. 87.
6. W. B. Shelley, J. C. McConahy, and E. N. Hesbacher, *J. Invest. Dermatol.*, 15(5):343-344 (1950).
7. D. M. Jenkinson and G. S. Walton, *Vet. Rec.*, pp. 8-12, Jan. 5, 1974.
8. W. E. Rahm, W. F. Strother, J. F. Crump, and D. E. Parker, *Ann. Otol., Rhinol. Laryngol.*, 71:116-123 (1962).
9. M. Comeau and R. Brummett, *Laryngoscope*, 88:277-285 (1978).
10. A. S. Rapperport, D. L. Larson, D. F. Henges, J. B. Lynch, T. G. Blocker, and R. S. Lewis, *Plast. Reconstruc. Surg.*, 36:547-552 (1965).
11. D. H. Kling and D. Sashin, *Arch. Phys. Ther. X-Ray Radium*, 18:333-338 (1937).
12. J. Russo, Jr., A. G. Lipman, T. J. Cornstock, B. C. Page, and R. L. Stephen, *Am. J. Hosp. Pharm.*, 37:843-847 (1980).
13. L. P. Gangarosa, N. H. Park, C. A. Wiggins, and J. M. Hill, *J. Pharm. Exp. Ther.*, 212(3):377-381 (1980).
14. S. LeDuc, *Electric Ions and Their Use in Medicine*. Rebman, London, 1908.
15. A. Strohl, J. Verne, J. C. Roucayrol, and P. F. Ceccaldi, *C. R. Soc. Biol.*, 144:819-824 (1950).
16. L. von Sallmann, *Am. J. Ophthalmol.*, 25:1292-1300 (1942).
17. P. R. Harris, *J. Orthopaed. Sports Phys. Ther.*, 4(2):109-112 (1982).
18. F. G. Delacerda, *J. Orthopaed. Sports Phys. Ther.*, 4(1):51-54 (1982).
19. S. S. Riar, R. C. Sawhney, J. Bardhan, P. Thomas, R. K. Jain, and A. K. Jain, *Andrologia*, 14(6):481-491 (1982).
20. L. P. Gangarosa, N. H. Park, B. C. Fong, D. F. Scott, and J. M. Hill, *J. Pharm. Sci.*, 67(10):1439-1443 (1978).
21. B. Kari, *Diabetes*, 35(2):217-221 (1986).
22. R. L. Stephen, T. J. Petelenz, and S. C. Jacobsen, *Biomed. Acta*, 43(5):553-558 (1984).
23. C. A. Webster, *CRC Crit. Rev. Clin. Lab. Sci.*, 18(4):313-338 (1983).

24. P. Tyle, in *Proceedings of the Bio-Expo '86*, the American Commercial and Industrial Conference and Exposition in Biotechnology. Butterworth, Stoneham, MA, 1986, pp. 583-594.
25. R.H. De Jong, in *Problems in Anesthesia, A Case Study Approach* (M. B. Ravin, ed.). Little, Brown, Boston, 1981, pp. 129-140.
26. T. Rosendal, *Acta Physiol. Scand.*, 5:130-151 (1942-1943).
27. D. F. Echols, C. H. Norris, and H. G. Tabb, *Arch. Otolaryngol.*, 101:418-421 (1975).
28. M. Comeau and J. Vernon, *Arch. Otolaryngol.*, 98:114-120 (1973).
29. R. Harris, in *Therapeutic Electricity and Ultraviolet Radioation* (S. Licht, ed.). Waverly Press, Baltimore, 1967, pp. 156-178.
30. L. P. Gangarosa, H. W. Merchant, N. H. Park, and J. M. Hill, *Methods Findings Exp. Clin. Pharmacol.*, 1:105-109 (1979).
31. H. A. Abramson, *J. Allergy*, 12:169-175 (1941).
32. A Globus, in *Bioelectric Recording Techniques*, Part A: *Cellular Processes and Brain Potentials* (R. F. Thompson and M. M. Patterson, eds.). Academic Press, London, New York, 1973, pp. 23-38.
33. T. Masada, U. Rohr, W. I. Higuchi, J. Fox, C. Behl, W. Malick, A. H. Goldberg, and S. Pons, in *39th National Meeting of Academy of Pharmaceutical Sciences Abstracts*, Minneapolis, 15(2):73 (1985).
34. R. R. Burnette and D. Marerro, *J. Pharm. Sci.*, 75:738-743 (1986).
35. E. P. O'Mally and Y. T. Oester, *Arch. Phys. Med. Rehabil.*, 36:310-316 (1955).
36. H. A. Abramson and A. Alley, *Arch. Phys. Ther.*, 18:327 (1937).
37. K. Harpuder, *Arch. Phys. Ther. X-Ray Radium*, 18:221-225 (1937).
38. O. Siddiqui, M. S. Roberts, and A. Z. Polack, *J. Pharm. Pharmacol.*, 37:732-735 (1985).
39. B. Jankelson, U.S. Patent 3,746,004 (1973).
40. W. J. Shriber, ed., *A Manual of Electrotherapy*, 4th ed. Lea & Febiger, Philadelphia, 1975, pp. 123, 131.
41. N. H. Bellantone, S. Rim, M. L. Francoeur, and B. Rasadi, *Int. J. Pharm.*, 30:63-72 (1986).
42. T. Suchi, *Jap. J. Physiol.*, 5:75-80 (1955).
43. R. Tapper, *J. Clin. Eng.*, 8(3):253-259 (1983).
44. R. Tapper, U.S. Patent 4,164,226 (1979).
45. R. Tapper, U.S. Patent 4,301,794 (1981).
46. Technical Insights, Inc., Fort Lee, New Jersey, *Drug Delivery Systems: A Technology Survey.* Chapter 7, pp. 154-162.
47. W. J. Jochem, A. R. Light, and D. Smith, *J. Neurosci. Method*, 3:261-269 (1981).
48. T. Ishikawa, S. Kuriyama, Y. Takaesu, H. Furuishi, Y. Okuzaki, S. Motomura, and Y. Musha, U.S. Patent 4,149,533 (1979).

49. R. Teitelman, *Forbes*, 135(3):148-149 (1985).
50. *Federal Register*, August 28, 1979, 44(168), 50520-50523; November 23, 1983, 48(227), 53052; and Code of Federal Regulations, 890.5525, 1985, p. 271.
51. A. B. Coyer, *Ann. Phys. Med.*, 2:16 (1954).
52. L. E. Bertolucci, *J. Orthopaed. Sprots Phys. Ther.*, 4(2):103-108 (1982).
53. D. C. Bonne, *Phys. Ther.*, 49(2):139-145 (1969).
54. B. S. Kwon, L. P. Gangarosa, N. H. Park, D. S. Hull, E. Fineberg, C. Wiggins, and J. M. Hill, *Invest. Ophthalmol. Vis. Sci.*, 18(9):984-988 (1979).
55. T. Petelenz, I. Axenti, T. J. Petelenz, J. Iwinski, and S. Dubel, *J. Clin. Pharmacol. Ther. Toxicol.*, 22(3):152-155 (1984).
56. J. M. Hill, L. P. Gangarosa, and N. H. Park, *Ann. N.Y. Acad. Sci.*, 284:604-612 (1977).
57. T. Cohn and S. Benson, *Arch. Phys. Ther. X-Ray Radium*, 18:583-587 (1937).
58. L. Martin and G. O. Eaton, *Arch. Phys. Ther. X-Ray Radium*, 18:226-237 (1937).
59. A. J. Schleuning, R. Brummett, and M. Comeau, *Trans. Am. Acad. Ophthalnol. Otol.*, 78:453-457 (1974).
60. L. R. Gangarosa, Sr., ed., *Iontophoresis in Dental Practice*, 1st ed. Quintessence, Chicago, 1983.
61. L. P. Gangarosa, *Methods Findings Exp. Clin. Pharmacol.*, 3(2):83-94 (1981).
62. S. B. Arvidsson, R. H. Ekroth, A. M. C. Hansby, A. H. Lindholm, and G. William-Olsson, *Acta Anaesthesiol. Scand.*, 28:209-210 (1984).
63. L. P. Gangarosa, N. H. Park, and J. M. Hill, *Proc. Soc. Exp. Biol. Med.*, 154:439-443 (1977).
64. L. P. Gangarosa, M. Haynes, S. Qureshi, M. M. Salim, A. Ozawa, K. Hayakawa, M. Ohkido, and P. E. Mahn, *Third International Dental Congress on Modern Pain Control*, Abstracts, 1982, p. 221.
65. L. P. Gangarosa and P. E. Mahon, *Ear Nose Throat J.*, 61:30-41 (1982).
66. A. H. Gordon and M. V. Weinstein, *Phys. Ther.*, 49(8):869-870 (1969).
67. J. Kahn, *Phys. Ther.*, 55(40):476-477 (1975).
68. J. Kahn, *Phys. Ther.*, 57(6):658-659 (1977).
69. C. D. Weir, *J. Laryngol.*, 81:1143-1150 (1967).
70. S. H. Rothfeld and W. Murray, *J. Urol.*, 97:874-875 (1967).
71. J. E. Marchand and N. Hagino, *Exp. Neurol.*, 78(3):790-795 (1982).
72. M. V. Weinstein and A. H. Gordon, *Phys. Ther. Rev.*, 38:96-98 (1958).
73. B. Csillik, E. Knyihar-Csillik, and A. Szucs, *Neurosci. Lett.*, 31:87-90 (1982).

74. I. Ulrich, *Schweiz Rundsch. Med.*, 69:617-619 (1979).
75. D. Kostadinov, I. Topalov, and I. Kiranov, *Kurortol. Fizioter.*, 10(1):20-22 (1973).
76. S. B. Sokolov, E. K. Sveshnikova, Y. A. Lavrentier, A. I. Pertsovsky, I. K. Ivanov, G. N. Panevskaya, and A. G. Zhuchkov, *Vopr. Kurortol. Fizioter. Lech Fizkult.*, 5:12-15 (1981).
77. A. N. Ostrokhovich and N. I. Strelkova, *S. S. Horsanov Zh. Neuropathol. Psikhiat.*, 82:34-38 (1982).
78. A. Martin, J. Swarbrick, and A. Cammarata, *Physical Pharmacy.* Lea & Febiger, Philadelphia, 1983, p. 428.
79. P. Tyle and S. G. Frank, in *Proceedings of the Medical Device and In Vitro Diagnostic Manufacturing Conference*, MD & DI Central, Cannon Communications, Santa Monica, CA, 1985, p. 89.
80. H. H. Schilkret, *J. Invest. Dermatol.*, 5:11-14 (1942).
81. J. W. Caudill, E. Romanowski, T. Araullo-Cruz, and Y. J. Gordon, *Curr. Eye Res.*, 5(1):41-45 (1986).
82. K. Okabe, H. Yamaguchi, and Y. Kawai, *J. Controlled Release*, 4:79-85 (1986).
83. P. Tyle, *Pharm. Res.*, 3(6):318-326 (1986).
84. M. W. Cornwall, *Phys. Ther.*, 61:359-360 (1981).
85. M. D. Lekas, *Otolaryng. Head Neck Surg.*, 87:292-298 (1977).
86. R. J. Popkin, *J. Invest. Dermatol.*, 16:97-102 (1951).
87. H. S. Schwartz, *Arch. Intern. Med.*, 95:662-668 (1955).
88. M. B. Moawad, *Dermatol. Monatsschr.*, 155:388-394 (1969).
89. M. Tannenbaum, *Phys. Ther.*, 60:792 (1980).
90. B. M. R. Hill, *Aust. J. Dermatol.*, 17:92-93 (1976).
91. K. Grice, H. Sattar, and M. Baker, *Br. J. Dermatol.*, 86:72-78 (1972).
92. F. Levit, *Arch. Dermatol.*, 98:505-507 (1968).
93. J. B. Sloan and K. Soltani, *J. Am. Acad. Dermatol.*, 15:671-684 (1986).
94. K. Midtgaard, *Br. J. Dermatol.*, 114:485-488 (1986).
95. E. Abell and K. Morgan, *Br. J. Dermatol.*, 91:87 (1974).
96. J. Gordan, T. P. Araullo-Cruz, E. Romanowski, L. Ruziczka, C. Balouris, J. Oren, K. P. Cheng, and S. Kim, *Invest. Ophthalmol. Vis. Sci.*, 28:1230-1234 (1986).
97. R. L. Stephen, *JAMA*, 256:769 (1986).
98. M. Braza, C. Peckman, and J. Baum, *Invest. Ophthalmol. Vis. Sci.*, 28:1033-1036 (1987).
99. O. Siddiqui, Y. Sun, J-C. Liu, and Y. W. Chien, *J. Pharm. Sci.*, 76:341-345 (1987).
100. J. E. Sanderson, R. W. Caldwell, J. Hsiao, R. Dixon, and R. R. Tuttle, *J. Pharm. Sci.*, 76:215-218 (1987).

15

Ophthalmic Drug Delivery Devices

ASHIM K. MITRA / Purdue University, West Lafayette, Indiana

I. INTRODUCTION

An ideal drug delivery system delivers a drug to an intended site of action at an appropriate therapeutic level for a desired period of time. The purpose is to achieve a desired pharmacological effect and to avoid untoward side effects from the drug. The fate of a drug following administration into a living system is partly dependent on the physicochemical properties of the drug and their effects on the absorption, distribution, metabolism, and elimination characteristics of the drug [1,2]. Therefore, the appropriate choice and design of therapeutic regimen and delivery system should be based on knowledge of the relationship between the physicochemical properties and the pharmacokinetic properties of the drug.

It is well established in the literature that the typical method of ophthalmic drug administration, which is the instillation of a drug solution or suspension into the cul-de-sac, is an extremely inefficient method of dosing. The availability of pilocarpine in the inner eye from an instilled solution is as low as or even less than 1% of an administered dose [3,4].

The bioavailability and relative pharmacological response obtained after the ocular instillation of a drug solution depends on the following general factors: (a) drug kinetics in the conjunctival cul-de-sac (precorneal), (b) the permeability of the cornea to drug species (corneal), and (c) the rate at which the drug is eliminated from the eye (postcorneal).

Drug molecules intended for therapeutic action in various eye pathologies will often have specific sites of action within the globe. For example, the receptor sites for miotics and mydriatics are located in the iris-ciliary body; and for sulfonamides, antibiotics, and steroids the site of action will sometimes be an infected or inflamed area within the eye. Thus, for a drug to reach an inner eye site of action, it must penetrate the cornea. The corneal membrane acts as a rate-limiting barrier to the productive absorption of ophthalmic drugs. A schematic diagram of a human eye is depicted in Fig. 1. Access to inner eye structures across the sclera or the conjunctiva is usually not considered productive, as any drug molecule penetrating the surface of the eye beyond the limbus will not enter the aqueous humor, but will be picked up in the capillary beds and carried into general circulation [5].

But in a recent study [6], the noncorneal route of absorption has been emphasized. The study suggested that intraocular penetration via the noncorneal route involves drug diffusion across conjunctiva and sclera and that neither reentry from the general circulation following drug absorption into the blood nor drug absorption by local vasculature can account for the observed results. The two compounds studied are inulin and timolol maleate—both of which appear to gain intraocular access (vitreous and iris) bypassing the anterior chamber.

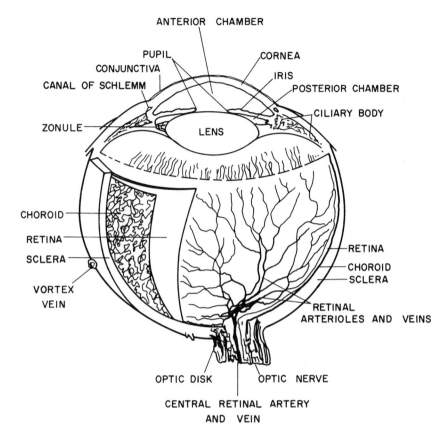

ANTERIOR CHAMBER

PUPIL
CONJUNCTIVA
CANAL OF SCHLEMM
ZONULE
LENS
CORNEA
IRIS
POSTERIOR CHAMBER
CILIARY BODY

CHOROID
RETINA
SCLERA
VORTEX
VEIN
RETINA
CHOROID
SCLERA
RETINAL
ARTERIOLES AND VEINS

OPTIC DISK   OPTIC NERVE

CENTRAL RETINAL ARTERY
AND VEIN

Fig. 1 Anatomical structure of the human eye.

Inulin, being a large molecular weight polar compound, has very low transcorneal permeability. Therefore, much of its intraocular access is achieved through noncorneal routes. Exploration of these sclera-conjunctival routes as sites for ocular absorption of poorly cornea-permeable molecules can provide interesting opportunities.

The penetration of drugs across the corneal membrane occurs from the precorneal tear film of precorneal space [7-9]. Thus, the mixing and kinetic behavior of drug disposition in the tears have a direct bearing on the efficiency of drug absorption into the inner eye. Non-productive drug loss includes the bulk drainage of the precorneal fluids, that is, the mixture of normal lacrimal fluid and the instilled drug solution, via the nasolacrimal drainage or turnover apparatus. Loss of drug by drainage away from the precorneal absorbing surface is the most significant of the mechanisms of drug loss [10,11]. From

Fick's laws of diffusion, it is known that the amount of any material diffusing per unit time per unit area (flux) across any membrane is a function of the concentration gradient across the membrane and the inherent ability of a molecule to diffuse across a membrane (diffusivity). The total mass of drug transported is, therefore, also a function of the total time over which the gradient is maintained [12]. It has been established that after a drug solution has been instilled topically into the eye, an administered dose is effectively removed from the absorbing corneal surface by the nasolacrimal turnover mechanism within 5 min of instillation [10,13]. As a result, ocular availability of the drug is significantly reduced, because of the limited contact time that a drug has with the absorbing corneal surface. The significance of nonproductive drug loss is twofold: (a) only a small fraction of the instilled drug reaches the intended site of action; and (b) the amount of drug ending up in the general circulation can represent a toxic systemic dose [16].

The productive absorption of most ophthalmic drugs results from the diffusional process across the corneal membrane. The efficiency of the absorption process is a function of the rate and extent at which the transport processes occur. The flux of any drug molecule across a biological membrane depends on the physicochemical properties of the permeating molecule and its interaction with the membrane. The extent to which the transport or absorption process occurs, as already mentioned, is also a function of the physiological mechanism of precorneal fluid drainage or turnover.

Two general approaches can be taken to improve the extent or efficiency of corneal drug absorption. The first approach, which aims at increasing the time of contact of an administered drug with the absorbing corneal surface by decreasing the effect of the drainage mechanism, has met with limited success.

Increase in contact time of instilled drug with the absorbing corneal surface has been achieved to some extent by adopting one or more of the following methods: viscosity-inducing agents, ointments, and reduction of administration volume.

A. Viscosity-Inducing Agents

The precorneal tear film is a fluid layer about 7 to 9 µm thick [15,16] that is spread over the corneal epithelium by a coacervate of mucin and stabilized by the superficial oily layer formed by meibomian gland secretion [17]. Utilization of viscous vehicles (e.g., solutions of methylcellulose, polyvinyl alcohol, can result in a 1.2- to 1.4-fold increase in the maximum miotic response—the profile of the area under the miosis versus time—as well as the duration of miotic effect after instillation of pilocarpine [18]. Increases in the amount of a drug in the tear film following instillation of a viscous solution are probably due to a slowing of the initial nonproductive drainage [19,20,22] and to the prolonged retention of the more viscous tear film [21]. Each of these results in a greater contact time for the drug to undergo productive absorption from the tear film.

B. Ointments

Ointments are often used as ophthalmic vehicles and can be classified into two types: the simple base (e.g., castor oil) and the compound base [23,24]. The compound bases are more often used, and the oil-in-water type of emulsion is particularly effective [23,25]. After instillation, these ointments separate into small droplets and remain in the cul-de-sac for a prolonged time acting as a drug depot [26].

C. Reduction of Administration Volume

Reduction of the instillation volume increases ocular drug availability because of the nature of the precorneal fluid turnover mechanism [10, 27].

The conjunctival cul-de-sac in both human and rabbit normally contains from 7 to 9 μl of tears [28,29], which is a result of the anatomical structure of the eye and its supporting tissues and, also, a function of normal tear fluid turnover rate, which is about 0.66 μl/min [10]. When the normal residual volume is perturbed, such as after the instillation of a dosing volume, the increased volume of fluid in the cul-de-sac is efficiently returned to the normal volume via the pumping action of the canaliculi associated with the blink movement [30]. Regardless of the instillation volume, a near-normal volume is reestablished within 5 min of dosing. The typical eye dropper used in delivering ophthalmic solutions delivers approximately a 50 μl volume of drug solution. If a comparison of ophthalmic availability is made between a drug delivered in a 50 μl installation volume to an identical amount of drug (but at a 10-fold greater concentration) contained in a 5 μl volume, the following hypothetical conclusion is obtained: where the 50 μl volume is instilled, on the order of 80% of the instilled fluid (and drug) is washed away from the absorbing corneal surface within 5 min. However, where 5 μl is instilled, only on the order of 30% of the instilled fluid (and drug) is washed away from the absorbing surfaces within the first 5 min. Experimental results obtained in evaluation of this concept demonstrated that the ocular availability of pilocarpine could be increased by a factor of 3, from approximately 1% to 3% by decreasing the drop size from 25 μl to 5 μl [27].

The second general approach that can be taken to improve the extent of efficiency of corneal absorption is to increase the rate of transport of the permeating drug across the corneal membrane without affecting the contact time. This can be achieved either by increasing the effective concentration or thermodynamic activity of the diffusing drug in the precorneal fluid or by changing the transport (permeability) characteristics of the drug across the corneal membrane.

D. Factors Affecting Corneal Transport

Three factors are considered responsible for determining the transport efficiency of a particular drug species across the corneal membrane:

1. The physicochemical properties of the drug substance (e.g., ionization constants, aqueous solubility, oil/water partition coefficients)
2. The formulation in which the drug is prepared (e.g., pH of the solution, types and concentrations of buffers, viscosity-inducing agents and stabilizers)
3. The corneal structure and integrity

In terms of transcorneal drug penetration, the cornea can be considered to consist of three primary layers (epithelium, stroma, and endothelium). A cross seciton of the cornea showing the respective drug absorption barriers is depicted in Fig. 2.

The epithelium and the endothelium contain on the order of a 100-fold greater amount of lipid material than the stroma [31]. Consequent-

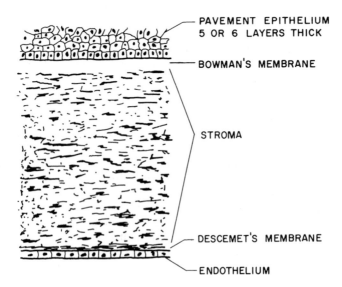

Fig. 2 Cross-sectional view of the corneal membrane depicting various barriers to drug absorption.

ly, depending on the physicochemical properties of a diffusing drug, the resistance offered by the individual layers varies greatly. Epithelium, being lipoidal, represents a diffusional barrier offering high resistance to ionic or other aqueous soluble or polar species. In contrast, compounds with relatively low polarity encounter a greater diffusional resistance in the hydrophilic stromal layer. This frequently cited concept of drug permeation across the corneal membrane, referred to as the differential solubility concept, was described by Kinsey [32]. This concept is particularly important relative to the transport of electrolyte drugs (i.e., ionizable weak acids and bases). Many drugs used in the treatment of eye diseases, such as pilocarpine, epinephrine, the amide local anesthetics, atropine, hematropine, and cyclopentolate, are weak organic bases. For reasons of dosage form stability (i.e., for minimizing chemical degradation), these drugs are commercially formulated at acidic pH. As a result, the drugs are delivered into the cul-de-sac largely in their ionized form. As such, they encounter considerable resistance relative to their partitioning into and diffusion across the lipoidal epithelial layer. Since the concentration of buffer in an ophthalmic formulation dictates the postinstillation time course of pH, it in turn dictates the time course of the state of ionization of pilocarpine in the precorneal fluid, which is changing as a function of time from the pilocarpinium ion to pilocarpine base. The extent of ionization of pilocarpine in the instilled solution affects the efficiency of pilocarpine absorption and the observed pharmacological response to the drug. When miosis-time profiles were obtained in rabbits after instillation of 25 µl of 1.0% pilocarpine nitrate solutions, which were buffered at a pH of 4.75 with different concentrations of citrate buffer, relative pharmacological response, as measured by the areas under the miosis-time profiles and the maximum observed pupillary diameter changes, decreased as the citrate buffer concentration was increased. A reduction in the miosis-time profile area of greater than fivefold was observed at the highest citrate concentration studied [33].

It is clear from the discussion above that topical administration of ophthalmic drugs will show a temporal pattern of pulse entry with a rapidly declining tear concentration, which usually follows apparent first-order behavior. Adequate therapy for glaucoma or for viral or bacterial infections of the inner eye structures depends on repetition of such pulse entries at a high frequency. In general, frequent drug administrations are accompanied by corresponding increases in local and systemic side effects. Continuous delivery of drugs in a controlled manner to the anterior chamber of the eye will eliminate the requirement for frequent drug administration, causing better patient compliance, and will result in extended duration of action, hence lower amount of total dose required, which in turn will minimize the local and/or systemic side effects. Continuous delivery would also avoid any prolonged period of underdosing, which often occurs between drug administrations. Such continuous drug entries allow for the practical use of short-half-life drugs. (Most drugs have half-lives around 20-30 min in the anterior chamber because loss of drug from aqueous humor is dependent mostly on the rate of aqueous removal from the chamber.) A number of ocular drug delivery devices have been developed, and most of them attempt to reach an ideal zero-order input. A number of such devices will be discussed in this chapter.

II. OCULAR INSERTS

A. Membrane-Controlled Devices

Diffusion of drugs from a reservoir through a rate-controlling membrane can result in a controlled zero-order release over a specific span till the drug reservoir is depleted. Such a device has been developed for the antiglaucoma drug pilocarpine (Ocusert) (Fig. 3). The rate-controlling membrane is composed of ethylene vinyl acetate, a copolymer that is biocompatible with eye tissues. A mixture of pilocarpine free base and alginic acid makes up the drug reservoir. Two strengths are available, Ocusert Pilo 20 and Pilo 40. The drug release rates are 20 and 40 µg/hr, respectively, over a duration of 7 days, although a higher release rate is obtained in the first day because of the leaching of the pilocarpine from the polymer membrane (Fig. 4). From the second day onward, a steady state concentration gradient is maintained and a continuous near-zero-order release is obtained. A higher release rate (40 µg/hr) is obtained by incorporating di(2-ethylhexyl)phthalate as a flux enhancer into the membrane. Macoul and Pavan Langston

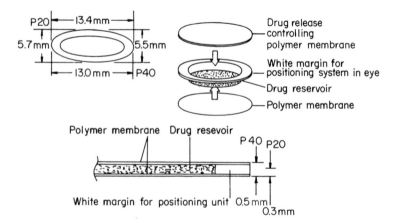

Fig. 3 Schematic diagram of an Ocusert controlled release drug delivery device.

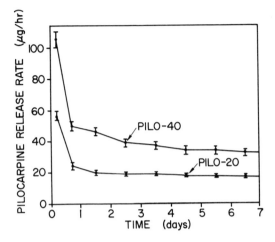

Fig. 4 In vitro release rates from pilocarpine ocular therapeutic systems.

[34] evaluated the effectiveness of the Ocusert delivery device in 29 patients with open-angle glaucoma. Patients placed the system in the cul-de-sac once a week. They retained it well and tolerated its continuing use without appreciable difficulty. Intraocular pressure was controlled satisfactorily. Side effects from the ocular therapeutic system were minimal or absent.

The pilocarpine Ocusert system enables the glaucoma patient to be treated effectively with one-fourth to one-eighth the dose required with pulsating eyedrop therapy. Therefore, continuous control of intraocular pressure can be gained with minimal visual disturbances.

Pilocarpine free base is freely water soluble as well as relatively hydrophobic, with an octanol/water partition coefficient of 2.0 at 25°C [35]. The use of pilocarpine free base in the Ocusert system allowed the use of relatively hydrophobic ethylene vinyl acetate copolymer, which caused very little water uptake into the core and subsequently very little osmotic pressure development.

B. Implantable Silicone Devices

For local treatment of intraocular tumors a silicone rubber device has been developed. This system has been used in experimental animal tumor models, particularly in rabbit eye tumor model. A useful antineoplastic agent 1,3-bis-(2-chloroethyl)-1-nitroso urea (BCNU) has been delivered with the aid of this device to the anterior segments of the rabbit eyes implanted with Brown-Pearce epithelioma and Greene

melanoma. The BCNU treatment using such silicone devices resulted
in tumor regression with much reduced systemic toxicity.

The system is comprised of two sheets of silicone rubber (Silastic
500-1, 0.13 mm thick) glued at the edges with silicone adhesive to form
a balloonlike sac through which a silicone tube (0.3 mm diameter) is
inserted (Fig. 5). The BCNU solution is released at a constant rate
through the silicone rubber by diffusive processes. In vitro experiments showed that a release rate of 200 to 300 μg/hr was achievable
for the length of time limited by the amount of drug in the device (Fig.
6). After total depletion of the drug reservoir, the balloon can be
refilled with drug solution. This device was implanted into the episcleral tissue of rabbits with Brown-Pearce epithelioma as shown in
Fig. 7.

Evaluation was made relative to the effectiveness of BCNU treatment
by comparing the tumor growth on treated and control eyes, by weighing the eyes before and after treatment, and by comparing the histopathological changes between treated and untreated eyes. In all cases,
sustained delivery of BCNU to the anterior chamber delayed tumor
growth. However, a combination of low intravenous dose and local
BCNU administration was most effective for the treatment of Greene
melanoma.

The rate of release of drugs through such polymeric membranes
can be expressed by a simple steady state expression:

$$\frac{1}{A}\frac{dx_t}{dt} = \frac{DK}{h}\Delta C \qquad (1)$$

where dx_t/dt represents the rate of drug release, A is the cross-sectional area of diffusion, D is the apparent diffusivity of the permeating
species across the silicone membrane, K is the apparent partition co-

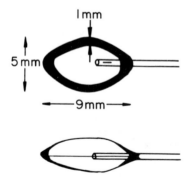

Fig. 5 Schematic diagram of an expandable silicone implant. [From
M. F. Refojo, et al., *J. Bioengin.*, 2:437 (1978).]

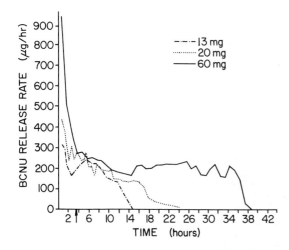

Fig. 6 Release of BCNU at 37°C from silicone balloons injected with 0.15 ml of BCNU solution in ethanol. The arrow indicates the point at which the alcohol had diffused out of the balloon. [From M. F. Refojo et al., *J. Bioeng.*, 2:437 (1978).]

efficient between the water and polymer phases, and ΔC is the concentration gradient across the membrane. Ueno et al. [36] studied the release of BCNU from a number of silicone and silicone-nylon hybrid devices and attempted to correlate the release rate with the wall thickness and surface area of the device. It must be emphasized that a silicone-nylon device releases BCNU through the silicone side only. The data in modified form are summarized in Table 1, which clearly shows that a predictable release rate could be obtained from a known wall thickness and exposed surface area of the device. Such silicone devices have significant potential for local controlled delivery of antibacterial, antineoplastic, or antiviral agents to the anterior chamber of the eye.

C. Implantable Infusion Systems

Patients suffering from dry-eye require frequent instillation of artificial tear preparations. A new method has been developed by Karesh and Nirankari [37] for the continuous infusion of these solutions. So far the device has been tested successfully in an animal (mongrel dog) model. In this procedure, the canalicular system is intubated with fenestrated Silastic tubing, which is subcutaneously tunneled and then attached to a miniaturized and computerized pumping device (ASGC Auto Syringe Pump; Travenol Laboratories, Inc., Hooksett, New Hamp-

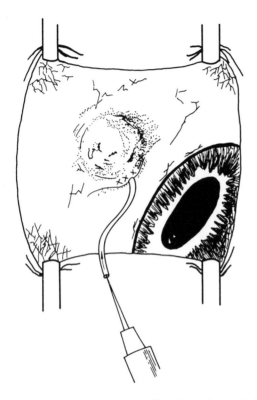

Fig. 7 Silicone device fixed on the episcleral tissue at the pars plana. BCNU injected through the tube of the device. [From H. S. Liu, et al., *Invest. Ophthalmol. Vis. Sci.*, 18:1061 (1979).]

shire). This makes it possible for a predetermined volume of solution to be automatically and continuously delivered. Using this technique, artificial tear solution (Tears Naturale, Alcon Laboratories, Inc., Fort Worth) was instilled at a rate of 1.75 µl/min, a rate approximating the normal basic tear secretion rate (0.5-2.2 µl/min). This treatment resulted in a 14% increase in tear flow from preoperative values. Such a tear flow rate represents a 74% increase in tear secretion rates for patients with keratoconjunctivitis sicca. None of the experimental animals developed subcutaneous infections, dacryocystitits, or corneal ulcers. By taking advantage of the normal anatomy of the lacrimal drainage system, this new technique (a) does not compromise the conjunctival cul-de-sac or the salivary system, (b) avoids the inconvenience of external devices, and (c) allows for the automatic instillation of predetermined volumes of artificial tear solutions.

TABLE 1 BCNU Release Rates from Silicone and Silicone-Nylon Hybrid Devices of Different Wall Thicknesses and Surface Areas

Number of observations	Wall thickness (mm)	Surface area (mm^2)	BCNU release rate ($\mu g/hr$)[a]
32		34.6	979 ± 101
14	0.13	58.4	1439 ± 57.7
14		115.0	2639 ± 126
33		31.8	459 ± 53.2
18	0.25	51.8	772 ± 73.8
15		107.0	1246 ± 87.5
15		33.4	338 ± 16.3
47	0.52	52.0	390 ± 77.9
33		120.0	747 ± 45.7
38	0.13 (0.05)[b]	17.4[c]	602 ± 41.3
33	0.25 (0.10)[b]	13.2[c]	284 ± 32.1

[a] Mean ± SD.
[b] Thickness of nylon.
[c] Surface area of silicone sheeting only.
Source: Modified from Ref. 36.

Another drug delivery pumping device is the Infusaid, which is also an implantable continuous infusion system (Infusaid Corporation, Sharon, Massachusetts). Since the device can be refilled in vivo, long-term infusion is possible. The energy requirement for the pumping action is met by an expanding fluid (a fluorocarbon in gas-liquid equilibrium) at body temperature [38].

When such a device was implanted in the lumbar region of a rabbit and injected with 0.5% fluorescein, a continuous delivery into the rabbit eye through a tube implanted into the superior conjunctival fornix was observed for 6 weeks [39]. With the Alzet minipump (a generic osmotic minipump developed by Alza Corporation, Palo Alto, California), drug delivery at a continuous rate is possible for only 2 weeks and the device is not replenishable in vivo. From that standpoint, Infusaid appears to have some advantage over the Alzet minipump. However, the Alzet minipump has much smaller dimensions and can be used in small animals.

III. FUTURE DIRECTIONS

An unusually high number of ocular conditions are either induced or aggravated because of overtreatment with drugs locally. Repeated instillation can cause mechanical injury, corneal pigmentation, as well as sensitivity reactions of the conjunctiva and eyelid. Side effects such as miosis with pilocarpine or mydriasis with atropine or sympathomimetic amines can cause local visual disturbances. Cholinesterase inhibitors such as alkyl phosphates and ecothiophate iodide can be absorbed through the conjunctiva, the mucous membranes of the nose, or the lacrimal passages and may give rise to characteristic systemic pharmacological responses. Ocular therapies with such classes of drugs can be significantly improved by interventions with ophthalmic drug delivery devices.

Currently, ocular antiviral therapy with agents like 5-iodo-2'-deoxyuridine, trifluorothymidine, and other antimetabolites require drug instillation every hour during the day and every 2 hr during the night. Besides being cytotoxic, these agents have both mutagenic and oncogenic potential. Therefore, such treatment modalities should be intervened with controlled release devices to minimize the toxic potential and to enhance therapeutic effectiveness. Iontophoretic devices have been utilized for evaluating herpes simplex (HSV) infection and reactivation as well as epinephrine distribution and concentration in full-thickness corneas and in trigeminal ganglia of rabbits [40]. Infectious virus was recovered from 58% of epinerphrine-induced eyes 24 to 96 hr after iontophoresis. Iontophoretic delivery of sulfa drugs in pyocyaneous infections has been reported to be 3 to 12 times greater in the cornea and 3 to 15 times greater in the aqueous humor than that resulting from diffusion alone [41]. (Also see Chapter 14, Iontophoretic Devices.)

Frequent local instillations of antibiotics or sulfonamides provide an unusually high drug concentration at the corneal epithelial surface. Since a high concentraiton of these agents is required at the infected intraocular sites, their recommended dosing interval is frequently between 1 and 2 hr. Controlled release devices could be more useful in these cases. Although drug delivery devices are seldom used in ophthalmology, the need for such devices in various ocular pathological conditions is undeniable. The unpopularity of ocular devices may partly stem from the fact that such devices have to be put in place and taken out from under the eyelid periodically. Moreover the device can move around in the precorneal space, resulting in some discomfort and visual disturbances. However, a device that is of the right size and shape could be designed to stay in the lower cul-de-sac firmly. If the material used for the construction of the device is degraded by the tear film, the need to remove it from the cul-de-sac will not arise. Therefore, improvement in design, construction, and bioerodible polymer technology can bring about a significant change in the use of ocular drug delivery devices.

ACKNOWLEDGMENT

The preparation of this chapter was supported in part by research grant EY-05863 from the National Eye Institute, National Institutes of Health.

REFERENCES

1. M. Gibaldi and D. Perrier, *Pharmacokinetics*, Vol. 15, Dekker, New York, 1982.
2. J. G. Wagner, *Fundamentals of Clinical Pharmacokinetics*. Drug Intelligence Publishing, Hamilton, IL, 1979.
3. T. J. Mikkelson, S. S. Chrai, and J. R. Robinson, *J. Pharm. Sci.*, 62:1648 (1973).
4. T. J. Mikkelson, S. S. Chrai, and J. R. Robinson, *J. Pharm. Sci.*, 62:1942 (1973).
5. D. M. Maurice, in *The Eye*, Vol. 1, *Vegetative Physiology and Biochemistry* (H. Davson, ed.). Academic Press, New York, 1969, p. 541.
6. T. F. Patton and I. Ahmed, *Invest. Ophthalmol. Vis. Sci.*, 26:584 (1985).
7. D. M. Maurice, *Int. Ophthalmol. Clin.*, 20(3):7 (1980).
8. J. E. Harris, in *Symposium on Ocular Therapy*, Vol. 3 (I. H. Leopold, ed.). Mosby, St. Louis, 1968, p. 96.
9. M. G. Doane, A. D. Jensen, and C. H. Dohlman, *Am. J. Ophthalmol.*, 85:383 (1978).
10. S. S. Chrai, T. F. Patton, A. Mehta, and J. R. Robinson, *J. Pharm. Sci.*, 62:1112 (1973).
11. S. S. Chrai, M. C. Makoid, S. P. Eriksen, and J. R. Robinson, *J. Pharm. Sci.*, 63:333 (1974).
12. J. Crank, *The Mathematics of Diffusion*, 2nd ed. Clarenden Press, Oxford, 1975, p. 2.
13. J. W. Sieg and J. R. Robinson, *J. Pharm. Sci.*, 65:1816 (1976).
14. T. F. Patton and M. Francoeur, *Am. J. Ophthalmol.*, 85:225 (1978).
15. N. Ehlers, *Acta Ophthalmol. Suppl.*, 81 (1965).
16. S. Mishima, *Arch. Ophthalmol.*, 73:233 (1965).
17. F. J. Holly, *Int. Ophthalmol. Clin.*, 13:73 (1973).
18. S. S. Chrai and J. R. Robinson, *J. Pharm. Sci.*, 63:1218 (1974).
19. M. Sugaya and S. Nagataki, *Jap. J. Ophthalmol.*, 22:127 (1978).
20. C. A. Adler, D. M. Maurice, and M. E. Petersen, *Exp. Eye Res.*, 11:34 (1971).

21. D. A. Benedetto, D. O. Shah, and H. E. Kaufman, *Invest. Ophthalmol. Vis. Sci.*, 14:887 (1975).
22. T. F. Patton and J. R. Robinson, *J. Pharm. Sci.*, 64:1312 (1975).
23. N. Ehlers, in *Drugs and Ocular Tissues* (S. Dikstein, ed.). Karger, Basel, 1977, p. 23.
24. J. S. Robin and P. P. Ellis, *Surv. Ophthalmol.*, 22:335 (1978).
25. M. Klien, *Arch. Clin. Exp. Ophthalmol.*, 129:413 (1933).
26. J. W. Sieg and J. R. Robinson, *J. Pharm. Sci.*, 64:931 (1975).
27. T. F. Patton, *J. Pharm. Sci.*, 66:1058 (1977).
28. S. Mishima, A. Gasset, S. D. Klyce, Jr., and J. L. Baum, *Invest. Ophthalmol.*, 5:264 (1966).
29. N. Ehlers, *Acta Ophthalmol. Suppl.*, 81 (1965).
30. D. M. Maurice, *Int. Ophthalmol. Clin.*, 13:73 (1973).
31. D. G. Cogan and E. D. Hirch, *Arch. Ophthalmol. N.Y.*, 32:276 (1944).
32. V. E. Kinsey, in *Physiology of the Eye*, 4th ed. (F. H. Adler, ed.). Mosby, St. Louis, 1965.
33. A. K. Mitra and T. J. Mikkelson, *Int. J. Pharm.*, 10:219 (1982).
34. K. L. Macoul and D. Pavon-Langston, *Arch. Ophthalmol.*, 93(8): 587 (1975).
35. A. K. Mitra, Passive and facilitated transport of pilocarpine across the corneal membrane of the rabbit. Ph.D. dissertation, University of Kansas, 1983, pp. 98-110.
36. N. Ueno, M. F. Refojo, and L. H. S. Liu, *J. Biomed. Mater. Res.*, 16:699 (1982).
37. J. W. Karesh and V. S. Nirankari, *Invest. Ophthalmol. Vis. Sci.*, 27:1286 (1986).
38. Implantable infusion system (model 300), *Users Manual.* Infusaid Corp., Sharon, MA.
39. P. G. Rehkopf, B. J. Mondino, S. I. Brown, and D. B. Goldberg, *Invest. Ophthalmol. Vis. Sci.*, 19:428 (1980).
40. E. C. Dunkel and D. Pavon-Langston, *Curr. Eye Res.*, 6(1): 75-86 (1987).
41. L. von Sallmann, *Am. J. Ophthalmol.*, 25:1292 (1942).

16

Intrauterine Devices

AMIR H. ANSARI / Shadyside Hospital and Pittsburgh Institute of
Reproductive Medicine, Pittsburgh, Pennsylvania and Medical College
of Georgia, Augusta, Georgia

FRANK M. STURTEVANT / G. D. Searle & Co., Skokie, Illinois

I. INTRODUCTION

Historically, the description of intrauterine devices (IUDs) and pessaries
can be traced back to Hippocrates. In more recent times, the era of
intrauterine contraception dates from 1909 to 1934 and the experiences
of Richter [1] with a ring of silkworm gut, of Pust [2] with silkworm
gut attached to a glass button, and of Gräfenberg [3] and Ota [4] with
silver rings. Nevertheless, acceptance by the medical profession was
not forthcoming until the advent of antibiotics and inert plastics.

The first plastic IUDs to gain acceptance were the Lippes loop [5] and the Margulies Spiral [6], followed by variations leading to the popular but ill-fated Dalkon shield [7], which was removed from the market in 1974. Despite their effectiveness, the plastic IUDs had nonetheless failed to gain total acceptability by consumers and, to some extent, by physicians for the following reasons:

Relatively high incidence of spontaneous expulsion
Associated menstrual dysfunction, mainly in the form of abnormal
    prolonged uterine bleeding, resulting on occasion in anemia
Associated endometritis and occasional pelvic inflammatory diseases
    (PID)
Occasional unwanted pregnancies

II. MEDICATED INTRAUTERINE DEVICES

To abate the aforementioned side effects, and most importantly to increase efficacy of the device in pregnancy prevention, a new generation of devices was introduced. These IUDs were the "medicated" devices, and because they delivered biologically active materials, they were treated by regulatory agencies as "new drugs" [8]. The most popular device came to be the copper-releasing IUD [9,10], first marketed in 1974. This concept was based on the original observations of Zipper [11,12] that copper enhanced contraceptive effectiveness. It is presumed that this effect of the metal is exerted locally, as copper levels become elevated in the endometrium [13,14], but not in the blood or other organs [13-16].

Besides the improved effectiveness, it appears that the copper IUDs have lower expulsion rates [17] and an incidence of pelvic inflammatory disease and associated infertility that is not markedly different from that expected in the sexually active female population [18-21]. This latter point is difficult to establish for several reasons: (a) there are no studies of copper IUDs specifically designed to compare PID incidence to that in a control group of sexually active, noncontracepting, nonpregnant women with similar exposure to pathogens; (b) the incidence of PID in the general female population of reproductive age is known sketchily at best; (c) all epidemiological studies have involved non-IUD users who employed other methods of contraception, which confer protection against PID to a certain extent; and (d) the bulk of the literature on IUDs and PID employs varying definitions of PID and classifies cases based on clinical diagnosis, which is notoriously unreliable.

The other major category of medicated IUDs consists of those releasing steroids such as progesterone [22,23] or levonorgestrel [24]. It has been generally believed that these devices have two main advantages over nonmedicated IUDs:

Sinificant decrease in the amount of menstrual flow [23,24]
Reduced incidence of unwanted pregnancy

Whether the addition of a steroid, with its smooth muscle relaxing effect, in actuality decreases the rate of spontaneous expulsion has not
been established with certainty at this time.

It should be emphasized that steroid release from this type of IUD
is considered to be the mechanism of action for reduction of unwanted
pregnancies, the steroid exerting an effect on the endometrium and
on the cervical mucus as well. An early accelerated release rate eventually levels off, providing a more constant release rate. This is the
explanation offered for the high rate of associated abnormal uterine
bleeding, particularly the intermenstrual spotting and bleeding observed in the first few months following device insertion [25]. The
gradually decreased rate of steroid release following insertion of these
IUDs is believed to be the result of (a) total decrease in the amount
of available steroids within the device, and (b) fibrin coating of the
device by the endothelial lining of the uterus.

One disadvantage of the progesterone-releasing IUD is the necessity for annual replacement [23]; however, the levonorgestrel device
is claimed to have a lfietime of 7 years [24].

A. Side Effects

In general, the usually encountered complications and side effects with
nonmedicated IUDs (perforation, infection, pain and cramping, etc.)
are similarly present with the medicated IUDs. Additionally, depending on the type of medicated IUD, metallic versus steroid, certain unusual reactions and side effects have been encountered. In particular,
systemic dermatitis has been reported in association with the copper
IUD, with skin manifestations disappearing after the device is removed.
Alterations in lipid and carbohydrate metabolism, which had been the
subject of intense investigational study during the use of oral proges-
tational compounds, have equally received the attention of several investigators during the period of time the steroid-impregnated IUD is
within the confines of the uterine cavity. Whether the specific design
of the medicated IUD has a direct bearing on the effect of IUD for con-
ception control or whether it is the amount of material with which it
is impregnated is a subject that has not been sufficiently explored
at this time.

III. CONCLUSIONS AND COMMENTS

In contrast to nonmedicated devices, medicated IUDs may have the
following advantages and superiority:

Reduced incidence of unwanted pregnancy
Reduced incidence of spontaneous expulsion
Decreased amount of menstrual flow (in the case of steroid-bearing IUDs)

A potential anti-infection effect of the medicated IUDs has not been established with certainty at this time and needs further exploration. Finally, it should be mentioned that due to strict governmental regulation and the current medicolegal atmosphere in some countries, there has been an abrupt halt in further development and research in this area of contraception, which has so far been proved to be a safe and effective method.

REFERENCES

1. R. Richter, *Dtsch. Med. Wochenschr.*, 35:1525 (1909).
2. K. Pust, *Dtsch. Med. Wochenschr.*, 49:952 (1923).
3. E. Gräfenberg, Die intrauterine Methode der Konzeptionsverhütung, *Proceedings of the Third Congress of the World League For Sexual Reform.* Amsterdam, 1929, pp. 116-125.
4. T. Ota, *Jap. J. Obstet. Gynecol.*, 17:210 (1934).
5. J. Lippes, A study of itnra-uterine contraception: Development of a plastic loop, *Proceedings of the Conference on Intra-uterine Contraceptive Devices, New York.* International Congress Series No. 54, Excerpta Medica, Amsterdam, 1962, pp. 69-75.
6. L. Margulies, Permanent reversible contraception with an intra-uterine plastic spiral (Perma-Spiral), *Proceedings of the Conference on Intra-uterine Contraceptive Devices, New York.* International Congress Series No. 54, Excerpta Medica, Amsterdam, 1962, pp. 61-68.
7. H. J. Davis, *Am. J. Obstet. Gynecol.*, 106:455 (1970).
8. L. Yin, in *Intrauterine Contraception: Advances and Future Prospects* (G. I. Zatuchni, A. Goldsmith, and J. J. Sciarra, eds.). Harper & Row, New York, 1985, p. 52.
9. H. J. Tatum, *Contraception*, 6:179 (1972).
10. J. Newton, J. Elias, and J. McEwan, *Lancet*, 2:951 (1972).
11. J. S. Zipper, H. J. Tatum, L. Pastene, M. Medel, and M. Rivera, *Am. J. Obstet. Gynecol.*, 105:1274 (1969).
12. J. A. Zipper, H. J. Tatum, M. Medel, L. Pastene, and M. Rivera, *Am. J. Obstet. Gynecol.*, 109:771 (1971).
13. R. E. Ranney, E. F. Nutting, P. L. Hackett, L. A. Rancitelli, J. L. Daniel, W. J. Clarke, and R. G. Wheeler, *Fertil. Steril.*, 28:80 (1975).
14. K. Hagenfeldt, *Contraception*, 6:37 (1972).

15. A. J. Moo-Young, H. J. Tatum, A. O. Brinson, and W. Hood, *Fertil. Steril.*, 24:848 (1973).
16. S. O. Anteby, H. A. B. Bassat, S. Yarkoni, Y. Aboulafia, and E. Sadovsky, *Fertil. Steril.*, 29:30 (1978).
17. D. A. Edelman, G. S. Berger, and L. Keith, *Intrauterine Devices and Their Complications*. G. K. Hall, Boston, 1979, p. 20.
18. F. B. O'Brien, W. C. Stewart, and F. M. Sturtevant, *Contraception*, 27:111 (1983).
19. N. C. Lee, G. L. Rubin, H. W. Ory, and R. T. Burkman, *Obstet. Gynecol.*, 62:1 (1983).
20. J. R. Daling, N. S. Weiss, B. J. Metch, W. H. Chow, R. M. Soderstrom, D. E. Moore, L. R. Spadoni, and B. V. Stadel, *New Engl. J. Med.*, 312:937 (1985).
21. D. W. Cramer, I. Schiff, S. C. Schoenbaum, M. Gibson, S. Belisle, B. Albrecht, R. J. Stillman, M. J. Berger, E. Wilson, B. V. Stadel, and M. Seibel, *New Engl. J. Med.*, 312:941 (1985).
22. B. B. Pharriss, R. Erickson, J. Bashaw, S. Hoff, V. A. Place, and A. Zaffaroni, *Fertil. Steril.*, 25:915 (1974).
23. Y. Gibor, in *Medicated Intrauterine Devices* (E. S. E. Hafez and A. A. van Os, eds.). Nijhoff, The Hague, 1980, p. 146.
24. M. Haukkamaa, H. Allonen, M. Heikkiltä, T. Luukkainen, P. Lähteenmäki, C. G. Nilsson, and J. Toivonen, in *Intrauterine Contraception: Advances and Future Prospects* (G. I. Zatuchni, A. Goldsmith, and J. J. Sciarra, eds.). Harper & Row, New York, 1985, p. 232.
25. C. G. Nilsson, T. Luumkkainen, J. Diaz, and H. Allonen, *Contraception*, 25:345 (1982).

17

Intranasal Delivery Devices

ALEX BELL* / Perfect-Valois UK Ltd., Aylesbury, Buckinghamshire, United Kingdom

*Current Affiliation: Valois S.A., Le Neubourg, France

I. INTRODUCTION

The nasal delivery route has been known for many years as a means of administering therapeutically active materials. There is some evidence to suggest that our ancestors even as far back as the Stone Age had discovered the beneficial effects of inhaling the vapors from their steaming herbal brews.

In most recent times there has been an increased interest (mainly in academic circles) in delivery by this route, particularly for systemically active compounds that are either inactivated when administered orally by gastrointestinal effects or hepatic first-pass metabolism, or are too large to be absorbed efficiently transdermally. The nasal route has been approached as a potential noninvasive alternative to many forms of parenteral therapy, having demonstrated effective bioavailability along with the obvious advantage of easy self-administration. Among the types of compounds that have received particular interest are vaccines (influenza, measles), antimicrobials (interferons), hormones (LHRH and its analogs, oxytocin, insulin), and cardiovasculars (β-adrenergic blockers, vasodilators) [1]. The majority of products utilizing this means of administration that have reached the market to date, however, have done so mainly for their localized effects. For as well as providing an attractive potential site of administration for systemic absorption, the useful localized administration of compounds such as corticosteroids, antihistamines, and decongestants, which exhibit certain unwanted systemic effects when given orally or parenterally, has been recognized for many years.

As more interest is generated within industrial circles for delivery by this means, more and more development scientists are going to be faced with the question: *Which nasal delivery system is best suited to my compound, and how best can I evaluate its efficiency?*

Today the two most commonly chosen delivery systems available for nasal administration are based around either metered-dose aerosol valve devices (pressurized) or metered-dose pump devices (nonpressurized). The former are usually nonaqueous systems, and the latter usually aqueous. This chapter outlines some of the major performance and selection criteria to be considered when evaluating these devices to determine which type best suits the requirements of a compound and its application. Figure 1 shows devices of both types.

II. HOW DO THESE DELIVERY DEVICES OPERATE?

A. The Metered-Dose Aerosol Valve

Although device designs will vary depending on manufacturer, their basic principle of operation remains the same. The aerosol delivery system relies almost solely on the inherent properties of its propellant

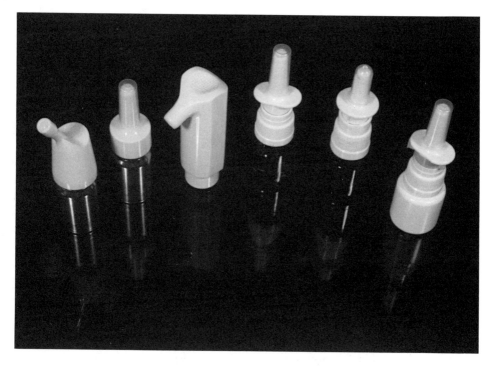

Fig. 1 A selection of aerosol valve and pump nasal delivery systems.
Three aerosol presentations (left) and three pump presentations (right).

system to provide the energy required to produce the sprayed dose.
The pack contents are held under the vapor pressure of the propellant
system.

At the rest or closed position (Fig. 2a), the product flows freely
into the metering chamber via the slots in the valve housing and the
narrow portion of the lower stem. On actuation of the device, the
wide portion of the upper stem engages the lower stem seal, thereby
isolating the dose within the metering chamber. Further depression
allows the passage of the stem orifice into the dosing chamber and thus
enables the dose to be released from the dosing chamber into the stem
and via the actuator into the nose (Fig. 2b).

B. The Metered-Dose Pump

Here again designs will vary from manufacturer to manufacturer but
basic principles remain similar. The metered-dose pump system relies
entirely on the mechanical energy imparted to the device by depression
of the actuator to achieve the sprayed dose (Fig. 3).

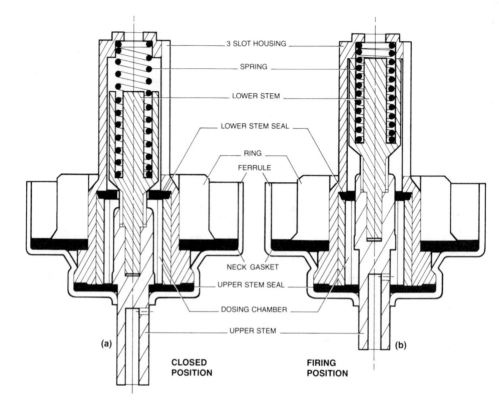

Fig. 2 Schematic diagram of an aerosol metering valve (Valois DF10) showing (a) the valve in the normal or rest position, and (b) the valve after dose delivery.

III. SELECTION AND PERFORMANCE CRITERIA

Factors and constraints in assessing the type of delivery system to be adopted for a particular application initially involve physicochemical considerations, as well as device performance and compatibility.

A. Physicochemical Considerations

The first stage of any dosage form development is to evaluate by preformulation study the physicochemical characteristics of the compound to be formulated relevant to the dosage form to be developed. For the two systems we are considering, the following areas should be evaluated:

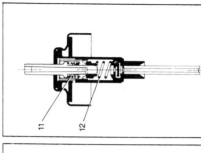

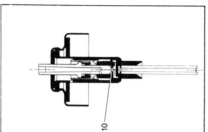

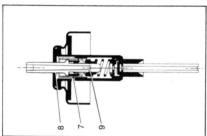

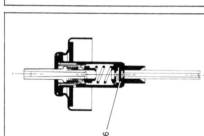

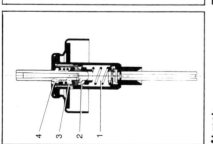

At rest:
The dosage chamber (1) is filled with liquid. The actuator must be pressed several times to prime the pump. At rest, the pump is sealed at positions 2, 3 and 4.

Pressurising:
Finger pressure on the actuator pushes the clapper (6) onto its base to form a tight seal which leads to an increase in pressure of the liquid in the dosage chamber.

Spraying:
As the liquid can not be compressed, the piston (7) is blocked in its downward movement. Continuing movement of the actuator forces the stem (8) down. The stem orifice (9) is thus disengaged from the piston and moves into the dosage chamber. The liquid is then sprayed.

Lowering position:
Spraying is completed. The mechanism is blocked at position 10.

Suction:
Under the pressure of the spring (11), the piston returns to its original position. This in turn isolates the stem orifice from the dosage chamber. The "return" spring (12) pushes all moving parts back to their rest position. The vacuum created by this movement raises the clapper and sucks up the liquid to fill the dosage chamber.

Fig. 3 Schematic diagram of a metering pump (Valois VP3) showing and describing the sequential mode of operation to effect dose delivery.

481

1. Solubility in appropriate solvents (i.e., water, aerosol propellants, and alcohols). In most cases aerosol delivery systems are either suspensions of the compound in the nonpolar aerosol propellant or solutions in alcohol/propellant mixtures. Pump systems are generally solutions or suspensions based on water or water/alcohol mixtures.

2. Degradative sensitivity of the compound and its solutions or suspensions. Reactions to heat, light, pH, moisture, oxygen, shear, and other conditions should be covered.

3. Protection of biological materials of certain types by carrier proteins. Special measures may be necessary to maintain biological activity. These carriers must be found to be compatible with the solvent systems under evaluation. Vaccines, interferons, and other proteins or macromolecules are of particular interest.

4. In vivo pharmacokinetic studies. If optimal conditions for compound absorption (e.g., pH, tonicity, viscosity, concentration, excipients), have already been derived, these may well influence or determine the system that is most appropriate for use. These characteristics are discussed in greater detail in another chapter.

B. Device Performance, Compatibility, and Selection

A preferred formulation approach will probably have been determined by physicochemical considerations (or political/economic and marketing considerations).

The selection of a delivery device to best suit this formulation approach will be based on four main criteria:

Dose performance
Device compatibility
Device integrity
Quality of manufacture

Dose Performance

Dose performance criteria for both valve and pump systems will be similar in many respects in that from both types of device a consistently accurate, discrete metered volume of product is required from each actuation throughout the entire life of the pack. For each system, therefore, dose performance needs evaluation throughout each dose delivered from the device (Figs. 4 and 5), from representative samples from within a batch (Figs. 6 and 7), and from representative samples from several batches (Fig. 8). Performance aspects to consider when evaluating these parameters include accuracy and reproducibility of dose delivered intradevice, interdevice, and batch to batch. For both valve and pump systems, clear and distinct emptying or tailing-off characteristics are desirable, and for pump systems a rapid and complete priming of the full dose delivered.

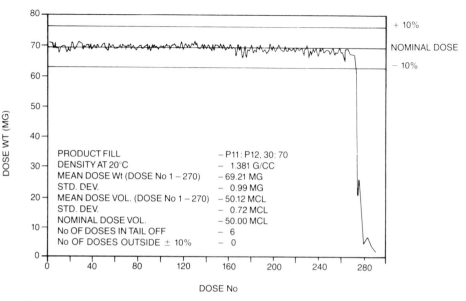

Fig. 4 Metered-dose nasal aerosol valve device (Valois DF10/50 mcl) dose performance: sequential dosing of product until pack is empty, with each dose weight monitored.

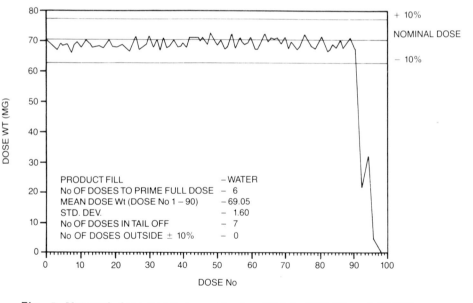

Fig. 5 Metered-dose nasal pump device (Valois VP3/70 mcl 18 PH) dose performance: sequential dosing of product until pack is empty, with each dose weight monitored.

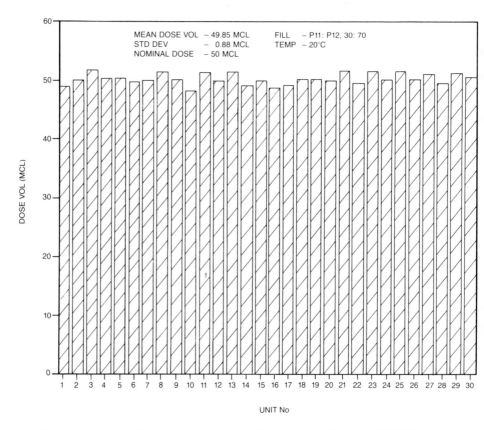

Fig. 6 Metered-dose nasal aerosol valve device (Valois DF10/50 mcl) dose performance characteristics of 30 random samples from within a batch showing individual mean dose weights and overall mean and standard deviation.

This type of dose performance assessment should also form part of the physical stability evaluation of the pack to ensure the maintenance of performance throughout shelf life conditions.

Device Compatibility

Compatibility of the selected formulation approach with the device and its component materials can be considered from two angles:

Material leaching out of the device and its components into the formulation—extractives

Material being lost from the formulation into or onto the device components—absorption and adsorption

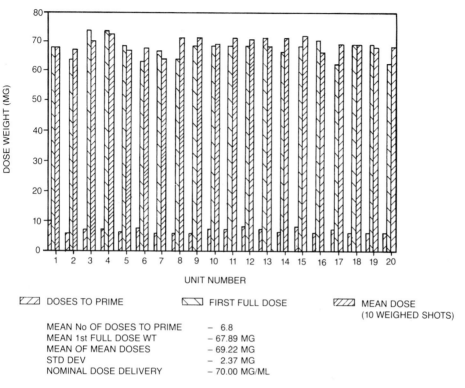

MEAN No OF DOSES TO PRIME   – 6.8
MEAN 1st FULL DOSE WT   – 67.89 MG
MEAN OF MEAN DOSES   – 69.22 MG
STD DEV   – 2.37 MG
NOMINAL DOSE DELIVERY   – 70.00 MG/ML

Fig. 7 Metered-dose nasal pump device (Valois VP3/70 mcl 18PH) dose performance characteristics of 20 random samples from within a batch, showing number of doses to prime a full dose, weight of first full dose, and mean dose weights from 10 individually weighed doses.

(The first of these usually gives most cause for concern, as extractives are usually very much an unknown quantity, from both the compositional and toxicological points of view.)

Extractives

The main potential source of extractable matter present in any device is that which comes from the elastomeric sealing materials within the device. These, depending on the elastomer manufacturer, will contain varying levels of materials such as plasticizers, which will be capable of extraction into the formulation (dependent in degree on the solvents present and the temperature).

Ideally a sealing material for pharmaceutical applications will show the following characteristics: (a) low levels of extractives, particularly

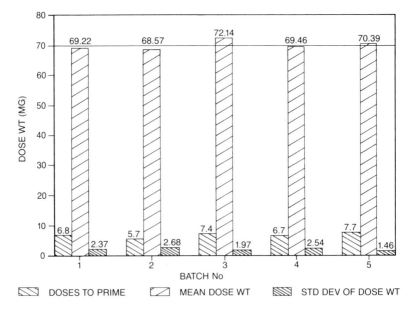

Fig. 8 Metered-dose nasal pump devices (Valois VP3/70 mcl): dose characteristics of several batches, showing overall mean number of doses to prime a full dose, mean dose weight, and standard deviation on the mean dose weight.

in the solvent systems on which the formulation is based, (b) extractives in a low-toxicity form (manufacturer using only materials permitted under FDA guidelines), (c) reliable and consistent quality, in both dimensional and physicochemical properties, and (d) consistent mechanical properties throughout the entire shelf life. To achieve the first of these characteristics, the major sources of extractives within the elastomer formulation need to be identified. These are usually found to be:

Plasticizers to aid processing and handling of the elastomer during
its manufacture
Organic impurities present on or in the "carbon black" used as a
filler in many rubber compounds, to provide a hardness and
rigidity to the final material

To overcome these main sources of extractives, an elastomer needs to be developed (from FDA-approved ingredients) to help satisfy criterion b, in which no plasticizers are used and no "carbon black" is present.

In practice this is achieved by replacing the "carbon black" by precipitated silica fillers and calcinated clays, which are essentially impurity free. In removing the plasticizers, a specialized continuous curing process of manufacture needs to be adopted to ensure reliable, consistent quality of a material that is extremely difficult to process by conventional means.

Absorption and Adsorption

Although the plastic components in delivery devices tend not to provide much in the way of extractives into the formulation, they can however, along with the seals, show significant absorption or adsorption of ingredients within the formulation (i.e., active ingredients, preservative systems, and surfactants). Absorbed materials can alter the physical properties of components, elastomeric seals in particular, and it is therefore often advisable to study formulation effects on these materials in isolation as well as in the complete delivery device.

Device Integrity

It is essential, as with any primary package, that the delivery device maintain its integrity throughout its shelf-life contact with the product. For aerosol delivery devices that are sealed pressurized systems, device integrity can be monitored by reference to weight loss of the total pack with time. In aerosol delivery systems this weight loss relates to the leakage or permeation of propellant vapor through the assembled aerosol valve (Fig. 2), through the closure between valve and container, or even through the component parts of the valve itself. Loss of aerosol propellant vapor (preferentially the more volatile propellant component) will alter the overall formulation propellant composition and vapor pressure, resulting in a change in dose spray characteristics produced and concentration of product delivered.

For pump delivery systems, which are usually formulated with nonvolatile solvents to give a nonpressurized package, the device sealing integrity is usually monitored by weight loss of the pack after subjection to negative pressures in a vacuum chamber.

Monitoring of these parameters at regular storage intervals and conditions as part of the product stability program should provide confidence in the sealing integrity of the systems, provided well-defined and validated closing specifications are applied to the pack during its manufacture.

"Quality of Manufacture"

Manufacturing/quality control documentation and procedures, manufacturing environment, handling, shipment, and packaging are all quality-related aspects of production. A device therefore needs not

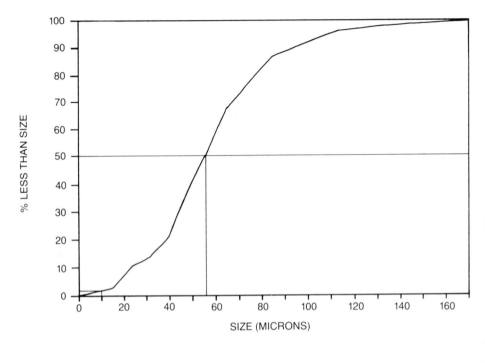

PRODUCT FILL	– WATER/ETHANOL 50:50
% BY WT < 10 MICRONS	– 1.4%
MASS MEDIAN DIAMETER	– 56 MICRONS
ACTUATOR TYPE	– 144 (GPC insert)

Fig. 9 Metered-dose nasal pump device. (Valois VP3/100 mcl): particle size analysis of the emitted spray as determined using a Malvern 2600 HSD particle size analyzer.

only to be of a good design and performance, it also needs to be manufactured and controlled by its supplier to the high standards expected by good pharmaceutical manufacturing practice.

IV. PARTICLE SIZE OF THE EMITTED SPRAY

For nasal delivery the particle size of the spray is of much less importance than for pulmonary applications.

In general terms, the larger the aerosol particle size distribution generated, the more efficient is its nasal entrapment and absorption in the anterior area of the nose beyond the nasal valve and in front of the ciliated epithelial region. Material deposited in the ciliated epithelial area is transported fairly rapidly to the nasopharynx, whence it is swallowed, in a similar manner to everyday airborne dust and pollutants. Very small particles (<10 µm) can potentially escape deposition in the nasal cavities and be inhaled [2], but in practice, particularly from the aqueous pump system, the amount of material within this size range is very small (Fig. 9). The actual particle size distribution attained from any device will be influenced by many factors within the delivery system, including nasal actuator geometry, solvent system, propellant system, formulation type (suspension/solution), surfactants (type and concentration), and dosage volume.

V. DISCUSSION

Regardless of which delivery device is chosen, be it valve or pump based, the basic performance and compatibility requirements from the delivery device must be addressed at an early stage in the development process. If these requirements are met and are successfully followed by long-term physical and chemical stability evaluations of the complete formulation package (which have not been discussed in any detail in this chapter), the product that reaches the marketing stage should merit confidence in its dose accuracy and consistency, both mechanically (by the delivery device) and physicochemically (by the formulation).

As interest in this means of administration grows, and as the development of excipient compounds to enhance absorption of active materials across the nasal mucosa continues, it is very likely that we will see many hitherto parenteral-only compounds reaching the market in nasal delivery systems. The benefits of such a move will be reflected in many areas: manufacturing costs, patient acceptance, self-administration, and reduced hospital outpatient care, to name but a few.

REFERENCES

1. Y. W. Chien and S. F. Chang, in *Transnasal Systemic Medications* (Y. W. Chien, ed.). Elsevier Science Publishers, Amsterdam, 1985, Chapter 1.
2. R. Masse and J. Bignon, Deposition des aerosols, *Proceedings of French Society for Aerosols in Medicine Conference 6th May 1982, Clermont-Ferrand, France*, pp. 105-150.

18

Sustained Release Drug Delivery Devices for Local Treatment of Dental Diseases

DORON STEINBERG and MICHAEL FRIEDMAN / The Hebrew University of Jerusalem, Jerusalem, Israel

I. INTRODUCTION

Dental diseases are recognized as a major public health problem through-out the world. Dental diseases can and do occur in all age groups, ethnicities, races, genders, and socioeconomic levels. Numerous epi-demiological studies show that dental diseases, tooth decay and diseases of the periodontum, are among the most common afflictions of mankind.

Studies conducted throughout the world have indicated the high prevalence of dental diseases [1,2]. Tooth decay is found most often in children, while gingivitis occurs in children, as well as in adults. Periodontal diseases progress with increasing age and constitute the major cause of tooth loss in adults.

The cost of treating tooth decay in the United States exceeds $2 billion annually, and complete treatment of the entire population would cost an additional $8 billion [3]. In 1977 approximately £250 million was spent on dental treatment at the England and Wales National Dental Service [4].

Pain, discomfort, and cosmetic considerations are added factors that also demonstrate the severity of the problems associated with den-tal diseases today. Hence, it is of the utmost importance to minimize and control dental diseases.

The most essential type of dental care begins at home. Daily oral hygiene plays a vital role in maintaining healthy teeth and gums. Clini-cal treatment and medication are also important aids in the upkeep of a healthy oral state. Since dental diseases may be chronic, long-term treatment is often necessary.

A significant pharmaceutical advantage is gained by targeting a particular drug to a desired site, thereby minimizing superfluous dis-tribution of the drug to other body organs. Improved local pharmaceu-tical delivery devices, which reduce the amounts of administered drugs and at the same time demonstrate the same or even better clinical re-sults, have numerous potential benefits over traditional treatments.

In this chapter we shall review the methods currently used in the treatment of tooth decay and periodontal diseases, while focusing on new drug delivery devices.

II. DENTAL CARIES

A. Etiology

Dental caries is a microbiotic disease causing destruction of the tooth tissues. There are three important factors in the creation of a carious lesion: the microflora, the teeth, and the substrate. All these factors must converge over a sufficient period of time in order to effect the destruction of the tooth tissues (Fig. 1).

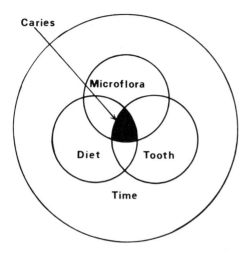

Fig. 1 Essential factors in the formation of a carious lesion.

Caries can be prevented by the manipulation of one of the above-illustrated factors: by reducing the number of cariogenic bacteria, by increasing the resistance of the teeth, by changing dietary habits, and by decreasing the time span that these three factors coexist.

The tooth enamel is composed of hydroxyapatite crystals, which give the tooth its characteristics of resistance and hardness. The hydroxyapatite crystals are susceptible to dissolution by acid. At a pH lower than 5.5 a demineralization process occurs in which an active carious lesion is opened. Certain ions, particularly fluoride, can replace hydroxyl group in the hydroxyapatite, resulting in the formation of a partially fluoridated hydroxyapatite. The fluoridated hydroxyapatite is now less susceptible to a low pH and thus to the demineralization process, moreover, in the presence of fluoride, a remineralization process is enhanced [5,6]. In addition to the effect of fluoride on the demineralization and remineralization process, it can interfere with several enzymatic pathways of bacteria, thus intensifying its anticariogenic effect [7].

Diet has a strong influence on the etiology of dental caries. High sugar consumption, mainly sucrose, results in a high incidence of caries [8,9]. The pH of the plaque drops rapidly after consuming certain food and drinks [10,11] due to acid production in the dental plaque.

The mouth in general is a good habitat for microbacterial development. Some of the potential cariogenic bacteria are already present as part of the natural flora of the mouth. However, due to changes in the oral environment, mainly the presence of carbohydrates, the existing microflora can become potentially cariogenic. Among the cariogenic bacteria are the *Streptococcus mutans*, which are aciduric as well as acidigenic bacteria. *Streptococcus mutans* bacteria are capable of producing extracellular polysaccharides, which play an important role in the accumulation and adherence of cariogenic bacteria to the tooth.

B. Fluoride Applications

Several therapeutic agents have proved effective in controlling dental plaque and in preventing tooth decay. One of the most commonly used agents is fluoride. Fluoride can be introduced systemically in the form of solid preparation, liquid preparation, or as local delivery applications. Mouthwashes and toothpastes are among the most common local fluoride applications. Systemic administration of fluoride is important prior to the eruption of the teeth, while local application is more important after the eruption of the teeth.

Systemic Fluoride Administration

Fluoridation of community water is an economical method of delivering fluoride to the teeth. In many countries water fluoridation is a widely used means of fluoride administration to large populations. In areas where central water fluoridation cannot be achieved, localized fluoridation (e.g., schools) can be used alternatively. The main disadvantage of water fluoridation is in controlling the optimal intake of fluoride. For example, in the winter, because personal water consumptions tends to be low, one's fluoride consumption is in turn low. Moreover, water consumption, hence fluoride intake, differs from one individual to another. In addition to the problem of varying dosages, water fluoridation generates legal and social controversies [12].

  Alternative methods of systemic fluoride application are tablets and drops. The main disadvantages of these systemic fluoride supplements are the risk of fluoride overdose leading to toxicity, the compliance of the patients, and the inconveniences caused by a regular daily intake.

Local Delivery Applications

Mouth rinses, gels, and toothpastes are popular local delivery systems. One of the main disadvantages of these forms of dosage is the short retention time of the fluoride in the mouth. Substantial amounts of fluoride are deposited on the surface of the tooth after a topical application, but most of it leaches into the oral cavity shortly after the application. Mouth rinsing is an easy way of delivering an initially sufficient dosage of fluoride to the mouth. However, after rinsing with a 1000 ppm of fluoride, the amount of fluoride found in the mouth decreased rapidly during the first 15 min [13]. It was found that the clearance of fluoride was more rapid in the lower mandibular part of the mouth than in the upper labial part, generating a problem of unequal clearance from different parts of the mouth. Gels containing fluoride have the advantage of a longer retention time of fluoride in the mouth due to their high viscosity. A clinical study using fluoridated gel has shown a significant increase in the amount of fluoride retained on the enamel surface 60 days after the applications of the gel [14]. Since gels are applied in trays, they may not be a convenient method of delivering the drug. Moreover, the rheological properties of the gel might act as an obstacle for sufficient penetration of the gel into the interstitial regions.

Toothpastes containing fluoride are the most frequently used local delivery system of fluoride. Introducing fluoride to the enamel surfaces during toothbrushing might be an advantage due to the abrasive properties of the toothpaste. The exposure of the enamel surface to the fluoride may give rise to better anticariogenic results. It was shown that toothbrushing with fluoridated toothpastes resulted in reduction of caries [15].

Sustained Release Delivery Devices

The retention time of fluoride in the mouth is a dominant factor in extending the effectiveness of its therapeutic activity. It is essential that optimum levels of fluoride be present in the mouth for a prolonged period of time. The anticariogenic activity of fluoride may be improved by extending the direct contact of fluoride with the tooth and with the dental plaque.

Several suggestions for designing sustained release of fluoride in tablet form have been reviewed in the literature [16]. Although sustained release tablets may prove to be effective in monitoring the concentrations of fluoride within the therapeutic index, they still present the problem of inconvenience caused by daily intake and the superfluous overload of fluoride in the body. They, however, can be helpful in achieving the optimal concentration of fluoride to the denture.

Intraoral devices are yet another sustained release delivery system of fluoride. One approach of a local controlled delivery system is via fluoridated cement, used as an intracoronal restoration [17]. Fluoride, as stannous fluoride (SnF_2), was incorporated into different dental cements: polycarboxylate, zinc oxide, and zinc phosphate. In vitro experiments have shown that 70% of SnF_2 incorporated into polycarboxylate released a greater amount of fluoride than the other formulations. This formulation was tried in one subject for a period of 30 days. It has been found that during this trial period the levels of fluoride in the saliva were increased, while plaque scores were

decreased. After the removal of the cement, it was calculated that
no more than 57 mg of fluoride was released during the clinical trial.

A different device for locally controlled release of fluoride was
designed to be attached onto the tooth's surface. This controlled release device was composed of a copolymer hydrogel of hydroxyethyl
methacrylate (HEMA) and methyl methacrylate (MMA) in which sodium
fluoride was dispersed [18]. The outer layer of the core was composed
of the same copolymers but in different proportions. The core serves
as a reservoir due to its limited controlled release properties. The
outside layer was the membrane that determined the rate of release
of the fluoride. The devices were designed to release 0.02 to 1.0 mg
of fluoride per day during a period of 30 to 180 days.

Clinical studies were performed using a similar membrane-controlled
device composed of MMA and HEMA [19]. A membrane-controlled fluoride reservoir, approximately 8 mm long, containing 42 mg of fluoride
in the core, was attached to the buccal surface of the maxillary first
molar. The device was designed to release 0.5 mg of the fluoride per
day for 30 days. It was found that during the time in which the device remained in the mouth, the level of fluoride in the saliva was elevated, and there was an increase of fluoride in the plaque, while no
significant change was detected in the levels of fluoride in the urine
or serum. Also, no alteration in the prevalence of the oral microflora
was registered. During this study, 4 of the 11 subjects complained
about irritation from the device. Erythema or small ulcers were detected on the buccal mucosa opposite the device. It is not clear whether
the irritation was a result of the device or was caused by the fluoride
released.

To improve the aforementioned device, a modification was designed
[20]. The composition was the same as that used previously, but the
second device was shorter and thinner, and contained only 17.5 mg
of sodium fluoride. A nylon suture, in the center of the device, was
used to attach the device to the buccal mucosa of rats. The device
released 0.15 mg of fluoride per day. Rats fitted with the controlled
release device exhibited 63% fewer carious enamel lesions than animals
with no treatment. The rats with the controlled release device were
found to develop fewer carious enamel areas when compared to animals
receiving 10 ppm fluoride, administered in their drinking water. The
controlled-release device was found to be more effective than a minipump implanted subcutaneously in rats [21]. The minipump was intended to release 12 μl/day of 0.9 M sodium fluoride (approximately
200 μg of fluoride systemically per day). Fewer proximal and total
carious enamel area was found using the controlled release device compared to the minipump. In this study, it was also shown that the
amount of fluoride found in the saliva was significantly higher in rats
wearing the intraoral device. Thus it can be concluded that the efficacy of the intraoral device is higher than that of a systemic adminis-

tration when the same initial amount of fluoride is used and the contact time of fluoride with the enamel is prolonged.

Additional methods of prolonging fluoride release involve matrix sustained release devices. Fluoride is embedded in a polymer matrix, which regulates the release rate of the fluoride. Pellets containing either sodium fluoride or calcium fluoride were prepared by pressure from a mixture of ethylcellulose polymer and fluoride [22]. In vitro experiments in pseudo-steady-state conditions were conducted to determine the rate of fluoride release. The release rate of fluoride from pellets containing 5% calcium fluoride was 38.7 times lower than that for a 5% sodium fluoride pellet. Similarly, the release rate of fluoride from pellets containing 10% calcium fluoride was 40 times lower than that for a 10% sodium fluoride pellet. The addition of stearic acid to the sodium fluoride pellets decreased the release of fluoride by way of decreasing the porosity of the pellets. An increase in the amount of fluoride salt in the pellets resulted in an increase in the release constant. The release rate of a pellet containing 2% sodium fluoride was 0.7×10^{-1} (mg/0.2 cm^2/min$^{1/2}$) and for a 15% sodium fluoride the rate was three times as fast. In both the calcium and sodium fluoride pellets, the release rate constant showed a linear correlation with the amount of the square root of the fluoride concentrations. The release rate of fluoride in pellets loaded with different concentrations of sodium fluoride was found to be linearly correlated with the square root of the released time. These findings suggest that the release of fluoride from the ethylcellulose pellets follows the diffusion control model of a heterogeneous nondegradable matrix [23] described in Equaiton (1):

$$Q = \left[\frac{D\varepsilon}{\tau}(2A - \varepsilon C_s)C_s t\right]^{1/2} \qquad . \qquad . \qquad (1)$$

where Q is the amount of drug released after time t per unit of exposed area, A the concentration of the drug in the matrix, D and C_s the diffusibility and solubility, respectively, in the extraction fluid, and ε and τ the porosity and tortuosity of the matrix, respectively. A clinical application of such a device can be achieved through direct adhesion of the pellets to teeth or to orthodontic appliances.

In another application fluoride was embedded in a filmlike device [24]. Different concentrations of sodium fluoride were incorporated into polydimethylsiloxane (silicone) fluid elastomer. The mixture was placed between two Teflon plates and was allowed to polymerize at room temperature. The release rate of sodium fluoride from the prepared film with 10% sodium fluoride was 0.010 (mg/hr$^{1/2}$ 3.5 cm^2). In vivo studies of orthodontic plates coated with the silicone polymer could not be conducted due to inadequate adherence of the film to the plates. Therefore, a different polymer, which could coat a plate, was used.

Different concentrations of sodium fluoride were incorporated into a ethylcellulose polymer dissolved in chloroform. To some of the formulations polyethylene glycol was added. The solution obtained was then used either for coating orthodontic plates or for casting films on a glass plate. In vitro kinetic studies of the released fluoride revealed a linear correlation between the amount of fluoride released and the square root of time. This linear correlation was found in the cast films as well as in the coated orthodontic plates. The rate at which the fluoride was released decreased with time and was found to be in linear correlation with the square root of fluoride concentration. The release rate data were in accordance with Higuchi's homogeneous planar mechanism [23] as described in Equation (2):

$$Q = [D(2A - C_s)C_s t]^{1/2} \qquad (2)$$

where Q is the amount of drug released per unit area, D the diffusion coefficient of the drug in the matrix, C_s, the solubility of the drug in the matrix, A represents the concentration of the drug in the matrix, while t is time.

By increasing the thickness of the film, the duration of the released drug was prolonged; however, the change in thickness did not alter the rate of release as may be concluded from Equation (2). The release rate constant of films, with the same thickness, containing 5% w/w sodium fluoride was 0.012; for films containing 10 and 15% sodium fluoride, it was found to be 0.019 and 0.026, respectively. The addition of polyethylene glycol enhanced the release of fluoride from the films.

Clinical studies were conducted on children undergoing orthodontic treatment [25]. The palatal part of the upper orthodontic plate was coated with 10% sodium fluoride suspended in ethanol solution of ethylcellulose. Significant increase of fluoride in the saliva was observed after the first 3 days. After the fourth day, the amount of fluoride returned to its initial level. According to the in vitro studies described above [24], fluoride duration may be achieved by adding layers of the coating solution to the plates. This increase in the thickness of the coating will therefore result in a prolonged release of the drug.

C. Antibacterial Treatment

Since tooth decay is a bacterial disease, antibacterial treatment seems to be an optimal method of therapy. Antibacterial agents were found to be effective in plaque reduction due to the susceptibility of the plaque bacteria to the antibacterial agent [26]. When added as supplements to animal food, penicillin, erythromycin, and tetracycline were shown to control plaque formation and dental caries [27,28]. However, due to numerous undesirable side effects of prolonged administration of antibacterial agents, the use of a systemically prolonged administration is not practical, despite its promising results. Therefore, topical administration of antibiotics and antibacterial agents is a preferable alternative.

Several topical applications are being used to minimize the general distribution of antibacterial agents in the body: mouth rinses, toothpastes, gels, and ointments are among the most common applications. Various antibacterial agents in different concentrations are used in these formulations [29]. In most instances, plaque score improvement is temporary. After the cessation of the treatments, the bacteria tend to return to their initial levels. The oral clearance of the agents applied in the above form is rather quick, resulting in a short retention time of the drug in the oral cavity. Since tooth decay is a chronic infection, therapy must be continuous to maintain good results.

Sustained Release Devices

Local administration of a drug to the mouth is a preferred method of application to a systemic route. As previously discussed, a local delivery application that prolongs the release of the drug in the mouth has great clinical advantages. It has been proved that the longer the drug is present in the oral cavity, the better the anticariogenic effect that can be obtained. Therefore, a sustained release application that can supply the drug for a prolonged period of time at suitable levels is an optimal means of application. Topical antibacterial sustained release devices for the prevention of dental caries are not yet popular nor developed. Hence, there is limited information currently available about research in this particular field.

A sustained release device composed of ethylcellulose, polyethylene glycol, and chlorhexidine as an active agent was applied as a coat to a removable partial acrylic denture [30]. The average chlorhexidine applied was calculated to be 51.6 mg. The patients were instructed not to execute any hygienic procedures, including brushing the dentures. Low plaque index was observed during the 12 days of the trial. Five days after the removal of the coating from the plates, the plaque index had returned to its initial level. The embedded chlorhexidine and the sustained release of the chlorhexidine masked its bitter taste. Only one subject had complained about a bitter sensation during the first 24 hr of the trial. No other side effects of chlorhexidine, such as discoloration or staining of the teeth, were detected. In another study [31], ethylcellulose and chlorhexidine in ethanol was applied directly to the buccal and lingual surfaces of the teeth by means of a soft brush and then dried with a stream of air. Plaque index was recorded over a 3 day period. In the first 2 days, a significant reduction of plaque index was observed. On the third day, plaque scores returned to their initial levels. A similar effect was noted when a removable orthodontic appliance was coated [32]. Plaque formation was significantly reduced during the first 4 days of this study. On the sixth day the plaque score had returned to near the average level.

Chlorhexidine and other antibacterial agents were used in a sustained release varnish intended to be applied on the teeth. The varnish was composed of chlorhexidine in 10% of Sumatra benzoin tincture poured into molds and allowed to air-dry [33]. In vitro results of a release of 10% w/w chlorhexidine from such a device showed a burst release in the first day, followed by a constant and moderate release rate. The total overall release of chlorhexidine from this device was only 30% of the loaded drug, of which about half was released within the first day.

Erythromycin incorporated in the same formulation exhibited a rather different release profile. Although only about 50% of the loaded drug was available for release, a more moderate release rate was noted. In the first day, approximately 10% of the loaded drug was released, followed by a gradual release.

Kinetic studies of the release of chlorhexidine and erythromycin have revealed two different mechanisms of release as proposed by the authors. It was suggested that the release of chlorhexidine followed a zero-order rate of release, since the release of chlorhexidine was constant. The release rate of erythromycin was found to be first order, since its release profile was similar to an exponential curve. When applying to the teeth the above formulation of varnishes and other formulations using penicillin as an active agent, a decrease in the amount of *Streptococcus mutans* in the mouth was observed [34]. However, when the coated teeth were overlayed with a supplemental coat of polyurethane, *Streptococcus mutans* were eliminated for weeks after the treatment. This study acts as a landmark in the research of elimination of the cariogenic bacteria *Streptococcus mutans* from the mouth by means of a local sustained release delivery system.

III. PERIODONTAL DISEASES

A. Etiology

Periodontal disease is an inflammatory response in which the structural supports of the tooth are destroyed.

The term "periodontal disease" broadly defines several diseases associated with the periodontum. Changes in the microflora, histopathological variations, clinical symptoms, and the location of the inflammation help to further delinate periodontal disease. Gingivitis, the moderate stage of the disease, caused by an accumulation of supragingival plaque, is characterized by swelling, light bleeding, and redness of the marginal gingiva. Gingivitis is associated with a change in the microflora, shifting from a Gram-positive anerobic flora to a more Gram-negative one [35]. Periodontitis, a more severe stage of periodontal disease, results in the resorption of the alveolar bone and detachment of the periodontal ligaments supporting the tooth.

One of the clinical features of periodontal disease is the formation of a periodontal pocket, which is a pathologically deepened sulcus (Fig. 2). In a normal sulcus, the gap between the gingiva and the tooth is normally between 1 and 3 mm deep. However, during periodontitis, the depth of the pocket usually exceeds 5 mm. Progressive pocket formation leads to the destruction of the supporting periodontal tissues, followed by high mobility and exfoliation of the tooth. Periodontitis is characterized by a dramatic change of the microflora; the number of Gram-negative bacteria can increase to 70% of the total flora, most of it being anaerobic rods.

There are numerous types of bacteria affiliated with periodontal disease: *Bacteriodes gingivalis, Bacteriodes melaninogenicus, Fusobacterium,* and *Capnocytophaga* [35]. The occurrence of motile bacteria, particularly rods and spirochetes, is an important microbiological parameter of periodontal disease [36,37]. These bacteria, as well as others, play an important role in the pathogenicity of the diseases. Collagenase and other enzymes originating from bacteria can destroy the connective tissue and ligaments of the periodontum. Toxins of the bacteria contribute to the progress of periodontal diseases [38]. In addition to the above-mentioned virulence factors, the bacteria and

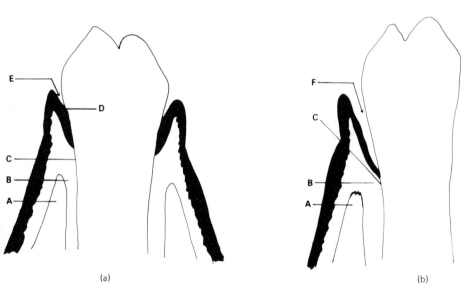

(a)   (b)

Fig. 2 (a) Healthy periodontum and (b) periodontal pocket: A = alveolar bone, B = periodontal ligaments, C = cementum, D = cementum-enamel junction, E = sulcus, and F = periodontal pocket.

their by-products act as chemotactic agents. This results in the migration of polymorphonuclear cells, evoking an inflammatory response by activating the immunological system [39].

Periodontal treatment aims to cure inflamed tissue, to reduce the number of pathogenic bacteria, and to eliminate the diseased pocket. Different clinical methods are currently being utilized. Mechanical procedures such as scaling, root planing, and surgery are the common methods of treatment. Chemotherapy, in addition to mechanical therapy, may be another way to cure periodontal diseases. Systemic administration of antibiotics or anti-inflammatory agents may also be helpful. Growing attention has been given to topical and local drug delivery systems as an alternative or as an adjunct way of treating periodontal diseases.

B. Conventional Therapy

Scaling, curettage, and root planing are among the most commonly used procedures in elimination of the periodontal pocket. Scaling is a mechanical means of removing the calculus and the plaque. Curettage involves clearing the inflamed soft tissue. Root planing is the removal of necrotic tooth tissue on the root surface. When elimination of the pocket cannot be achieved by these methods, surgery is used to remove the necrotic tissue and to reduce the pocket's depth.

C. Systemic Drug Administration

Because periodontal diseases are associated with bacteria, antibacterial treatment seems to be an appropriate method of improving the condition of the inflamed tissues. However, the overall benefit of systemic administration of antibiotics in periodontal treatment is debatable. In vitro experiments have showed that several antimicrobial agents are characterized by a low minimal inhibitory concentration for oral anaerobic bacteria [40,41]. Some antibacterial agents are highly effective against periodontal bacteria. The susceptibility of several antibacterial agents was tested on 193 strains of bacteria, most of them isolated from subgingival plaque. Penicillin G at 2 U/ml was found to be active against 98% of the isolated bacteria. Metronidazole was active against more than 90% of the anaerobic bacteria, while tetracycline demonstrated a variable effect against different bacterial isolates.

Clinical studies have been conducted on the effects of antibiotics on periodontal disease. In studies on adult periodontitis, the effect of systemic administration of tetracycline was evaluated [42-44]. It was found that when tetracycline is used as an adjunct to conventional therapy, it does not exhibit a superior effect over the conventional therapy alone. In another study [45] minocycline, a semisynthetic derivative of tetracycline, was used in a split-mouth trial. Half the mouth received scaling and root planing, while the other half served as a control. A 200 mg dosage of minocycline per day was administered for a period of 7 days. The results indicated that the minocycline-scaled group had a marked improvement in gingival condition and a marked reduction in pathological bacteria. The sites that received minocycline without any scaling exhibited an improvement in the inflamed gingiva, although with slightly less reduction in the pathological bacteria. A comparative study of metronidazole with or without treatment of root planing was conducted on patients with periodontal disease [46]. One week of administration of metronidazol significantly reduced the proportion of the anaerobic bacteria associated with the disease for a term that lasted up to 6 months. Clinical improvements such as reduction in the depth of the pocket were observed as well.

Although systemic administration of antibiotics might be valuable in the healing process of periodontal disease as a means of treatment, it cannot be used over a long period of time. Many undesirable side effects may arise due to a prolonged intake of systemic antibiotics, lowering the benefit/risk ratio to a point at which this kind of treatment is no longer acceptable.

D. Local Delivery Application

One method of minimizing the distribution of therapeutic agents in the body is through a local delivery drug system. Many antibacterial agents are applied directly to the mouth for treatment of periodontal diseases.

Mouth rinses constitute a widely used method. Chlorhexidine in a mouthwash, at the concentration of 0.2%, was found to be very effective in controlling supragingival plaque and gingivitis [47,48]; however, these rinses are found to have a very limited effect on periodontitis with pocket formation [49].

To achieve drug penetration into deep periodontal pockets, a direct irrigation method was used [50]. A 0.2% solution of chlorhexidine was applied by syringe into the periodontal pockets of patients with severe periodontal disease. In a clinical study, two groups were compared. One group received chlorhexidine irrigation for 2 consecutive days, while the other received water irrigation. A decrease in the number of pathogenic bacteria was then observed in the chlorhexidine-irrigated group. However, 5 days after the intercervicular rinses were administered, there were no significant differences between the two groups. These results indicate a good short-term effect of chlorhexidine irrigation, yet a poor prolonged effect.

Continuous chlorhexidine irrigation of deep periodontal pockets has proved to be more effective than short-term application [51]. Periodontal pockets were irrigated daily with a solution of 0.2% chlorhexidine gluconate for a period of 28 days. A meaningful reduction in the inflammation was noted at levels significantly below the baseline for a further 28 day period, without any additional irrigation.

E. Sustained Release Devices

Local delivery application is one way of targeting a drug to a desired site. However, to prolong the therapeutic levels of the drug at the site, a local sustained release device is required. The periodontal pocket is a defined site surrounded by tissues, which nonetheless allows relatively easy access when inserting a delivery device inside. The periodontal pocket is an area conducive to treatment with a local sustained release device. The goals to be achieved by the use of an intrapocket device are to release a therapeutic agent inside the pocket and to maintain sufficient levels of the drug for a stated period of time.

Several requirements should be met when inserting a sustained release device inside a periodontal pocket. The periodontal pocket is naturally irrigated with gingival crevice fluid (GCF). In subjects with periodontal disease, a mean rate of GCF flow at individual sites is approximately 150 μl/hr [52]. Generally, a high flow of GCF will result in a faster rate of diffusion of the drug from the control release reservoir, while a low flow rate retards this depletion. Consequently, the high flow rate of GCF will cause a fast evacuation of the already released drug from the pocket to the mouth, thereby depleting the concentration of the drug in the pocket. Therefore, the rate of release should be higher at the initial stage of release, to achieve an immediate therapeutic level of the drug in the pocket. The next stage of release should maintain the therapeutic levels in the pocket and thus, a moderate release profile is required. Another parameter to be considered is the drug's absorbency. A poorly absorbent drug that has low penetration through the mucosal tissues enables the drug's level to reach higher concentrations and prolongs higher levels in the pocket.

The size and depth of the periodontal pocket play an important role in the formulation of the intrapocket device. Since the average depth of a pocket is between 6 and 8 mm, the therapeutic drug device cannot be large. Thus, it is required that small dosage of the active agent in the device should be highly effective as a therapeutic agent. Antibacterial drugs should be highly specific against the pathogenic bacteria in the pocket. The development of resistant strains of bacteria might occur, due to the long duration of an antibacterial agent in the periodontal pocket. The drug of choice, then, should not cause the development of resistant bacterial strains.

In addition, a local delivery device for periodontal disease calls for a pharmaceutical application that would be readily accepted by the patient. Due to the degree of vanity that humans exhibit regarding the mouth, a device cannot be exposed beyond the gingival margin, nor can it be bulky. A device should not cause any interference to the normal daily oral hygiene, which includes toothbrushing and dental flossing. Moreover, the device need not generate a problem in terms of the patient's dietary patterns. As the inflamed periodontum is a sensitive tissue, the applied device should have physical characteristics that facilitate a swift insertion into the pocket, thereby causing minimal pain and discomfort to the patient.

One way to introduce a therapeutic agent inside a periodontal pocket is via hollow fiber devices. Different lengths of cellulose-based, hollow fibers were loaded with 20% solution of chlorhexidine gluconate. In vitro results [53] showed a release of the drug within the first day, in a fiber 1 cm long, as well as in a fiber 4 cm long. The release rates of the drug through an unsealed end to a sealed end were compared, and were found to exibit similar profile rates of release. These results indicated that the evacuation of the drug was through the walls of the tubes rather than through the opened ends. However, an in vivo study [54] showed that the tubes retrieved after 7 days in the periodontal pocket inhibited the growth of *Staphylococcus aureus* on an agar blood plate. A remarkable clinical improvement was recorded after the tube was kept in the pocket for 7 days: gingival fluid flow was notably reduced; less bleeding on probe was observed; and a relief of discomfort was reported.

Another research study was conducted on cellulose acetate hollow fibers, this time loaded with a 20% solution of tetracycline. The hollow fibers (outer diameter of 250 μm) were placed for 2 days in periodontal pockets deeper than 6 mm [55]. A control group was given a root planing and scaling treatment. Clinical parameters and changes in the microflora were evaluated every 7, 14, 28, and 37 days from the onset of the treatment. Microbiological counts showed a reduction in the number of spirochetes and motile rods in both groups tested. However, the decrease in the proportion of the spirochetes was greater in the control group as compared to the group that had the fibers inserted. A reduction in the pocket depth was observed in the hollow fiber group as well as in the control group, although the reduction in the pocket depth was almost twice as much in the latter. A study on the release rate of tetracycline from hollow fibers in vivo has demonstrated a high release rate [56]. About 95% of the drug was released 2 hr after the hollow fibers were inserted into the pockets. The quick rate of release from these devices indicates that the hollow fibers serve as a good reservoir for a drug, but as a poor rate-limiting apparatus, permitting too rapid depletion of tetracycline.

The monolithic fibers represent a modification of the hollow fiber devices [57]. Various polymers (polyethylene, polypropylene, polycaprolactone, polyurethane, and cellulose acetate propionate) were melted and then spun at high temperatures. After tetracycline was added, the molten material was cooled into a fiber form. The fibers prepared in this procedure were approximately 0.5 mm in diameter and contained 322 µg of tetracycline per centimeter. In vitro release of tetracycline from fibers of this type was completed within one day. Fibers composed of ethylene vinyl acetate polymer were unique in providing a gradual in vitro release over a period of 9 days. However, when inserted in the periodontal pocket, the half-time concentration of ethylene vinyl acetate fibers was 13 hr. To prolong the duration of the drug in the periodontal pocket, the inserted fibers were covered with periodontal dressing and maintained for 10 days. A 12 month posttreatment study showed reduction in pocket depth and gain of attachment [58].

A different pharmaceutical approach for delivery and release of a drug in the periodontal pocket is a slablike device (Fig. 3). A slab dosage form has several physical properties that can be of great importance in inserting a local delivery device inside a periodontal pocket. The dimensions and the shape of the slab (length, width, and thickness) can be adjusted to resemble the dimensions of the pocket. This results in minimal interference of the existing periodontal ligaments. Insertion of a slab is a rather quick and easy method for placing a device in the pocket using limited force. The slab's flexibility allows for a smooth insertion with little discomfort to the patient (Fig. 4). Moreover, a slab device can be inserted deep into the pocket, with no part exposed above the marginal gingiva.

One type of a slab form for treatment of periodontal disease is an ethylcellulose film [59]. Ethylcellulose polymer was dissolved in chloro-

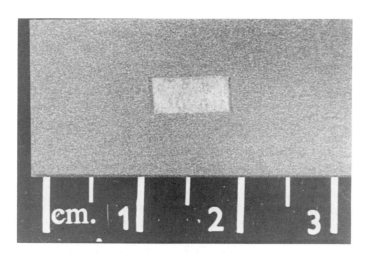

Fig. 3 An ethylcellulose film containing a drug, to be inserted into a periodontal pocket.

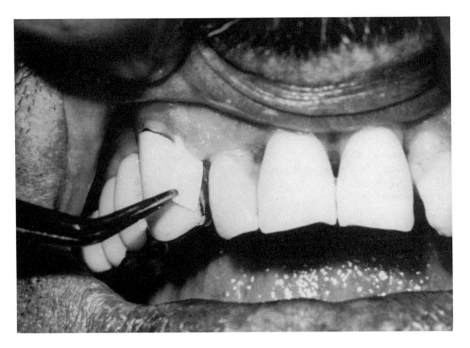

Fig. 4 Insertion of an ethylcellulose film into a periodontal pocket.

form or in ethanol solution. Chlorhexidine was then added and the
solution was mixed for several hours. Additives such as polyethylene
glycol were added. The solution obtained was poured into molds and
allowed to evaporate. The dried film was then cut into strips. The
films, incorporated with different concentrations of chlorhexidine,
sustained the release of chlorhexidine from the matrix. In vitro studies of an ethanol-cast film, containing 5% chlorhexidine acetate, released
the drug over a period of 10 days. Films cast from chloroform with
5, 10, and 20% loads of chlorhexidine, released 20, 30, and 60% of the
drug, respectively, after a period of 205 days. Films containing 5%
chlorhexidine have demonstrated a high correlation coefficient (0.998)
between the square root of time and the amount of the drug that has
been released. This result suggests that the release of chlorhexidine
occurs according to a planar homogeneous diffusion model, as previously described in Equation (2).
     It has been shown that ethylcellulose films containing metronida-
zole can act as sustained release devices [60]. The in vitro release
of films containing metronidazole was compared in two different leaching media. Ethylcellulose films containing 30% of metronidazole and
10% of polyethylene glycol 3000 released about 90% of the drug after 24

hr in water. When the leaching medium was changed to buffer (pH 2), only 70% of the drug was released after the same period of time. A similar release profile was obtained using a film containing 40% metronidazole. The release rate of the drug into water was slower than the release into buffer of pH 2.

These studies emphasize the important role played by the leaching medium with respect to the rate of release. The kinetic release of the metronidazole films, supplemented with polyethylene glycol, followed the heterogeneous diffusion model as described in Equation (1). In vivo study on the release rate of the films above demonstrated a release profile similar to that which was found when the leaching medium was water, indicating a high correlation of the in vivo study to the in vitro one.

Polyethylene glycol is a hydrophilic polymer that has been found to enhance the release of chlorhexidine and metronidazole when supplemented into ethylcellulose films. The release rate constant of metronidazole films supplemented with 10% polyethylene glycol was almost five times as much as the rate constant of films without polyethylene glycol (0.14 and 0.67 mg/hr$^{1/2}$·cm^2, respectively) [60]. Films containing polyethylene glycol 3000 have proved to be more permeable due to rapid evacuation of the polyethylene glycol 3000 into the extracted media. The high porosity of the film reduces the effective path length of the released drug (Fig. 5). Consequently, the overall result of polyethylene glycol 3000 in ethylcellulose film is the enhancement of the release of the incorporated drug [61,62].

In an in vivo kinetics study [63], it was found that a film cast from ethanol released approximately 80% of chlorhexidine within 3 days. Film cast from chloroform with an addition of polyethylene glycol 3000 released approximately 50% of chlorhexidine after 6 days inside the periodontal pocket. In a microbiological follow-up study it was found that periodontal pockets treated with ethylcellulose film containing chlorhexidine demonstrated a marked reduction in the relative numbers of spirochetes and motile rods. After 14 days, spirochete counts were relatively high, almost returning to the pretreatment level. Replacing the ethylcellulose film every 3 days for a period of 9 days has proved to prolong clinical and microbiological improvements [64]. An increase in the pocket depth was noted immediately after the removal of the film, probably due to the mechanical separation of the junctional epithelium by the film. However, the treated pockets exhibited a reduction in probing depth at 3 and 11 weeks posttreatment. A long-term follow-up was conducted on the microflora of the pockets as well. A marked reduction in the percentage of spirochetes and motile rods was observed at 11 weeks posttreatment, as well as a reduction in the total anaerobic counts.

Another type of film reported in the literature is an acrylic strip. A mixture of the polymer, monomer, and different concentrations of

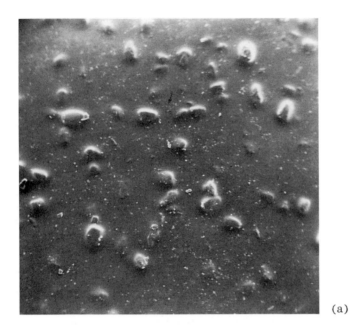

(a)

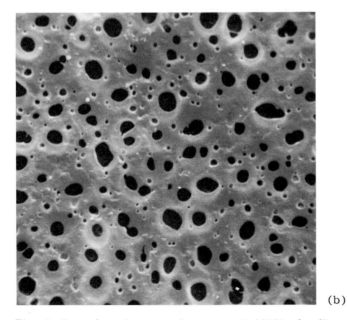

(b)

Fig. 5 Scanning electron microscopy (×2000) of a film containing 30% polyethylene glycol (a) before and (b) after the leaching of the hydrophilic component.

chlorhexidine were placed under high pressure. The molten disks were then cut into strips [53]. In vitro release of chlorhexidine from the strips demonstrated a burst effect on the first day followed by a moderate rate of release in the succeeding days. In some of the formulations, the release of chlorhexidine continued for 14 days. Similar results were obtained from acrylic strips loaded with different drugs, such as metronidazole and tetracycline. The periodontal microflora had been altered after a 2 day and a 3 day treatment with the acrylic strips. Strips containing either tetracycline, metronidazole, or chlorhexidine demonstrated a decrease in the number of motile rods, notably spirochetes [65]. In a long-term study, acrylic strips containing 40% metronidazole were placed in periodontal pockets for a duration of one week and then replaced each week for a period of 4 weeks. Significant improvement was noted during the treatment period and persisted afterward for an additional 8 weeks [66]. The clinical results did not differ substantially from the results obtained from a control group, which received daily irrigation of 0.2% chlorhexidine for four consecutive weeks. As regards the bleeding parameter, the metronidazole group was found to be superior to the chlorhexidine irrigation group.

In a similarly designed study [67], four different drug applications were compared: acrylic strips, dialysis tubes (both containing metronidazole), self-irrigation with chlorhexidine solution, and root planing. Periodontal pockets that received a treatment of 0.5% metronidazole in the dialysis tubes and the group that received a treatment of 40% metronidazole in the acrylic strips showed a reduction in the number of spirochetes. A low percentage of spirochetes was observed for an additional period of 3 months. The chlorhexidine irrigation group also demonstrated a reduction in the percentage of spirochetes and a rapid reduction in the number of motile rods. The group that received only root planing exhibited a less dramatic effect.

All the devices reviewed above are nondegradable, necessitating their removal from the periodontal pocket after evacuation of the drug. A degradable controlled release device would have several advantages over the nondegradable; for example, the elimination of a return visit to the periodontist to extract the device from the pocket would represent a great time-cost factor. A degradable device, moreover, would not be an obstacle during reattachment of the periodontal tissues to the tooth, thereby offering minimal interference in the reduction of the pocket depth. Another potential advantage of degradable devices is that they could be implanted in a tissue after surgery, whereupon the drug could be released and the device could degrade without any further manipulation to the suture. A factor that needs to be taken into account when considering degradable devices is the problem of toxicity. The degradable components of the device would have to be irrigated or absrobed from the site without causing any tissue irritation.

A hydroxypropylcellulose-based film containing several antibacterial agents was found to be a resorbable carrier device for use in
periodontal pockets [68]. In vitro studies of the release of tetracycline
and chlorhexidine from such films have demonstrated an almost complete release of the drugs from the films after 2 hr. In the process
of dissolving, the hydroxypropylcellulose peaked at 3 hr, followed by
a more gradual dissolving rate in the following 20 hr. In vivo studies
of these inserted strips in periodontal pockets have shown a retention
of tetracycline for 24 hr postinsertion in the gingival cervicular fluid.
A marked reduction in bleeding upon probing was noticed at the pockets
where chlorhexidine strips were applied. A significant reduction in
the relative proportion of *Bacteriodes asaccharolyticus* and a reduction
in the pocket depth was observed when compared to the control group.
Although this study is a pioneering effort in the development of a degradable sustained release device in the periodontal pocket, the short
duration time of the drug in the pocket site is a disadvantage of this
device.

IV. CONCLUSIONS

Dental diseases are among the most widely spread afflictions of modern
times. The first and most important factor in fighting tooth decay
as well as periodontal diseases is care that takes place in the home.
Better active agents and improved drug delivery systems serve to
assist home care in treating and healing dental disease. Because dental diseases are associated with the presence of bacteria, an antibacterial approach as a treatment method seems to be appropriate.
    The aim of today's pharmaceutical technology lies in targeting a
drug to the desired organ or site, with the aim of minimizing its overall distribution in the body, thereby limiting any undesired effects of
the drug. Only a small fraction of the drug that is administered per
os does reach the periodontal pocket [69]. Repeated dosages of tetracycline can keep sufficient therapeutic levels of the drug in the pocket
for a long period [70]. The simplest way of targeting a drug is by
initially placing it in the desired site. The localized nature of tooth
decay, and particularly periodontal pockets, is such that access is
facilitated and the surrounding organs are undisturbed. Thus, they
are ideal sites for treatment with a local delivery device.
    Periodontal disease and tooth decay are recurring and chronic
diseases and for both, time is a vitally important factor in their progression. Therefore, the drug's duration in the site is a dominant
factor in the healing process. Extending the presence of the drug
at the site results in clinical improvements. A sustained release of
antibacterial agents from a device placed in the oral cavity thus has
advantages over a systemic application.

Local sustained release devices offer many advantages: (a) the means of controlling and monitoring the desired drug levels in the site, (b) a useful means of delivering to the oral cavity a drug that is not absorbed into the gastrointestinal system (e.g., chlorhexidine), (c) the achievement of higher concentrations of the drug as compared to serum levels after per os administration, and (d) the means of masking an unpleasant taste and avoiding staining within the oral cavity.

The primary advantage of a local sustained delivery system stems from the lower ratio of the drug administered to the drug concentrations found in the desired sites. Levels of fluoride in saliva found in children drinking fluoridated water are 0.01 to 0.05 ppm [71]. The same range of levels is achieved by using a sustained release device, as demonstrated by Harary and Friedman [25] and others. According to Hirschfeld et al. [30], 51.6 mg of chlorhexidine incorporated into a sustained release device resulted in reduced levels of plaque for 12 days. To achieve similar results using a daily mouthwash, 480 mg of chlorhexidine was required (10 ml twice a day of a 0.2% chlorhexidine solution). Goodson et al. [58] have calculated the amount of tetracycline administered in a systemic form in comparison to a local sustained released device. According to this study, only 2.4 mg per tooth was needed for 10 days of treatment, which was 460 times less than that of a parallel systemic adminsitration.

There are several properties of the drug that may be beneficial in the design of a local sustained delivery device. First, a drug that is poorly absorbed by mucosal tissues is more slowly depleted from the desired site; thus, the resulting concentrations minimize the initial levels of the drug in the reservoir. Second, adsorption onto the tooth enamel, while not changing the antibacterial effect, results in a secondary release phase of the drug, thereby prolonging the drug's duration in the site. Tooth surfaces tend to adsorb chlorhexidine and tetracycline, thus prolonging their effect.

A sustained release drug that offers a one-time application has an advantage over repeated applications. The repetition of a drug can generate a problem in terms of patient compliance. Handicapped, disabled, and geriatric patients may find sustained released delivery devices a more suitable way of application. In xerothemic patients, it is of great importance to maintain levels of anticariogenic agents in the mouth for as long as possible.

The mechanism by which the drug is released from the device, as well as the factors that influence the release rate of the drug from the device, are fundamental elements in the study of sustained release systems. Better understanding of the drug release mechanism is essential in designing and improving sustained release devices.

Although the research concerning sustained release devices in the treatment of dental disease is still young, it has attracted much attention. There is great potential in the treatment offered by local sustained release devices in dentistry, and the research has proved this to be a promising alternative method of treatment.

REFERENCES

1. R. C. Page and H. E. Schroeder, *Periodontitis in Man and Other Animals, A comparative Review.* Karger, Basel, 1982.
2. D. E. Barmes, *J. Clin. Periodontal.*, 4:80 (1977).
3. J. P. Carlos, ed., *Prevention and Oral Health.* U.S. Department of Health, Education and Welfare [now Health and Human Services] Publication No. NIH 74-707. Government Printing Office, Washington, DC, 1974.
4. L. M. Silverstone, N. W. Johnson, J. M. Hardie, and R.A.D. Williams, *Dental Caries, Aetiology, Pathology and Prevention.* Macmillan, London, 1985, p. 6.
5. E. C. Moreno, M. Kresak, and R. T. Zahradnik, *Caries Res.*, 11 (Suppl. 1):142 (1977).
6. L. M. Silverstone, *Caries Res.*, 11 (Suppl. 1):59 (1977).
7. I. R. Hamilton, *Caries Res.*, 11 (Suppl. 1):262 (1977).
8. E. Newburn, *Int. Dent. J.*, 32(1):13 (1982).
9. E. Newburn, *Odontol. Rev.*, 18:373 (1967).
10. W. M. Edgar, B. G. Bibby, S. Mundroff, and J. Rowley, *J. Am. Dent. Assoc.*, 90:418 (1975).
11. D. Neff, *Caries Res.*, 1:78 (1967).
12. G. L. Waldbott, *Fluoridation, the Great Dilemma.* Coronado Press, Lawrence, KA, 1978.
13. J. A. Weatherell, M. Strong, C. Robinson, and J. P. Ralph, *Caries Res.*, 20:111 (1986).
14. P. Hotz, *Helv. Odontol. Acta,* 16:32 (1972).
15. S. B. Heifetz and H. S. Horowitz, in *Fluorides and Dental Caries* (E. Newbrun, ed.). Charles C. Thomas, Springfield, IL, 1986, p. 50.
16. C. McKnight Hanes, and P. J. Hanes, *J. Am. Dent. Assoc.*, 113:431 (1986).
17. T. D. Swanson and N. Tinanoff, *J. Oral Rehabil.*, 11:53 (1984).
18. D. B. Mirth, *Pharmacol. Ther. Dent.*, 5:59 (1980).
19. D. B. Mirth, R. J. Shern, C. G. Emilson, D. D. Addelry, S. Li, I. M. Gomez, and W. H. Bowen, *J. Am. Dent. Assoc.*, 105(5): 791 (1982).
20. D. B. Mirth, D. D. Adderly, S. M. Amsbaugh, E. Monell-Torrens, S. Li, and W. H. Bowen, *J. Am. Dent. Assoc.*, 107(1):55 (1983).
21. D. B. Mirth, D. D. Adderly, E. Monell-Torrens, S. M. Amsbaugh, S. Li, and W. H. Bowen, *Caries Res.*, 19:466 (1985).
22. M. Friedman, *Arch. Oral Biol.*, 26:131 (1981).
23. T. Higuchi, *J. Pharm. Sci.*, 52(12):1145 (1963).

24. M. Friedman, *J. Dent. Res.*, 59(8):1392 (1980).
25. D. Harary and M. Friedman, *J. Pharm. Sci.*, 73(1):135 (1984).
26. E. Newbrun, *The Compendium of Continuing Education in Dentistry*, Suppl. 6, 1985, p. 1110.
27. R. J. Fitzgerald, *Antimicrob. Agents Chemother.*, 1(4):296 (1972).
28. R. J. Fitzgerald, *J. Am. Dent. Assoc.*, 87 (special issue):1006 (1973).
29. W. J. Loesche, in *Cariology Today* (B. Guggenheim, ed.). Karger, Basel, 1984, p. 293.
30. Z. Hirschfeld, M. Friedman, G. Golomb, and D. Ben-Yaacov, *J. Oral Rehabil.*, 11:477 (1984).
31. M. Friedman, L. Brayer, G. Golomb, and H. Hiller, *J. Controlled Release*, 1:157 (1984).
32. M. Friedman, D. Harari, H. Raz, G. Golomb, and L. Brayer, *J. Dent. Res.*, 64(11):1319 (1985).
33. T. E. Balanyk and H. J. Sandham, *J. Dent. Res.*, 64(12):1356 (1985).
34. H. J. Sandham, J. Brown, and K. H. Chan, *J. Dent. Res.*, 64 (special issue) (IADR abstr. No. 343):213, 1985.
35. J. Slots, *J. Clin. Periodontol.*, 6:351 (1979).
36. M. A. Listgarten and L. Hellden, *J. Clin. Periodontol.*, 5:115 (1978).
37. G. C. Armitage, W. R. Dickinson, R. S. Jenderseck, S. M. Levine, and D. W. Chambers, *J. Periodontol.*, 53(9):550 (1982).
38. J. Slots and G. Dahlén, *Scand. J. Dent. Res.*, 93:119 (1985).
39. D. R. Miller, I. B. Lamster, and A. I. Chasens, *J. Clin. Peridontol.*, 11:1 (1984).
40. P. J. Baker, J. Slots, R. J. Genco, and R. T. Evans, *Antimicrob. Agents Chemother.*, 24(3):420 (1983).
41. V. L. Sutter, M. J. Jones, and A.T.M. Ghoneim, *Antimicrob. Agents Chemother.*, 23(3):483 (1983).
42. M. A. Listgarten, J. Lindhe, and L. Hellden, *J. Clin. Periodontol.*, 5:246 (1978).
43. J. Slots, P. Mashimo, M. J. Levine, and R. J. Genco, *J. Periodontol.*, 50(10):495 (1979).
44. J. Lindhe, B. Liljenberg, and B. Adielsson, *J. Clin. Periodontol.*, 10:590 (1983).
45. S. G. Ciancio, J. Slots, H. S. Reynolds, J. J. Zambon, and J. D. McKenna, *J. Periodontol.*, 53(9):557 (1982).
46. W. J. Loesche, S. A. Syed, E. C. Morrison, B. Laughon, and N. S. Grossman, *J. Clin. Periodontol.*, 8:29 (1981).
47. H. Löe, C. R. Schiott, L. Glavind, and T. Karring, *J. Periodontal Res.*, 11:135 (1976).
48. L. Flotra, P. Gjermo, G. Rolla, and J. Waerhaug, *Scand. J. Dent. Res.*, 80:10 (1972).
49. L. Flotra, *J. Periodont. Res.*, 8 (suppl. 12):41 (1973).

50. M. Weinstling and G. Tynelius-Bratthall, *J. Periodont. Res.*, 19: 202 (1984).
51. L. L. Soh, H. N. Newman, and J. D. Strahan, *J. Clin. Periodontol.*, 9:66 (1982).
52. J. M. Goodson, in *Medical Applications of Controlled Release*, Vol. 2 (R. S. Langer and D. L. Wise, eds.). CRC Press, Boca Raton, FL, 1984, p. 115.
53. M. Addy, L. Rawle, R. Handley, H. N. Newman, and J. F. Coventry, *J. Periodontol.*, 53:693 (1982).
54. J. Coventry and H. N. Newman, *J. Clin. Periodontol.*, 9:129 (1982).
55. J. Lindhe, L. Heijl, J. M. Goodson, and S. S. Socransky, *J. Clin. Periodontol.*, 6:141 (1979).
56. J. M. Goodson, A. Haffajee, and S. S. Socransky, *J. Clin. Periodontol.*, 6:83 (1979).
57. J. M. Goodson, D. Halborow, R. L. Dunn, P. Hogan, and S. Dunham, *J. Periodontol.*, 54:575 (1983).
58. J. M. Goodson, P. E. Hogan, and S. L. Dunham, *J. Periodontol.*, Suppl. Special Issue, 81 (1985).
59. M. Friedman and G. Golomb, *J. Periodon. Res.*, 17:323 (1982).
60. G. Golomb, M. Friedman, A. Soskolne, A. Stabholz, and M. N. Sela, *J. Dent. Res.*, 63(9):1149 (1984).
61. Y. Samuelov, M. Donbrow, and M. Friedman, *J. Pharm. Sci.*, 68:325 (1979).
62. M. Donbrow and M. Friedman, *J. Pharm. Pharmacol.*, 27:633 (1974).
63. A. Soskolne, G. Golomb, M. Friedman, and M. N. Sela, *J. Periodont. Res.*, 18:330 (1983).
64. A. Stabholz, M. N. Sela, M. Friedman, G. Golomb, and A. Soskolne, *J. Clin. Periodontol.*, 13:783 (1986).
65. M. Addy and M. Langeroudi, *J. Clin. Periodontol.*, 11:379 (1984).
66. F.I.S. Yeung, H. N. Newman, and M. Addy, *J. Periodontol.*, 54:651 (1983).
67. J.G.L. Khoo and H. N. Newman, *J. Periodontn. Res.*, 18:607 (1983).
68. T. Noguchi, K. Izumizawa, M. Fukuda, S. Kitamura, Y. Suzuki, and H. Ikura, *Bull. Tokyo Med. Dent. Univ.*, 31:145 (1984).
69. J. M. Gordon, C. B. Walker, J. C. Murphy, J. M. Goodson, and S. S. Socransky, *J. Clin. Periodontol.*, 8:117 (1981).
70. J. M. Gordon, C. B. Walker, J. C. Murphy, J. M. Goodson, and S. S. Socransky, *J. Periodontol.*, 52:609 (1981).
71. P. Grøn, H. G. McCann, and F. Brudevold, *Arch. Oral Biol.*, 13:203 (1968).

Part Four
VETERINARY USAGE DEVICES

19

Ectoparasitic Devices

LILIAN CHONG KWAN / SmithKline Beckman Animal Health Products,
West Chester, Pennsylvania

I. INTRODUCTION

Biting and blood-sucking parasites feed on animal hosts. Their life cycle ranges from 2 weeks for horn flies to several months for ticks [1,2]. Some of them, such as fleas, thrive in warm and humid environments while others, such as lice, can live through cold winters [1,3]. To eradicate the pest infestation, animals are treated topically with insecticide sprays, dips, dusts, emulsions, pour-ons and spot-ons [2,4,5]. The treatment can be repeated as frequently as every 2 to 3 weeks in each season [6]. To reduce the frequency of treatments, the residual insecticide activities from various topical preparations must be lengthened. Long-acting ectoparasitic devices were developed for this purpose and to provide convenient, safe, and effective means of pest control. This chapter reviews several ectoparasitic devices available to livestock producers and pet owners.

II. DEVICES FOR PET ANIMALS

Fleas and ticks are blood-sucking parasites that live on and off their warm-blooded hosts, such as dogs and cats. Flea bites, if left untreated, can lead to increasing skin irritation and flea hypersensitivity [7]. These pests were also reported to be the transmitters of diseases to other animals and to humans [8,9]. Therefore, infestation of fleas and ticks on pet animals must be controlled.

    These pests have different life cycles. The flea is a wingless insect that has an egg-to-adult life cycle range of $2\frac{1}{2}$ weeks in a warm and humid environment to 20 months in a cold environment [10]. The tick is an arachnid with a hard skin. It has an egg-to-adult life cycle of 4 months or more [2] and is more difficult to kill. To control the pests' infestation on pet animals effectively, a suitable delivery system is needed to deliver the insecticide slowly for a period of several months. The flea and tick collar is a device that was developed to meet this requirement.

A. Flea and Tick Collars

Fleas and ticks prefer to concentrate in or migrate from the neck area of their hosts [1]. An ectoparasitic device attached to the neck area of the animal will provide a suitable means of delivering the insecticide to the principal site of pest infestation. Insecticide collars such as those shown in Fig. 1, initially developed by Folckemer, Hanson, and Miller in 1967 [12], were designed to control fleas and tick bites on pet animals. Other collars were developed later by Grubb and Baxter in 1974 and Miller and Morales in 1976 [13,14].

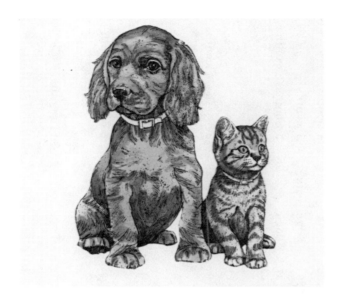

Fig. 1 Flea and tick collar on pet animals. (Courtesy of Zoecon Corporation, Dallas.)

The collars are made of plasticized polyvinyl chloride or polyurethane and impregnated with insecticides. The active ingredients, which are slowly released from the polymer matrix over a long period of time, are primarily carbamates (propoxur, carbaryl) or organophosphorus compounds (dichlorvos, diazinon, stirofos). Examples of these collars are summarized in Table 1 and shown in Fig. 2. The collars are effective for 3 to 11 months.

B. Delivery Systems

Three basic types of collar are available commercially: vapor-release, dust-release, and liquid-release collars. The differences in their delivery characteristics are described below.

Vapor-Release Collars

A volatile liquid insecticide such as dichlorvos or naled [7,15,16] is impregnated in the plasticized polymer resin. The insecticide vapor is distributed throughout the polymer matrix and is slowly released from the collar [11]. The atmosphere around the neck area of the animal is saturated with insecticide vapor that kills the fleas and ticks but is safe for the animal. Some of the vapor is lost through dilution

TABLE 1 Examples of Flea and Tick Collars

Product name	Manufacturer	Active ingredient	% Active	Animal species	Kills fleas/ticks for
Vapor-release collars					
Zodiac Stardust or clear	Zodiac Pet Products, Div. of Zoecon	Dichlorvos (DDVP)	9.3	Dogs	3 months/—
Vivopets	C-Vet	Dichlorvos	4.65	Cats	3 months/—
			18.6	Dogs, cats[a]	3 months/—
Grow	Sterling Animal Health Products	Dichlorvos Related compound	8.37 0.63	Dogs	3 months/2 months
Liquid-release collars					
Escort	Schering	Diazinon	15.0	Medium/small dogs, cats	5 months/4 months
Catovel	Beecham Animal Health	Diazinon	15.0	Cats	4 months/—[b]
Canovel	Beecham Animal Health	Diazinon	15.0	Dogs	4 months/—[b]
Escort Plus	Schering	Diazinon w/fatty acid	11.0	Large dogs, cats	5 months/1 month
Dermaton	Coopers Animal Health	Chlorfenvinphos	15.0	Dogs	$6\frac{1}{2}$ months/4 months

Dust-release collars

Product	Manufacturer	Active ingredient	%	Animal	Duration
Zodiac 4 month	Zodiac Pet Products, Div. of Zoecon	Carbaryl	8.5	Cats	4 months/—
Zodiac	Zodiac Pet Products, Div. of Zoecon	Carbaryl	16.0	Puppies	4 months/1 month
Vaporette Super II	Vaporette/Pet'm, Div. of Zoecon	Carbaryl	8.5	Cats	4 months/3 months[c]
Vet-Kem 4 month	Vet-Kem, Div. of Zoecon	Carbaryl	8.5	Cats	4 months/—
Zodiac 5 month	Zodiac Pet Products, Div. of Zoecon	Propoxur	9.4	Dogs, large dogs, cats	5 months/5 months
Vet-Kem	Vet-Kem, Div. of Zoecon	Propoxur	9.4	Dogs, large dogs, cats	5 months/5 months
Zodiac Breakaway	Zodiac Pet Products, Div. of Zoecon	Propoxur	9.4	Cats	5 months/5 months
Vet-Kem Breakaway	Vet-Kem, Div. of Zoecon	Propoxur	9.4	Cats	5 months/5 months
Duration 6	Schering	Chlorpyrifos	3.0	Cats	6 months/6 months
Duration 11	Schering	Chlorpyrifos	8.0	Dogs	11 months/7 months
Zodiac 11 Month	Zodiac Pet Products, Div. of Zoecon	Chlorpyrifos (Dursban)	8.0	Dogs	11 months/7 months

TABLE 1 (continued)

Product name	Manufacturer	Active ingredient	% Active	Animal species	Kills fleas/ticks for
Vet-Kem Dursban	Vet-Kem, Div. of Zoecon	Chlorpyrifos (Dursban)	8.0	Dogs	11 months/7 months
Hartz 2 in 1 Long Lasting	Hartz Mountain	Stirofos (Rabon)	13.7	Puppy	5 months/5 months
Hartz 2 in 1 Plus	Hartz Mountain	Stirofos (Rabon)	13.7	Cats, dogs	5 months/5 months
Zodiac 7 Month	Zodiac Pet Products, Div. of Zoecon	Phosmet (Prolate)	15.0	Dogs	7 months/7 months
Vet-Kem Paramite	Vet-Kem, Div. of Zoecon	Phosmet	15.0	Dogs	7 months/7 months

[a]Not for use on Persian cats [27].
[b]From Ref. 27.
[c]Brown dog ticks

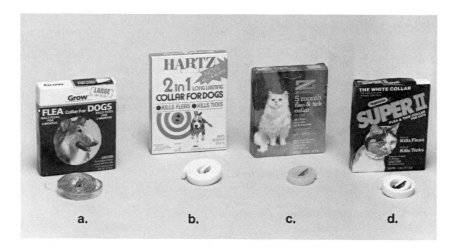

a. b. c. d.

Fig. 2 Examples of flea and tick collars. (a) Grow flea collar for dogs.
(Sterling Animal Health Products, a division of Sterling Drug, Inc.,
New York.) (b) Hartz 2 in 1 Long Lasting Collar for Dogs. (Hartz
Mountain Corporation, Harrision, New Jersey.) (c) Zodiac 5 month
flea and tick collar for cats. (Zodiac Pet Products, a division of Zoecon
Corporation, Dallas.) (d) Vaporette Super II flea and tick collar for
cats. (Vaporette/Pet'm, a division of Zoecon Corporation, Dallas.)

of the air around the animal. Consequently, the insecticide becomes
less effective in controlling these pests in other areas of the animal's
body.

Dust-Release Collar

Powdered insecticide, such as phosmet, stirofos, carbaryl, or propoxur
[7,11,17], is impregnated in the plasticized polymer resin. The insecticide slowly migrates through the polymer matrix and forms a powdery
dust on the surface of the collar. The dust is spread to other areas
of the animal's body by means of the animal's behavior (e.g., sleeping
in a curled position) [7,11].

The migration rate of stirofos (Rabon) is further controlled by a
phase change in the active ingredient [11]. The insecticide forms
needlelike polymorph II below 44°C (Fig. 3) and can migrate continuously to the surface of the collar. To reduce or inhibit the migration
of the insecticide during storage, the collar is heat treated briefly
between 55 and 65°C before storage. Rabon is converted to the platelet-
like polymorph I, which does not migrate readily. To reactivate the
collar, the user should stretch, rub, or otherwise disturb the surface

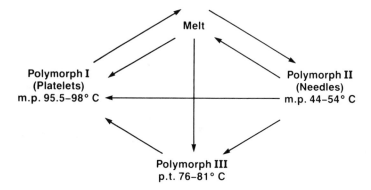

Fig. 3 Polymorphic forms of stirofos (Rabon). (From Ref. 11.)

of the collar to facilitate conversion to polymorph II, which then migrates continuously through the polymer matrix (Fig. 4).

Liquid-Release Collar

A nonvolatile liquid insecticide such as chlorfenvinphos or diazinon is impregnated in the collar. The liquid insecticide migrates from the polymer matrix and distributes to other parts of the animal's body through "wicking" [7]. With this type of collar the extent of insecticide distribution also depends on the animal's activity.

C. Discussion

Several investigators have evaluated the effectiveness of flea and tick collars in controlling pest infestations on dogs and cats. Fox et al. [18,19] and Pope [20] reported that dichlorvos collars provided good control of ticks (80% reduction of tick populations) for 7 weeks. Stiro-

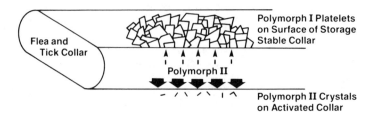

Fig. 4 Diagrammatic representation of release characteristics of stirofos (Rabon) from a plasticized solid thermoplastic resin. (From Ref. 11.)

fos collars [20] showed excellent control (100% reduction) of ticks for
10 weeks. Miller et al. [21] reported that collars containing 16% carbaryl exhibited good flea control for 16 weeks in dogs and up to 19
weeks in cats. Collars containing 9.4 to 10% propoxur [20,21-23]
provided good to excellent flea control in dogs for 10 to 13 weeks,
and good tick control for about 7 weeks. Baker and Miller [24] reported that collars containing temephos were 100% effective against
fleas during the first 2 weeks of use. Thereafter, they exhibited 80%
control for 36 weeks in dogs and up to 90% control for 41 weeks in cats.

Some studies [25-27] showed that the flea collar alone is inadequate in controlling flea hypersensitivity for extended periods of time.
Furthermore, the volatile liquid insecticide can develop skin irritation
around the neck area of the animal [11]. Despite these drawbacks,
the collar remains a very popular delivery system for controlling pest
infestations on pet animals. Pet owners prefer the convenience of the
insecticidal collars to other delivery systems. Melman and Hutton [7]
have recommended the use of flea collars on cats for preventive purposes.

III. DEVICES FOR LIVESTOCK ANIMALS

Pest bites from blood-sucking parasites, such as stable flies, horn
flies, lice, and ticks, can cause constant skin irritation and annoyance
to livestock [28]. Untreated pest bites can lead to weight losses and
reduction in feed efficiency and milk and egg production of livestock.
Quality of carcasses, hides, and wools of these animals can be significantly reduced. In some cases, severe infestation can lead to anemia
or even death of livestock. The parasites can also transmit infectious
diseases such as pinkeye and anaplasmosis in cattle. In the United
States, damage caused by insect pests results in an annual loss of
hundreds of millions of dollars to livestock producers. Horn flies alone
can cost cattle producers $730 million per year in lost production [28].
Therefore, insect pests must be controlled to reduce infestation and
increase livestock productivity.

Livestock pests behave differently [28]. Stable flies live on and
off their hosts and prefer to feed on the legs of cattle. Horn flies
spend most of their adult life on cattle and like to gather on the backs
and withers of these animals. Spinose ear ticks are small parasites
that live inside the ear and are difficult to detect. Lice feed on their
host for most of these lives and thrive in winter months, unlike other
pests. Face flies, which are non-blood-sucking parasites, prefer to
feed on animal protein secretions such as tears and saliva.

Periodic administration of insecticide sprays, dips, pour-ons, or
spot-ons is frequently used to control insect pests on livestock [5].
To reduce the frequency of treatments and labor costs, a suitable de-

livery device is needed to provide prolonged residual insecticide activity on animals. Several drug delivery devices were developed to meet these requirements and are reviewed below.

A. Dust Bags

Dust bags provide a convenient means of applying insecticides topically to livestock animals two or more times daily. They offer low labor costs and a minimum of equipment investment [1]. For examples of insecticide dust bags, see Figs. 5 and 6 and Table 2.

An insecticide dust, which is loaded into a porous inner bag [5, 29], is discharged through the lower and side parts of the inner bag. The inner bag is protected with a flexible weather-resistant cover such as a piece of vinyl-impregnated canvas [1]. The flip-top dust bag (Anchor Laboratories) is fitted with a steel hanger bar to prevent it from sagging, turning sideways, or rolling away from the animal during use.

To ensure that cattle receive the insecticide dust several times a day, the bag is suspended in areas frequented by the cattle [1,30]:

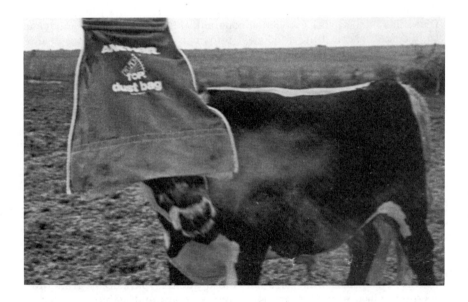

Fig. 5 Anchor flip-top dust bag kit. (Courtesy of Anchor Laboratories, Inc., a division of Boehringer Ingelheim Animal Health, Inc., St. Joseph, Missouri.)

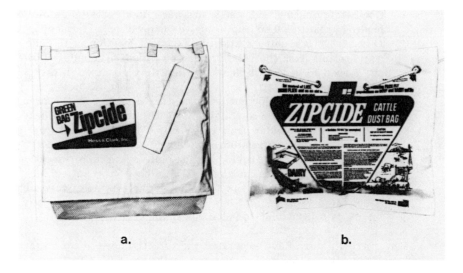

Fig. 6 Zipcide dust bags: (a) Green Bag Zipcide cattle duster and
(b) Zipcide cattle dust bag. (Courtesy of Rhone-Poulenc, Inc., Hess
and Clark Division, Ashland, Ohio.)

TABLE 2 Examples of Insecticide Dust Bags

Product name	Manufacturer	Active
Permectrin Flip-Top Dust Bag Kit	Anchor Laboratories, division of Boehringer Ingelheim Animal Health	0.25% Permethrin
Co-Ral Flip-Top Dust Bag Kit	Anchor Laboratories, division of Boehringer Ingelheim Animal Health	1.0% Coumaphos (Co-Ral)
Rabon Flip-Top Dust Bag Kit	Anchor Laboratories, division of Boehringer Ingelheim Animal Health	3.0% Stirofos (Rabon)
Zipcide Cattle Dust Bag	Hess and Clark, division of Rhone-Poulenc	1.0% Coumaphos (Co-Ral)

1. Good locations for beef cattle are barn door exits or gateways leading from the feed supply or the mineral or water feeder (Fig. 7a). For dairy cattle, an excellent location is the alleyway leading from the milking barn or in loafing sheds. Cows are forced to receive a dusting when they go through the passageway.

2. A suitable location for cattle on pasture or range is the area where the cattle like to congregate. For example, the dust bag can be suspended from tree limbs (Fig. 7b), poles, or an overhead structure where the cattle can receive dusting by free choice. To provide an adequate sprinkle of insecticide dust on the face and back of an animal, the bottom of the bag must be hung 4 to 6 in. below the topline of the animal. A 10 pound Zipcide dust bag can treat 60 animals twice daily for 65 days [30] and reduces labor cost considerably.

Many investigators have evaluated the effectiveness of insecticide dust bags for controlling insect pests on cattle [31-39]. Dust bags containing 1.0% coumaphos, 3.0% stirofos, 5% fenthion, 5% phosmet, or 3% crotoxyphos are shown to provide good to excellent control of horn flies. Loomis [39] reported that cattle could take up to 2 weeks to become accustomed to the administration of insecticides from the dust bags.

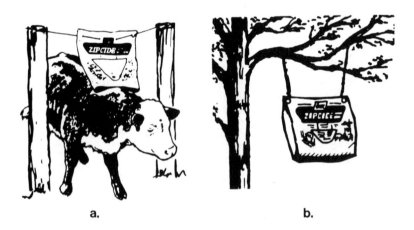

a.   b.

Fig. 7 Two ways to hang a dust bag: (a) in an entrance or alleyway leading to a food or water feeder and (b) from a tree limb. (Courtesy of Rhone-Poulenc, Inc., Hess and Clark Division, Ashland, Ohio.)

B. Back Rubbers and Face Flyps

Back rubbers [40-42] are made of special fiber wicking packed into double-thick acrylic and polyester sleeves. Hog-rubs (Fig. 8) and Cow Life-Cattle Rubs (Fig. 9) are available from P. H. White, Jr. Back rubbers are suspended between two poles and saturated with an insecticide solution. Examples of insecticide preparations for use with the back rubbers are listed in Table 3. The preparations are usually emulsifiable concentrates diluted with mineral oil or diesel fuel. The 5 ft Hog-rub can hold up to 1.5 gal of insecticide solutions, while the 10 ft Cow Life-Cattle Rub holds about 4 gal of an insecticide solution. The rub acts as an oil reservoir of the insecticide. As the animal passes under it, the insecticide is released by "wicking" through the rubbing action. Burns et al. [43], Kinzer [37], and Kessler and Berndt [38] reported that the back rubbers are effective in controlling horn flies in cattle. The rubs can also provide protection against pinkeye and can control lice and mange in hogs. The rubs need refilling every 4 to 8 weeks depending on the size of the herd. This device offers substantial labor savings and provides an economical means of pest control.

Face flyps (Figs. 10 and 11) are often used with the Cow Life-Cattle Rub to control face flies. They are made of DuPont orlon fabric and act as wicks for movement of the insecticide from the rub [44]. Face flyps are suspended about 2 ft below the rub. As the animal passes under them, the face flyps are dragged across the face of the animal and leave behind a good coat of insecticide on the animal's face.

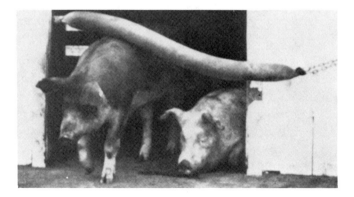

Fig. 8 Hog-Rub. (Courtesy of P. H. White, Jr., Dyersburg, Tennessee.)

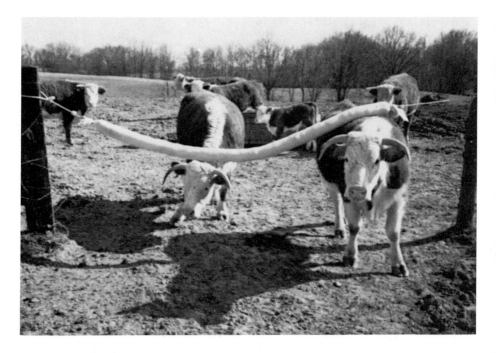

Fig. 9 Cow Life-Cattle Rub. (Courtesy of P. H. White, Jr., Dyersburg, Tennessee.)

TABLE 3 Examples of Insecticide Preparations for Use with Back Rubbers and Fly Bullets

Product name	Manufacturer	Active
Ciovap	SDS Biotech, division of Fermenta	Crotoxyphos 10%, dichlorvos (Vapona) 2.3%
Co-Ral E.C.	Cutter Animal Health	Coumaphos 11.6%
Permectrin II	Anchor Laboratories, division of Boehringer Ingelheim Animal Health	Permethrin 10.0%
Ravap	SDS Biotech, division of Fermenta	Stirofos 23%, dichlorvos (Vapona) 5.3%

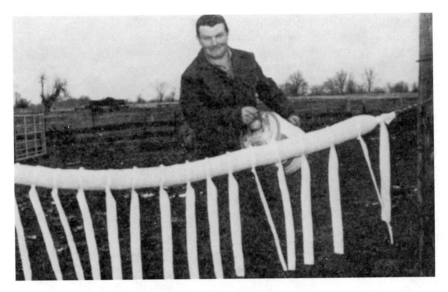

Fig. 10 Cow Life-Cattle Rub with Face Flyps. (Courtesy of P. H. White, Jr., Dyersburg, Tennessee.)

C. Fly Bullets

Fly bullets saturated with an insecticide solution can provide added protection against pinkeye in cattle [42]. They are made of DuPont orlon and acrylic fiber (Fig. 12) and are usually hung near creep openings or mineral feeders. They can hold about a pint of insecticide solution with diesel fuel or mineral oil as the carrier. The device provides fly control as well as protection for pinkeye at a negligible cost.

D. Ear Devices

Ear Strips

In 1970 Harvey and Brethour [45] developed ear strips made of polymeric resins and impregnated with dichlorvos to control horn flies in cattle. One example of an ear strip, the Permectrin strip (Fig. 13), contains 10% permethrin and is used to control horn flies, face flies, Gulf Coast ticks, and spinose ear ticks in beef and dairy cattle. It is also used on horses to control horn flies, face flies, and eye gnats [46]. The strip is attached to an ear tag or halter with the cable tie provided.

The insecticide migrates to the surface of the device and is spread to the animal's body by self-grooming and animal movement, probably

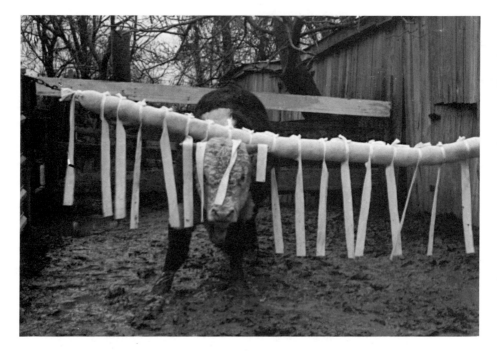

Fig. 11 Face Flyps. (Courtesy of P. H. White, Jr., Dyersburg, Tennessee.)

similar to the action of flea and tick collars. Kopp and Meyer [47] reported that strips containing 10% permethrin provided good control of flies. Gladney et al. [48] reported that ear strips impregnated with dichlorvos could control Gulf Coast ticks for about 2 weeks.

Tapes

Ectiban insecticide tapes manufactured by Coopers Animal Health (Fig. 14) offer an alternative means of attaching an insecticide delivery device to the ears of cattle. The tape, with a self-adhesive backing, is wrapped around the "neck" of an ear tag (Fig. 15 and Ref. 49). The insecticide is stored in two glass ampules inside the tape. To activate the tape, thumb pressure is applied to break the ampules and the insecticide is slowly released through the slits at the bottom of the tape. Ectiban tape containing 1.2 g of permethrin can control horn flies and face flies for 5 months [49].

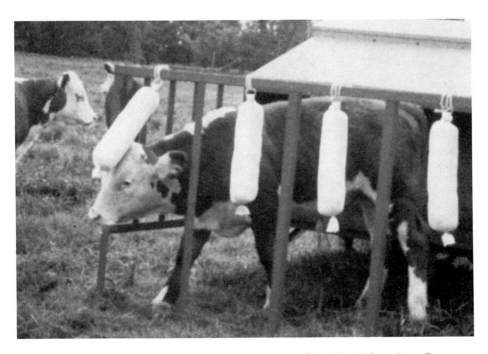

Fig. 12 Fly Bullets with Creep. (Courtesy of P. H. White, Jr., Dyersburg, Tennessee.)

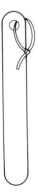

Fig. 13 Permectrin ear strip. (Courtesy of Anchor Laboratories, Inc., a division of Boehringer Ingelheim Animal Health, Inc., St. Joseph Missouri.)

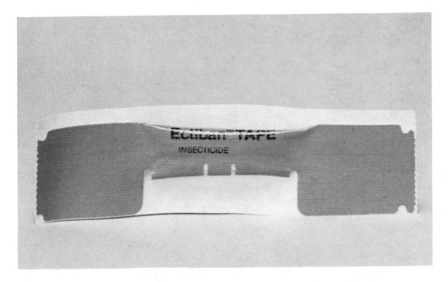

Fig. 14 Ectiban tape. (Courtesy of Coopers Animal Health, Inc., Kansas City, Missouri.)

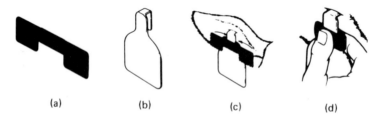

(a)   (b)   (c)   (d)

Fig. 15 Attachment of Ectiban tape (a) to an ear tag (b). First the paper backing is removed from the tape. Then the tape is applied, with the release slits down, to the narrow neck of an ear tag (c). Next the tape is wrapped around the "neck" of the tag and the ends are sealed with the self-adhesive flaps. Finally (d), the tape is activated by pressing lightly with thumb to break the ampules containing Ectiban. (Courtesy of Coopers Animal Health, Inc., Kansas City, Missouri.)

Ear Tags

Insecticide ear tags were developed for beef and dairy cattle as an improvement to ear strips and tapes. They have a larger surface area and can deliver more insecticide to provide season-long pest control [50,51]. The tag is attached to the flat part of an animal's ear (Fig. 16) with the Allflex tagging system (Allflex Tag Company).

The tags contain insecticides dissolved in a polymer matrix such as plasticized polyvinyl chloride or polyurethane [31,52-54]. The polymer formulation is formed into the desired shape by injection molding [55]. For examples of various insecticide ear tags, see Fig. 17 and Table 4.

Impregnated insecticide is released slowly from the monolithic device to the surface of the tag. It migrates gradually to the neck and the rest of the animal's body by way of animal movement and self-grooming [56]. Diffusion of an active agent from a polymeric slab to the surface can be expressed by the Baker and Lonsdale equation [57], which is based on Fick's law of diffusion. For the first 60% of desorption, fraction of solute released from the slab varies with the square root of time t:

$$\frac{M_t}{M_\infty} = 4 \left(\frac{D\sqrt{t}}{\pi \, 1^2} \right) \tag{1}$$

where

$$0 \leqslant \frac{M_t}{M_\infty} \leqslant 0.6$$

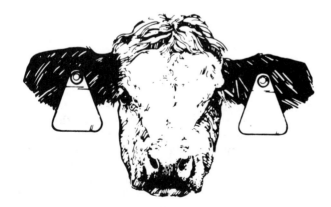

Fig. 16 Atroban insecticide ear tags attached to cattle. (Courtesy of Coopers Animal Health, Inc., Kansas City, Missouri.)

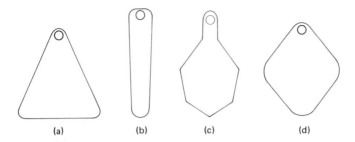

Fig. 17 Examples of insecticide ear tags: (a) Atroban insecticide ear tag (Coopers Animal Health, Inc., Kansas, Missouri). (b) Permectrin ear tag (Anchor Laboratories, Inc., a division of Boehringer Ingelheim Animal Health, Inc., St. Joseph, Missouri). (c) Ectrin insecticide cattle ear tag (Fermenta Animal Health Company, Painesville, Ohio). (d) Ear Force tag (Bio-Ceutic, a division of Boehringer Ingelheim Animal Health, Inc., St. Joseph, Missouri).

and

M_t = cumulative amount of solute released at time t
M_∞ = total amount of solute released at infinite time (i.e., initial amount of solute present in the formulation)
D = diffusion coefficient (cm^2/time) of the solute
l = half the thickness of the slab

For the last 60% of desorption, fraction of solute released varies exponentially with time:

$$\frac{M_t}{M_\infty} = 1 - \frac{8}{\pi^2} \exp - \left(\frac{\pi^2 \, Dt}{l^2} \right) \tag{2}$$

where $0.4 \leqslant M_t/M_\infty \leqslant 1.0$

Miller et al. [58] determined the desorption and release rates of different insecticides from the ear tags. Among those investigated were tags containing 8% fenvalerate (Ectrin), 10% permethrin (Atroban), and 5 and 10% decamethrin. Figures 18 and 19 show the desorption of these insecticides from the ear tags. The release rates of the insecticides were determined from the first derivative d (M_t/M_∞)/dt and are shown in Figs. 20 and 21. The release rate of 8% fenvalerate is slower than that of 10% permethrin, and the difference may be partly due to the unequal thickness of the ear tags. Fenvalerate ear tags are

TABLE 4 Examples of Insecticide Ear Tags

Product name	Manufacturer	Active
Ear Force	Bio-Ceutic, division of Boehringer Ingelheim	10% Permethrin
Ectrin	SDS Biotech, division of Fermenta	8% Fenvalerate
Permectrin	Anchor Laboratories, division of Boehringer Ingelheim	10% Permethrin
Atroban	Coopers Animal Health	10% Permethrin
Expar	Coopers Animal Health	10% Permethrin
Guardian	American Cyanamid	7.5% Flucythrinate

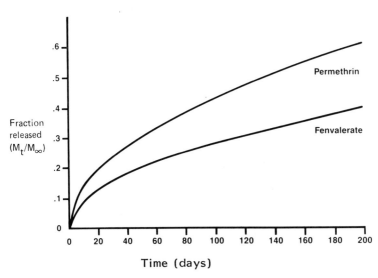

Fig. 18 Fraction of permethrin (Atroban) and fenvalerate (Ectrin) released from ear tags. (From Ref. 58.)

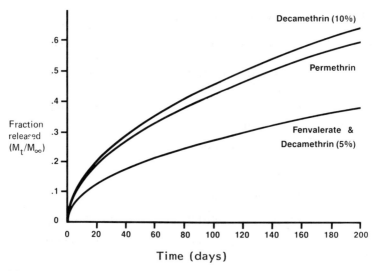

Fig. 19 Fraction of pyrethrins released from ear tags. (From Ref. 58.)

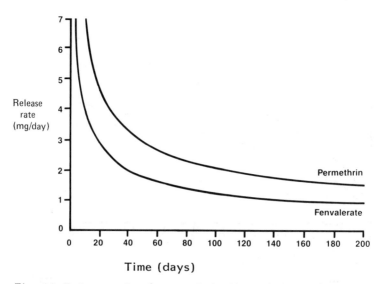

Fig. 20 Release rate of permethrin (Atroban) and fenvalerate (Ectrin) from ear tags. (From Ref. 58.)

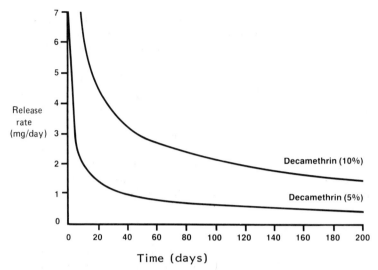

Fig. 21 Release rate of 5 and 10% decamethrin from ear tags. (From Ref. 58.)

2194 ±7 μm thick, compared with 1254 ±2 μm for the permethrin device. Figure 21 also shows that doubling the drug loading more than doubled the release rate. The diffusion coefficient D calculated for the 10% decamethrin coefficient is almost triple the value determined for the 5% decamethrin: D values are 15.97×10^{-7} cm^2/day and 5.86×10^{-7} cm^2/day, respectively, for 10 and 5% decamethrin. Miller et al. [58] reported that the minimum effective delivery rates for the ear tags were estimated to be 1.0 mg/day for 8% fenvalerate and 1.9 mg/day for 10% permethrin. The study also showed that the ear tags had lost their effectiveness even when more than 50% of the pesticide remained in the device.

Many investigators have reported that insecticide ear tags can provide good to excellent control of flies and ticks for a prolonged period. Ear tags containing 8% fenvalerate [47,53,59-68], 10% permethrin [47,52,53,63,69], 8% cypermethrin [70-72], 13.7% stirofos [53,63, 73-75], or 1.5% deltamethrin [69] can control horn fly infestations at 90 to 100% levels for a period of 12 to 20 weeks. The control of face flies varies more extensively with the chemical insecticide in the ear tag. Control ranges from 50 to 90% for a period of 5 to 21 weeks [52, 60,63,64,68,69,70,72,73]. Ear tags containing 15% stirofos, 3% deltamethrin, 10% chlorpyrifos, or 8% fenvalerate can reduce tick populations 80 to 90% for a period of 11 weeks [76,77]. The fenvalerate tags were effective for beef cattle, dairy cows, and calves [62,64]. The cypermethrin tags can reduce incidence of summer mastitis [78].

In recent years the resistance of horn flies to pyrethroids has increased in some parts of the country [79]. A new approach to pest management is to alternate the insecticide devices seasonally between pyrethroids and organophosphorus compounds. Ernst [80] reported that new ear tags have been marketed recently by Ralston-Purina and Fearing Corporation to control horn flies more effectively. Dual-Gard ear tags (Ralston-Purina) contain permethrin and chlorpyrifos impregnated in a plastic resin with a synergist, piperonyl butoxide. Duo Deckem ear tags (Fearing) contain permethrin and piperonyl butoxide in a replaceable reservoir disk. The disk has a membrane system that maintains a thin film of the insecticide on its surface. With this device the insecticide is delivered at a constant rate for up to 6 months. The effectiveness of the new device is still being evaluated.

E. Bands and Tail Tags

Insecticide-impregnated bands and tail tags were developed as alternatives to ear tags [81]. Beadles et al. [56] showed that an oil-based dye solution attached to bands and tail tags can spread to various parts of the animal's body to different degrees. Neck bands transfer the dye from behind the ears to the front of the shoulders (Fig. 22a), while ear tag or halter application spreads it to the side of the head, neck, and shoulders (Fig. 22b). The dye solution migrates from the leg bands to lower legs, dewlap, and lower belly (Fig. 22c). Tail tags were shown to spread the dye solution to the greatest extent to the posterior end of the animal (Fig. 22d). Therefore, it is feasible to select a specific insecticide device to control target pests for better efficacy. Gladney [48,82] and Ahrens [54,77] and their colleagues reported that neck bands, leg bands, and horn bands impregnated with propoxur or stirofos could control Gulf Coast ticks satisfactorily. Miller [83], Beadles [84,85], and Hunt [86] and their co-workers showed that leg bands and tail tags impregnated with dichlorvos are effective for controlling horn flies and common cattle grub.

IV. CONCLUSION

Various ectoparasitic devices have been reviewed for the control of pests in pets and livestock animals. Each device delivers the insecticide differently according to the physical characteristics and residual activity of the active ingredient. The user needs to select the device carefully to suit individual needs.

Future development of the devices will focus on lengthening the residual activity from a single treatment and reducing the amount of insecticide needed for topical applications [51]. New delivery systems

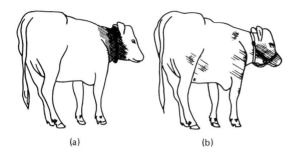

(a)   (b)

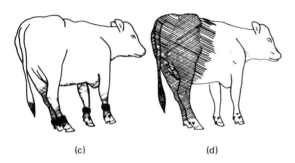

(c)   (d)

Fig. 22 Dye transfer from various devices to parts of the animal body: (a) from neck strap with dye-impregnated pad attached to outer surface, (b) from halter with dye-impregnated pads attached to the cheek straps and nose straps, (c) from leg bands with dye-impregnated pad attached to the outer surface, and (d) from dye-impregnated pad attached to a tail tag. (From Ref. 56.)

will be developed as animal farming practices change and new insecticides become available.

ACKNOWLEDGMENTS

The author expresses appreciation to Mrs. Frances McPherson for assistance to literature searches and to Mrs. Judy Cosgrove for assistance in preparation of the manuscript.

REFERENCES

1. *Flip-Top Dust Bag Kit.* Anchor Laboratories, Inc., a Division of Boehringer Ingelheim Animal Health, Inc., St. Joseph, MO, 1984.
2. *Product Reference Guide.* Vet-Kem, a Division of Zoecon Corporation, Dallas, 1985.
3. *Pet Owner's Guide to Inside Out Pet Hygiene.* Coopers Animal Health, Inc., Kansas City, MO, 1985.
4. R. O. Drummond, *Vet. Parasitol.*, 18:111 (1985).
5. D. G. Pope, in *Formulation of Veterinary Dosage Forms* (J. Blodinger, ed.). Dekker, New York, 1983, pp. 97-107.
6. J. A. Miller, S. E. Kunz, and D. D. Oehler, in *Controlled Release of Pesticides and Pharmaceuticals* (D. H. Lewis, ed.). Plenum Press, New York, 1980, pp. 311-318.
7. S. A. Melman and P. Hutton, *Compend. on Contin. Educ. Pract. Vet.*, 7:869 (1985).
8. M. Wilson, G. Bennett, and A. Proonsha, *Practical Insect Management, in Insects of Man, Household and Health.* Waveland Press, Prospect Heights, IL, 1977.
9. E.J.L. Soulsby, in *Fleas, in Helminths, Arthropods, and Protozoa of Domestic Animals,* 6th ed. Williams & Wilkins, Baltimore, 1968, pp. 383-389.
10. G. H. Muller, R. W. Kirk, and D. W. Scott, *Small Animal Dermatology.* Saunders, Philadelphia, 1983.
11. D. G. Pope, in *Animal Health Products Design and Evaluation* (D. C. Monkhouse, ed.). American Pharmaceutical Association, Academy of Pharmaceutical Sciences, Washington, DC, 1978, pp. 87-91.
12. F. B. Folckemer, R. E. Hanson, and A. Miller, U.S. Patent 3, 318, 769 (1967).
13. L. M. Grubb and J. K. Baxter, U.S. Patent 3, 852, 416 (1974).
14. A. Miller and J. G. Morales, U.S. Patent 3, 944, 662 (1976).
15. W. N. Beesley, in *Chemotherapy of Parasitic Diseases* (W. C. Campbell and R. S. Rew, eds.). Plenum Press, New York, 1986, pp. 564-565.
16. R. O. Drummond, in *Chemotherapy of Parasitic Diseases* W. C. Campbell and R. S. Rew, eds.). Plenum Press, New York, 1986, p. 579.
17. *Product Reference Guide.* Zodiac Pet Products, a Division of Zoecon Corporation, Dallas, 1986.
18. I. Fox, I. G. Bayona, and J. L. Armstrong, *J. Am. Vet. Med. Assoc.*, 155:1621 (1969).
19. I. Fox, G. A. Rivera, and I. G. Bayona, *J. Econ. Entomol.*, 62:1246 (1969).

20. *Unipet Flea and Tick Collar Technical Bulletin* V2247. Upjohn Company, 1975, from Ref. 11.

21. J. E. Miller, N. F. Baker, and E. L. Colburn, Jr., *Am. J. Vet. Res.*, 38:923 (1977).

22. I. G. Horak, *J. South Afr. Vet. Assoc.*, 47:17 (1976).

23. H. Fisch, R. A. Angerhofer, and J. H. Nelson, *J. Am. Vet. Med. Assoc.*, 171:269 (1977).

24. N. F. Baker and J. E. Miller, *Am. J. Vet. Res.*, 38:1187 (1977).

25. W. F. Randell, K. E. Bradley, and D. L. Brown, *Vet. Med. Small Animal Clin.*, 75:606 (1980).

26. L. Medleau and W. H. Miller, *Int. J. Dermatol.*, 22:378 (1983).

27. D. Grant, *In Practice* [British Veterinary Association, London], 6:121, 123, 125, 127 (1984).

28. *Coopers Insecticide Guide to Livestock Pest Control.* Coopers Animal Health, Inc., Kansas City, MO, 1985.

29. W. C. Cortner, Jr., U.S. Patent 3, 902, 461 (1975).

30. *How to Use the Zipcide Cattle Dust Bags.* Rhone-Pulenc, Inc., Hess and Clark Division, Ashland, OH.

31. R. E. Williams, E. J. Westby, K. S. Hendrix, and R. P. Lemenager, *J. Animal Sci.*, 53:1159 (1981).

32. T. L. Harvey and J. R. Brethour, *J. Econ. Entomol.*, 72:516 (1979).

33. J. B. Campbell, *J. Econ. Entomol.*, 69:711 (1976).

34. F. W. Knapp, *J. Econ. Entomol.*, 65:470 (1972).

35. B. W. Hayes, M. J. Janes, and D. W. Beardlsey, *J. Econ. Entomol.*, 65:368 (1972).

36. N. I. Greer, M. Murphy, and M. J. Janes, *Florida Entomol.*, 54:231 (1971).

37. H. G. Kinzer, *Vet. Med. Rev.*, No. 1, 83, 1971.

38. H. Kessler and W. L. Berndt, *J. Econ. Entomol.*, 64:1465 (1971).

39. E. C. Loomis, D. C. Cannon, C. W. Rimby, and L. L. Dunning, *California Agric.*, 23:8 (1969).

40. P. H. White, Jr., U.S. Patent 3, 677, 233 (1972).

41. *Hog-Rub.* P. H. White, Jr., Dyersburg, TN.

42. *Cow Life-Cattle Rub Bright Eyes and No Flies.* P. H. White, Jr., Dyersburg, TN.

43. E. C. Burns, G. R. McCoy, D. G. Melancon, L. I. Smart, J. M. Perkins, and T. O. McRae, *Proceedings of the Fifteenth Annual Livestock Producers' Day.* Louisiana State University, Baton Rouge, 1975, p. 258.

44. Face Flyps package insert. P. H. White, Jr., Dyersburg, TN.

45. T. L. Harvey and J. R. Brethour, *J. Econ. Entomol.*, 63:1688 (1970).

46. *Permectrin Ear Tags and Strips.* Anchor Laboratories, Inc., a Division of Boehringer Ingelheim Animal Health, Inc., St. Joseph, MO.

47. D. D. Kopp and H. J. Meyer, *North Dakota Farm Res.*, 40:19 (1983).
48. W. J. Gladney, M. A. Price, and O. H. Graham, *J. Med. Entomol.*, 13:579 (1977).
49. *Ectiban Tape.* Coopers Animal Health Inc., Kansas City, MO, 1985.
50. W. V. Miller, U.S. Patent 4, 195, 075 (1980).
51. R. O. Drummond, *Vet. Parasitol.*, 18:111 (1985).
52. F. W. Knapp and F. Herald, *Southwes. Entomol.*, 5:183 (1980).
53. E. C. Burns, S. M. De Rouen, J. C. Carpenter, Jr., L. I. Smart, and J. M. Perkins, *Louisiana Agric.*, 23:23 (1980).
54. E. H. Ahrens, *Southwest. Entomol.*, 2:8 (1977).
55. Ear Force Tags technical data sheet. Bio-Ceutic, a Division of Boehringer Ingelheim Animal Health, Inc., St. Joseph, MO, 1986.
56. M. L. Beadles, A. R. Gingrich, and J. A. Miller, *J. Econ. Entomol.*, 70:72 (1977).
57. R. W. Baker and H. K. Lonsdale, in *Controlled Release of Biologically Active Agents* (A. C. Tanquary and R. E. Lacey, eds.). Pleunm Press, New York, 1974, p. 15.
58. J. A. Miller, D. D. Oehler, and S. E. Kunz, *J. Econ. Entomol.*, 76:1335 (1983).
59. E. D. Janzen and H. H. Nicholson, *Can. J. Animal Sci.*, 64:204 (1984).
60. J. H. Burton, I. McMillan, and G. Surgeoner, *Can. J. Animal Sci.*, 64:113 (1984).
61. S. E. Kunz, H. G. Kinzer, and J. A. Miller, *J. Econ. Entomol.*, 76:525 (1983).
62. T. L. Harvey and J. R. Brethour, *J. Econ. Entomol.*, 76:117 (1983).
63. R. E. Williams and E. J. Westby, *J. Kansas Entomol. Soc.*, 55:335 (1982).
64. F. W. Knapp and F. Herald, *J. Econ. Entomol.*, 74:295 (1981).
65. T. L. Harvey and J. R. Brethour, *Prot. Ecol.*, 2:313 (1981).
66. C. D. Schmidt and S. E. Kunz, *Southwest. Entomol.*, 5:202 (1980).
67. E. H. Ahrens and J. Cocke, *J. Econ. Entomol.*, 72:215 (1979).
68. R. R. Gerhardt and B. A. Mullens, *Progress Report, Tennessee Farm and Home Science*, No. 105, 1978, p. 2.
69. R. E. Williams and E. J. Westby, *J. Econ. Entomol.*, 73:791 (1980).
70. J. E. Hillerton, A. J. Bramley, and N. H. Yarrow, *Br. Vet. J.*, 141:160 (1985).
71. J. C. Wilcox and R. A. Peers, *Trawsgoed Experimental Husbandry Farm. Annual Review*, Aberystwyth, Wales, U.K., 1983, 47 pp.
72. J. S. Liddel and R. Clayton, *Vet. Record*, 110:502 (1982).
73. D. J. Lewis and E. Block, *Can. J. Animal Sci.*, 62:1249 (1982).
74. C. Sheppard, *J. Econ. Entomol.*, 73:276 (1980).
75. J. E. Huston and D. I. Davis, *Southwest. Vet.*, 31:197 (1978).

76. R. B. Davey, E. H. Ahrens, and J. Garza, Jr., *J. Econ. Entomol.*, 73:651 (1980).
77. E. H. Ahrens and J. Cocke, *J. Econ. Entomol.*, 71:764 (1978).
78. G. Bertels and J. M. Robijns, *Vlaams Diergeneeskd. Tijdschr.*, 52:77 (1983).
79. S. Muirhead, *Feedstuff*, Nov. 3, 1986, p. 10.
80. D. Ernst, *Kansas Farmer*, July 6, 1985, p. 8.
81. J. A. Miller, S. E. Kunz, and D. D. Oehler, in *Controlled Release of Pesticides and Pharmaceuticals* (D. H. Lewis, ed.). Plenum Press, New York, 1980, pp. 311-318.
82. W. J. Gladney, *J. Econ. Entomol.*, 69:757 (1976).
83. J. A. Miller, S. E. Kunz, and M. L. Beadles, *Southwest. Entomol.*, 6:265 (1981).
84. M. L. Beadles, J. A. Miller, B. K. Shelley, and D. P. Ingenhuett, *Southwest. Entomol.*, 4:70 (1979).
85. M. L. Beadles, J. A. Miller, B. K. Shelley, and R. E. Reeves, *J. Econ. Entomol.*, 71:287 (1978).
86. L. M. Hunt, M. L. Beadles, B. K. Shelley, B. N. Gilbert, and R. O. Drummond, *J. Econ. Entomol.*, 73:32 (1980).

20

Rumen Retention Devices

ROBERT J. GYURIK / SmithKline Beckman Animal Health Products,
West Chester, Pennsylvania

I. INTRODUCTION AND PRINCIPLES

The animal health marketplace has provided many opportunities for the introduction of new drug delivery devices, and innovators have employed new and exciting elements from other fields for these systems. A major driving force for such innovation is the increasing need for labor-saving and convenience products. Labor costs are rising in both developed and developing countries, and the trend toward larger farms and more intensive methods of animal husbandry continues.

A. The Ruminant Animal

This chapter will focus on delivery systems that are retained in the "first stomach" or rumenoreticulum of the ruminant or grazing animal (primarily cattle and sheep). Due to the unique physiological characteristics of the digestive system of ruminants, as well as the highly specialized methods of animal husbandry that have evolved around them, these food-producing animals have offered and continue to offer many new opportunities for the development of delivery devices. First, some basic underlying principles governing the design and function of rumen retention devices (RRDs) must be explained.

Physiological Principles

Ruminant animals have evolved an anterior digestive organ called the *rumenoreticulum*, which functions as the initial site for the breakdown of less digestible cellulosic food sources. An active fermentation by symbiotic bacteria and protozoa accomplishes this. The fermentation metabolites as well as the microorganisms themselves are utilized by the animal to fulfill its own metabolic requirements for growth and maintenance. The rumenoreticulum can be envisioned as a "fermentation vat," typically 100 to 200 liters in the cow and 10 to 15 liters in the sheep. It has an entrance port at the proximal end of the esophagus through which food and buffering saliva enter and an exit sphincter through which the rumen contents enter the abomasum, or "true stomach," after passing through a "strainer," the omasum. The remaining digestive tract is similar to that of most other monogastric mammals (see Fig. 1) [1-3].

The rumenoreticulum provides a unique opportunity for the application of drug delivery systems; a device retained there by suitable means can serve as a platform for the long-term presentation of prophylactic or therapeutic medicaments. Principles governing the retention of RRDs will be discussed in detail in Section I.B.

Drug Delivery Opportunities

A variety of agents have been used in RRDs for either prophylactic or therapeutic purposes.

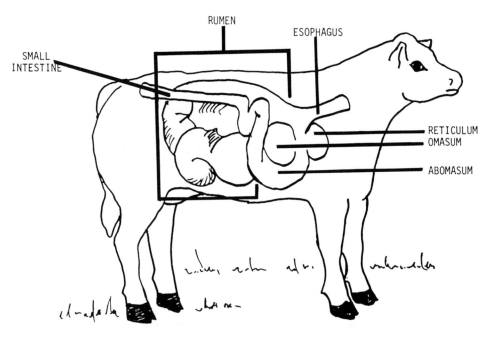

Fig. 1 Digestive system of the ruminant animal, showing the relative position of the digestive organs. An RRD density of greater than 2.5 g/ml ensures disposition of the RRD in the reticulum, the anteriormost organ. RRDs that depend on geometry for retention float freely throughout the expanse of the rumen. RRDs are administered orally by means of a specialized device called a balling gun.

Anthelmintics

Antiparasitic agents have recently provided the greatest opportunity for rumen retention devices. Special factors governing parasitic disease have contributed to the high level of activity in this area [7]. These will be covered in detail in Section II.

Nutrients (especially trace elements)

Trace elements were the first agents incorporated into rumen retention devices. Cobalt, selenium, copper, zinc, and iodine are the elements usually selected, either singly or in combination, for use in RRDs. Various locales have soils deficient in these essential elements, leading to disease conditions ranging from severely acute to chronic [4,5].

Growth Promoters

Agents that enhance the growth of ruminants at very low doses have been developed. These act by inhibiting the bacteria that adversely affect growth [6].

Antibiotics

The therapeutic use of antibiotics against disease-causing pathogens has been seen in boluses that degrade slowly in the rumen, releasing antibiotics over the course of several days for treatment of diseases such as calf scours (dysentery) or shipping fever.

Reasons for the Present Success of
Rumen Retention Devices

In addition to labor saving and convenience, the following reasons are important in generating a high level of interest in RRDs.

Avoidance of Handling Stress

Economic losses are sustained by the repeated handling of animals for treatment. These losses are difficult to quantify but may be considerable. Reducing the number of handling episodes results in economic benefit to the farmer that is realized as increased animal weight and lower overall death rates.

Optimization of Strategic Programs

RRDs incorporate husbandry practices that have been advocated by practitioners but are difficult to perform consistently in the field. This is especially true with anthelmintic treatment programs, which have developed to a very sophisticated level in many areas of the world. The epidemiology of parasitic infection involves complex interactions among the host animal, the environment, and the parasite. An *epidemiological benefit* of reduced pasture contamination results from anthelmintic therapy provided by appropriate treatment programs or drug delivery systems [7]. The beneficial effect of reduced reinfection may far outlast the individual life of the device or treatment. Some anthelmintic agents are also ovicidal in the parasite, thereby conferring an additional bonus of further reduction in the reinfection rate.

B. Principles Governing Design and Function of Rumen Retention Devices

RRDs fall into two basic categories, those that release drugs constantly throughout their lifetime in the rumen, *sustained release* devices, and those that release discrete doses in a pulsatile manner, *intermittent release* devices, as described in Sections II and III, respectively. RRDs are administered orally by means of a device called an esophageal balling gun, types of which have been described in the literature [8]; see also Figs. 1 to 4 in Chapter 21.

The unique anatomical and physiological features of ruminant animals necessitate special design features for RRDs. Two major problems an RRD must overcome are regurgitation and the harsh conditions within the rumen environment.

Regurgitation

Another function of ruminant animals that is of primary concern when RRDs are designed is that of *rumination*, commonly known as "chewing the cud." Rumination is a process wherein rumen contents that have been collected, cursorily chewed, and swallowed during grazing are regurgitated and remasticated at the animal's leisure. In cattle a liter or more may be brought up the esophagus at a time. There are two basic ways to ensure against the regurgitation of an intraruminal device: by making it heavy enough (high density) to remain in the rumenoreticulum, or by utilizing a design geometry that will prevent passage back through the esophagus [9].

Density

If a device is sufficiently dense, it will remain in the anterior part of the rumenoreticulum in an area called the *reticulum*. This area collects heavy objects that may be inadvertently swallowed, such as nails, stones, and the like. The muscle walls of this organ are sufficiently tough to offer resistance to puncture by sharp objects, but large, sharp ones can cause reticulitis or "hardware disease," severe cases of which may result in death by penetrating the wall and the adjacent pericardium. It is therefore wise to avoid sharp detail on any RRD.

The minimum density to prevent regurgitation varies depending on whether the animal is housed or on pasture. Pastured animals need greater density because the motility of the rumen is greater in grazing animals than in those housed and receiving more refined diets. It is generally recognized that a density of 2.25 to 3.5 g/ml should be maintained to prevent regurgitation in grazing animals [8]. A density of 1.8 g/ml is probably sufficient for housed animals [22].

Geometry

Various geometries have been utilized to prevent regurgitation or passage of devices once they are in the rumenoreticulum. Devices have been designed to unfold once in the rumen (variable geometry), giving rise to a plethora of bulky shaped possibilities, including wings and unfolding sheets. To facilitate dosing, the eventual geometry is suppressed by digestible or soluble holdfasts, such as cellulosic or gelatin bands, which disintegrate after entering the rumenoreticulum. These various designs have been covered extensively in a previous review [8].

For retention, there are also two caveats to consider: (a) whatever a ruminant can swallow, it can potentially expel, and (b) sheep are known to regurgitate devices more easily than cattle. Regurgitation may be kept to a minimum by careful attention to correct design.

Rumen Environment

A good understanding of the very harsh environment within the rumen is necessary before one can design durable RRDs that will function reproducibly. Here is a brief summary of some of the factors to be considered; for further study, the reader is directed to some of the standard textbooks, which detail ruminant anatomy and physiology [1-3].

Rumen pH

Rumen pH may vary between 5 and 7 units in the healthy animal. This depends on the type of diet, primarily, and on the species or strain of animal. This is a very important consideration, since any device that is sensitive to changes in pH will not be consistent in its performance.

Rumen Atmosphere

The atmosphere within the rumen is anaerobic, the conditions strongly reducing. Hydrogen, methane, and carbon dioxide are the principal gases. Devices must be designed to withstand these conditions; also, in vitro studies may not be relevant to in vivo results if a device is sensitive to these conditions.

Rumen Microflora

The symbiotic microflora within the rumen have coevolved to effect the predigestion of highly intractable polysaccharides, mostly celluloses, that form the bulk of the ruminant diet. The microorganisms in return receive a comfortable environmental niche. The enzymes released by such microorganisms are capable of breaking down almost anything within the rumen, so very inert materials capable of withstanding these chemicals must be utilized in devices. Even many plastics will not last long in the rumen; polyethylene, polypropylene, and stainless steel are good choices for the surfaces of devices deployed therein. Again, in vitro models must be used with caution. It is indeed possible to maintain artificial rumens by continuous fermentation techniques in the laboratory, but only with great expertise and expenditure of effort. It is simpler to study the function of devices within the target animals themselves, especially through the use of rumen-fistulated study animals, which contain removable cannulae through which devices may be placed and removed.

Drug Resistance

Much has been written about the consequences of long-term anthelmintic therapy as it impacts the phenomenon of increased drug resistance by parasites. Overuse or abuse of chemotherapeutic agents has led to the development of resistance in worm populations, especially in the sheep-rearing areas of the Southern Hemisphere. Frequent or prolonged anthelmintic usage is clearly associated with the problem [15]; cross-resistance among classes of compounds has also been demonstrated [16]. Release of subtherapeutic levels of drug over extended periods of time may substantially increase the risk of selection pressure. Also, because of "tailing off," or declining drug levels with time, as is common with many of the slow release devices already mentioned, this risk may be augmented. Also, too frequent dosing by intermittent release methodologies, especially when the same drug is employed for each release, may carry this liability. Choice of the proper intervals and minimization of the number of releases should therefore be considered judiciously.

Regulatory Issues

Drug Residues

Ruminant animals, since they are raised primarily as a food source, present an additional consideration for the design of RRDs, that of residual drug in tissues. When drugs are administered to meat-producing animals, a waiting period called the *withdrawal time* is prescribed by the regulatory agencies, before which the meat may not be slaughtered for human consumption [17]. This withdrawal period varies depending on the drug and the dose used. An RRD must be designed so that the drug residues do not exceed the allowable levels at that time when the animal is intended for food. Otherwise, undesirably long withdrawal periods may be assigned to devices, impacting adversely their attractiveness in the marketplace. Two factors may contribute to having longer withdrawal times imposed on RRDs: "cutoff uncertainty" and bioaccumulation.

Cutoff Uncertainty: Any delivery system for which there is uncertainty concerning the time at which drug ceases to be administered to the animal may present a liability, depending on the magnitude of the uncertainty—the greater the uncertainty, the greater the penalty for the delivery system, paid in increased withdrawal time assessment.

Bioaccumulation: Drugs administered in a sustained release manner
or intermittently, if the intervals are too short, may accumulate in
tissues above the amounts realized when single-dose regimens are employed. This depends on the metabolism of the drug, and new residue
studies must be performed to determine whether this has happened.
Again, the penalty for increased accumulation is assessed by increasing
the withdrawal time [17].

Environmental Impact

RRDs must be designed with the potential adverse effects on the
environment in mind. Sustained release devices, since they chronically
challenge the ecosystem with low levels of biologically active chemical,
may adversely affect other organisms; this may be severe, especially
if the drug has a broad spectrum of activity. Intermittent release
devices may mitigate this liability, provided the number of releases
of drug is kept to the minimum necessary to achieve the desired effect.

II. SUSTAINED RELEASE DEVICES

It is necessary first to define some terms. Sustained release, prolonged
release, slow release, and continuous steady release are some of the
descriptives proposed for products that release relatively low, or subtherapeutic, amounts of drug over an extended period of time. The
aim of all these products is to deliver the active agents in as close
to zero-order kinetics as possible; however, there are varying degrees
of success. *Sustained release* is chosen as a general term for the devices discussed in this section, meaning the release of low levels of
medicament over an extended period of time. *Slow release* refers to
diffusion-controlled or matrix devices that deliver decreasing amounts
of active agent in proportion to the square root of time. *Continuous
release* refers to devices with predominantly internal control, such
as mechanical or osmotic, which come closest to the zero-order aims.
These terms are adapted from many possibilities present in the literature [9-11].

A. Slow Release Devices

Matrix Devices

Matrix devices consist of a compressed inactive carrier, or matrix,
within which is dispersed the active agent. Dissolution of the matrix
allows the slow release of the medicament. These devices are subject
to changes in the rumen environment, such as pH, abrasion, or type
of foodstuffs present. "Tailing off" or reduction in the levels of drug
as time progresses is a feature of these systems. Examples of this

type are the Spanbolet (SmithKline), which delivers sulfamethazine over 5 days for control of bacterioses in cattle and sheep (Fig. 2a), the Cronomintic bolus (Virbac) [19], which uses a polymeric matrix to deliver the anthelmintic levamisole over the grazing season to control roundworm infection, and the Rumensin bolus (Lilly), which uses a compressed polymer matrix confined within a steel tube, open at both ends and protected by a plastic shield, to deliver the growth efficiency enhancer sodium monensin to cattle over 150 days (Fig. 2c). The tube design may overcome the root-of-time problem by presenting a constant surface area of matrix to be eroded by ruminal fluid. This is possible provided erosion is uniform and no pitting occurs, and provided active agent does not diffuse within the matrix.

Diffusion Devices

Diffusion devices control the release of drug through diffusion from a stationary matrix, often through a semipermeable membrane. These devices rely on Fick's Law of diffusion, and drug delivery tails off as the drug concentration within the matrix depletes proportional to the square root of time. An example of an RRD with this mechanism is the morantel sustained release bolus (MSRB) or Paratect (Pfizer), which releases the anthelmintic agent morantel for control of parasites during the cattle grazing season (Fig. 2b) [12].

The RRDs listed above rely on density for retention.

B. Continuous Release Devices

Continuous release devices may be controlled by mechanical or osmotic means. These rely primarily on internal control, thus minimizing the problems imposed by variability of the rumen environment. Two types of continuous release device are currently being developed: the Laby device and the osmotic pump.

Laby Device

The Laby device (after the inventor) also called the Captec device (Captec), comprises a drug-containing polymer matrix within an impervious polyethylene capsule. The formulation, in the form of discrete tablets, is exposed at one end to a small orifice that contacts the rumen environment. Swelling of the tablet exposed at the orifice and subsequent breakdown by the rumen fluid releases the active principle. Pressure from behind the tablets provided by a spring ensures contact of a tablet with the orifice end, preventing rumen contents from interacting with any but the exposed surface. This design provides good control of release, approximating zero-order kinetics, with the amount of drug released determined by the composition of the tablet matrix and the diameter of the orifice.

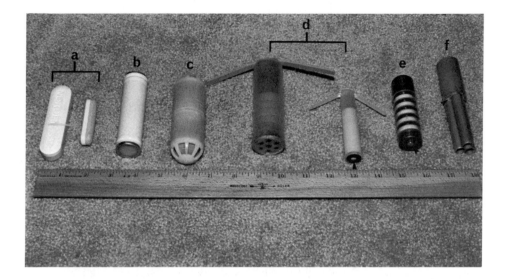

Fig. 2 Examples of rumen retention devices. (a) Two sulfamethazine Spanbolet boluses, the larger one for cattle, the other for sheep. The dark layer contains iron, which increases the density of the bolus. (b) Paratect bolus. The end shows one of the semipermeable membranes, which allow the drug to permeate into the ruminal contents. (c) Rumensin bolus. A cage at each end protects the matrix from direct abrasion by ruminal contents. (d) Two Captec devices, with wings in the unfolded position. The larger device is for cattle, the other for sheep. Note the orifice through which the drug and swollen matrix escape (arrow). (e) The Castex Multidose 130 device. Note the five white sections, which contain the anthelmintic agent. The magnesium spindle is visible at the bottom of the photo (arrow). The other end is the attached steel weight. (f) E-Bolus. Note the three adjacent tubes, which contain the anthelmintic agent. The other end contains weight. One of the conductive rubber electrodes for sensing ruminal contents is visible (arrow).

This device provides retention by the deployment of two "wings," which unfold after administration (Fig. 2d) [10,13].

Osmotic Pump

Details of the mechanism of the osmotic pump are provided in Chapter 4. The osmotically driven RRD for cattle is similar to those for human use, only larger. The cattle device, called the Alzet 2ML4 mini-osmotic pump (Alza) containing the antiparasitic agent Ivomec (Merck) has been developed recently, with steady state achieved in 7 to 14 days and continuing under approximately zero-order release kinetics for approximately 35 days [14]. Regurgitation is prevented by weighting to a density of 2.7 g/ml.

III. INTERMITTENT RELEASE DEVICES

Intermittent (also called pulsatile or pulse) release is the release from a device of discrete doses of active agent separated by intervals in which no drug is presented to the animal. "Intermittent" is the preferred general term here, since "pulse" connotes intervals of equal spacing, whereas "intermittent" implies no temporal restraint of this kind. There are applications in which it may be desirable to deliver doses with unequal spacings. Preferably full therapeutic doses are administered at appropriate times, so the device reproduces manual dosing regimes that have historically given good results after years of practical field experience, or have been justified by controlled husbandry studies.

Anthelmintic drug therapy has offered the greatest initial opportunity for intermittent release RRDs. In Section I.A we considered the epidemiological and economic factors that have made long-term therapy by RRD so attractive for parasite control. Recently, intermittent release devices have been introduced to address some of the issues presented in Section I.B, specifically in the areas of drug residues, environmental impact, and anthelmintic resistance buildup. Two different intermittent release devices are currently in the marketplace, one that operates by erosion and one that is controlled by electronic means. Both are retained in the rumen by suitable weighting to a density of at least 2.5 g/ml.

A. Castex Device

The Castex device, named for the company that began the development some time ago, was brought to the marketplace by a joint venture involving the Wellcome Foundation, Coopers, and Syntex. It is marketed under the tradenames Multidose 130 (Syntex) and Repidose 5 (Coopers) (Fig. 2e); these two products are of identical manufacture. Once the device is in the rumen, erosion of the central magnesium spindle releases each of five successive plastic segments that contain the anthelmintic agent oxfendazole, resulting in a dose of 750 mg for each pulse. The erosion is augmented by a galvanic action produced by reaction between the two dissimilar metals, iron and magnesium, which proceeds once the conductive ruminal fluid has begun to provide the conduit for electron transfer.

The interval between doses averages 23 days, but the erosion is pH dependent, which may contribute to some animal-to-animal variability.

A withdrawal period of 6 months has been recommended in the product
literature, possibly as a result of this uncertainty [18].

B. The Electronic Bolus

The E-Bolus (SmithKline Animal Health Products) is an intermittent
release RRD that releases three therapeutic doses of the anthelmintic
albendazole separated by 31 day intervals (Fig. 2f). Timing for the
device is controlled by a custom-integrated circuit, and power is provided by alkaline watch batteries. The drug, contained in each of
three adjacent tubes, is expelled at once by the action of a gas generator situated at the base of each tube. After immersion in the conductive ruminal fluid for a continuous 10 min period as sensed by two conductive rubber electrodes, the device turns itself on, shuts off the
external sensors, and begins counting for 31 days. After this time,
logic on the chip routes battery energy to the first gas generator,
which releases gas, predominantly carbon dioxide, sufficient to expel
the medication and a protecting rubber stopper. The device then re-
sets, counts an additional 31 days, routes energy to the second gas
generator, whereupon the second dose is released on day 62, and this
is repeated for the last release on day 93. Accuracy is provided by
a quartz crystal, so that precision of release is within 15 min for the
final release. An impervious casing of polypropylene protects the drug
and the electronics from ruminal fluid, and the device operates inde-
pendently of any changes within the rumen environment [20,21].

IV. CONCLUSION

Rumen retention devices are providing a valuable contribution to the
fields of veterinary medicine and animal husbandry. The ruminant
animal is particularly amenable to the application of new systems, and
one can expect new technologies to be applied to RRDs as the success
of the current market introductions becomes apparent. Animal health
drug delivery by devices will continue to prove to be an exciting area
for additional innovation in the future, leading to new advances in
livestock production that will revolutionize traditional concepts in the
years to come.

REFERENCES

1. J. E. Breazile, *Textbook of Veterinary Physiology.* Lea & Febiger,
   Philadelphia, 1971, Chapter 21.
2. R. Nickel, A. Schummer, and E. Seiferle, *The Viscera of Domestic
   Animals.* Sprinter-Verlag, New York, 1973, pp. 147-166.

3. R. Getty, in *Sisson and Grossman's The Anatomy of the Domestic Animals*, Vol. 1, 5th ed., C. Rosenbaum, ed., Saunders, Philadelphia, 1975, Chapter 29.
4. British Agricultural Research Council, *The Nutrient Requirements of Farm Livestock*, no. 2, *Ruminants*. Her Majesty's Stationery Office, London, 1965, pp. 99-104.
5. Agricultural Research Council, *The Nutrient Requirements of Ruminant Livestock*. Commonwealth Agricultural Bureaux, Slough, England, 1980, Chapter 6.
6. W. Haresign, *Recent Advances in Animal Nutrition*. Butterworths, London, 1983, pp. 163-178.
7. Association of Veterinarians in Industry, in *Perspectives in the Control of Parasitic Disease in Animals in Europe* (D. W. Jolly, ed.). Gresham Press, Old Woking, England, 1977, pp. 27-44.
8. D. G. Pope, in *Formulation of Veterinary Dosage Forms* (J. Blodinger, ed.). Dekker, New York, 1983, p. 73.
9. D. G. Pope, in *Formulation of Veterinary Dosage Forms* (J. Blodinger, ed.). Dekker, New York, 1983, pp. 90-95.
10. N. Anderson, *Vet. Parasitol.*, 18:59-66 (1985).
11. A. D. Donald, *Vet. Parasitol.*, 18:121-137 (1985).
12. F. H. M. Borgsteede, A. Kloosterman, D. Oostendorp, and H. Van Tarrij, *Vet. Parasitol.*, 18:39-49 (1985).
13. N. Anderson, R. M. Laby, R. K. Prichard, and D. Hennessy, *Res. Vet. Sci.*, 29:333-341 (1980).
14. D. G. Pope, P. K. Wilkinson, J. R. Egerton, and J. Conroy, *J. Pharm. Sci.*, 74(10):1108-1110 (1985).
15. Commonwealth Scientific and Industrial Research Organization, Division of Animal Health Australian Wool Corporation, in *Resistance to Nematodes to Anthelmintic Drugs* (N. Anderson and P. J. Waller, eds.). CSIRO, Glebe, Australia, 1985, p. 54.
16. Commonwealth Scientific and Industrial Research Organization, Division of Animal Health Australian Wool Corporation, in *Resistance to Nematodes to Anthelmintic Drugs* (N. Anderson and P. J. Waller, eds.). CSIRO, Glebe, Australia, 1985, p. 32.
17. G. Vettorazi, *Handbook of International Food Regulatory Toxicology*. SP Medical and Scientific Books, New York, 1980.
18. Product insert literature, Syntex Multidose 130* Bolus. Syntex, Palo Alto, 1986.
19. C. R. B. Virbac, German Off. Patent, 3 507 987 (1985).
20. B. Bagnall and R. Gyurik, U.S. Patent 4, 564, 363 (1986).
21. H. Wetzel, H. Pfeiffer, A. Jacob, R. Gyurik, and B. Bagnall, *Dtsch. Tieraerztl. Wochenschr.*, 93(9):437-438 (1986).
22. J. L. Riner, R. L. Byford, L. G. Stratton, and J. A. Hair, *Am. J. Vet. Res.*, 43(11):2028-2030 (1982).

21

Special Delivery Devices for Animals

PAUL K. WILKINSON, SERAP BÜYÜKYAYLACI, and JOEL R. ZINGERMAN / Merck Sharp & Dohme Research Laboratories, Division of Merck & Co., Inc., Rahway, New Jersey

I. INTRODUCTION

The success of any treatment program for animals, be it for prophylaxis or therapy, depends on the administration of the correct dose
of medication to the correct subject (single animal or group of animals)
at the appropriate time and frequency. Due to the variations in morpho-
logy and handling characteristics of the animals subject to drug treatment and the varied economic outlooks of different animal handlers
(pet owner or food producer), the veterinary drug manufacturer de-
velops numerous dosage forms and delivery systems for the same medicament. Along with the development of these varied dosage forms followed the development of specialized dosing devices and treatment
regimens. This chapter will consider the major dosage tools and devices utilized in veterinary practice. These discussions will highlight
any special physical characteristics of the drug delivery devices and
special requirements for animal handling as they interact during the
successful administration of drugs to animals.

II. SOLID ORAL MEDICATION

A. Conventional Oral Bolus Delivery Devices

Solid dosage forms for animals, better known as boluses, range in size
up to 4 in. and can weigh in excess of 40 g. Because of the potential
for obstruction, boluses of up to 2 in. in size are given to sheep, goats,
and calves, and the larger sizes are given to cattle. Horses generally
do not receive boluses because these animals are difficult to restrain
and can easily be incorrectly dosed by passage of the bolus into the
trachea instead of the esophagus. The bolus dosage form is discussed
in detail in Chapter 20, Rumen Retention Devices.
     A balling (or bolling) gun is used to administer the bolus dosage
form to large animals. Special balling guns called "pill poppers" are
used to administer solid dosage forms to dogs and cats. A novel gas
propelled apparatus for the oral administration of capsules to animals,
particularly ruminants such as sheep, has recently been patented [1].

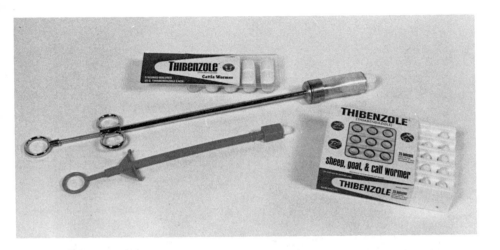

Fig. 1 Examples of balling guns and bolus products. Top: cattle balling gun with bolus inserted. (Courtesy of Ideal Instruments, Chicago.) Bottom: sheep balling gun with bolus inserted. (Courtesy of Merck & Co., Inc., Rahway, New Jersey.)

In its simplest form, the balling gun is basically a plunger-like device having a cup at the terminal end to hold the bolus or capsule to be administered (Fig. 1).

Dosing of large animals with a balling gun is relatively difficult compared to other methods of administration. Large animals must be restrained in a stanchion or by some other means prior to dosing. The bolus is then placed at the base of the tongue, and is delivered by positive displacement of the plunger of the balling gun or other release mechanism which is activated by the fingers. After the bolus is placed in the pharynx, it is allowed to be swallowed by a reflex action, and then passed into the ruminal sac as demonstrated in Fig. 2. There are a variety of balling guns ranging from devices of simple plastic composition, which may be included as a component of a commercial package of boluses, to the more durable stainless steel gun owned by animal handlers, farmers and professionals who administer boluses in higher frequency. Examples of various types of balling guns are shown in Fig. 3.

B. Sustained Release Oral Bolus Delivery Devices

The expanding arena of sustained or controlled release oral bolus delivery systems, used primarily for cattle, has seen the development of drug delivery systems which are larger, more expensive and generally

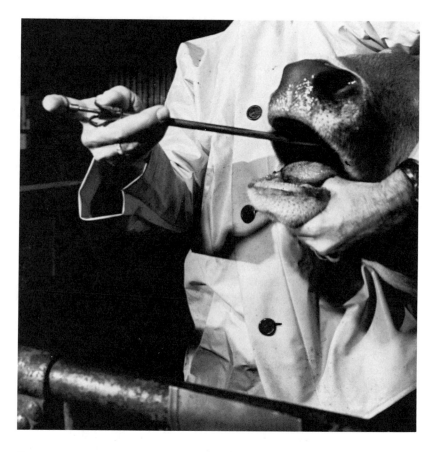

Fig. 2 Dosing cattle with a balling gun. Bolus is released at the base of the tongue. (Courtesy of Merck & Co., Inc., Rahway, New Jersey.)

more prone to damage during dosing than conventional compressed tablet type boluses. Sustained Release (SR) boluses, in the market place and in development, consist of multiple components with outer shells of varying composition (e.g., metal tubes with porous plastic endcaps, plastic tubing with and without external retaining wings, injection molded polymeric materials, etc.). The delivery control of these SR boluses may be electronic, osmotic, diffusional, or device disintegration in nature (see Chapter 20). Any damage to the delivery rate controlling mechanism renders the SR bolus useless.

Sustained release boluses are often administered with standard balling guns. Due to their large sizes, these boluses often extend beyond the protective bolus cup of standard balling guns. Depending

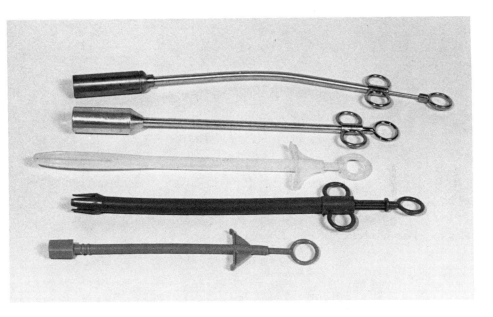

Fig. 3 Assortment of typical balling guns. Top: stainless steel professional model. (Courtesy of Ideal Instruments, Chicago.) Bottom: plastic models (limited lifetime). (Courtesy of Merck & Co., Inc., Rahway, New Jersey.)

on the skill of the animal handler and the cooperation of the animal under treatment, the SR bolus may sometimes be successfully administered without damage to the delivery rate controlling component of the bolus. To preclude or at least minimize the unacceptable potential for bolus damage due to chewing or biting of an inappropriately administered bolus, a specialized balling gun should be considered. While no single design is universally appropriate, the following considerations of user convenience and bolus safety are important (see Fig. 4).

1. *Overall length and weight.* The unit must be manageable in a one-handed operation; an overall length of 0.5 to 0.6 m is acceptable for cattle. It should be long enough to provide sufficient safety margin (distance from the teeth) for the user but not so long as to become unwieldy. With modern metal alloys, construction of a strong, lightweight gun is achievable. To ensure intraesophageal delivery of the SR bolus (i.e., beyond the molars), a bend in the shaft may be considered. This design concept is common in Europe even for standard balling guns. The purpose of the bend (160° at 5-10 cm from the bolus cup) is to assist in positioning of the gun in the mouth for bolus release

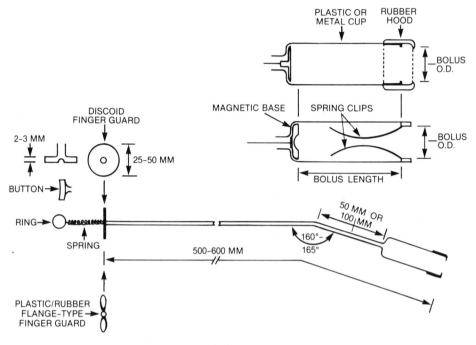

Fig. 4 Balling gun design for controlled release boluses.

into the esophagus. The bend roughly corresponds with the promi-
nence of the tongue and permits the handle of the gun to remain in a
plane parallel to the jaw line (see Fig. 5).

2. *Bolus Cup*. The bolus cup should be of sufficient size to totally enclose the SR bolus during the balling operation. There should
be a positive retention mechanism (i.e., magnetic, spring clips, or
shroud) to preclude the premature release of the SR bolus. The bolus
cup should be composed of a material sufficiently resilient to prevent
accidental crushing, tearing, or burring, of the bolus or the cup.
It should be easily lubricated to improve slip, which minimizes trauma
to the buccal and esophageal mucosa.

3. *Release Mechanism*. The release mechanism should result in a
positive displacement delivery, that is, the release mechanism must be
restrained in the ready position and the bolus must not be released
without movement (release) of the shaft or retaining clips. The standard release mechanisms (spring loaded plunger, trigger, moving shaft,
etc.) are suitable as long as premature release of the SR bolus can
be avoided.

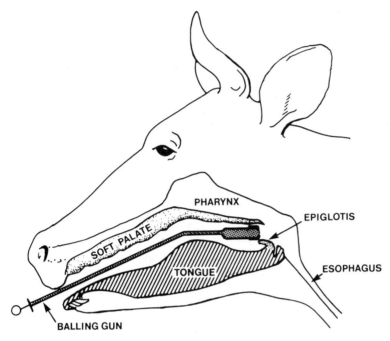

PHARYNX

EPIGLOTIS

SOFT PALATE

TONGUE

ESOPHAGUS

BALLING GUN

Fig. 5 Bolus administration technique for controlled release boluses.

To ensure the integrity of the SR bolus, extreme care should be exercised in handling the bolus before placement into an appropriately designed balling gun as well as during administration.

III. LIQUID ORAL MEDICATIONS

Solutions, emulsions, and suspensions are the major liquid dosage forms for oral administration to animals. The selection of one dosage form over the others depends on the physicochemical properties of the drug to be formulated, the type of action desired (immediate or sustained), and the animal to be treated.

The method of administration of liquid oral dosage forms primarily depends on the species of animal for which the drug treatment is intended. Equine are dosed by esophageal devices because they generally resist all dosing procedures. There exists a high potential for aspiration of the liquid medication with the drenching procedure. Young animals are commonly dosed by esophageal devices, as well as cattle, sheep and goats.

A. Esophageal Delivery Devices

Most commonly used esophageal delivery devices are stomach tubes of varying length, internal and external diameters, and composition. The usual tube size for equine administration is 1/2 to 5/8 in (12.5-16 mm) external diameter. Stomach tubes which are made of silicone rubber, polyvinyl chloride, Tygon, polyethylene, cloth reinforced red rubber, etc., must be flexible and strong enough to resist kinking. Silicone tubes maintain a constant degree of flexibility over a wide range of temperatures and reduce adherence to tissues or fluids due to their hydrophobic, nonwetting surfaces, and are preferred over other types of materials.

Once an appropriate stomach tube is identified, it is lubricated at one end, passed through the horse's nostril and down into the stomach for dosing. A funnel is placed at the other end of the tube, held above the horse's head and the medication is poured down the tube. For ease of administration, the medication needs to flow readily and cleanly through the tube. A dose consisting of an aqueous solution or suspension is preferred due to its ease of administration and rinsing of the dose with water to assure complete delivery. Administration of medication to a horse using a stomach tube is shown in Fig. 6.

Special techniques are required to insure that the stomach tube is inserted into the esophagus and not into the trachea. If it is passed only to the thoracic inlet, fluids may return up along the tube when there is a partial obstruction of the tube-opening by the esophageal wall. In such cases, there is a danger of the fluids entering the trachea. Following administration of the medication and the rinsing water, the contents of the tube should be blown out, and the end of the tube should be closed to prevent siphoning of fluids as the tube is being withdrawn from the stomach.

The flow of the product through tubing should be checked to assure that the animal will be treated in a reasonable period of time. A vertically suspended Tygon tube (6-1/2 ft long, internal diameter = 3/8 in.) can be used to test a product. As a rule of thumb, the maximum time of flow of 300 ml of product, through the tubing previously rinsed with water, should not exceed 60 sec. If flow rates are not satisfactory, viscosity adjustments may be necessary to achieve desirable flow rates.

B. Drenching Devices

Oral liquid medications are administered to cattle, sheep and goats using a method called drenching. Drenching can be done by using drenching syringes or drenching guns.

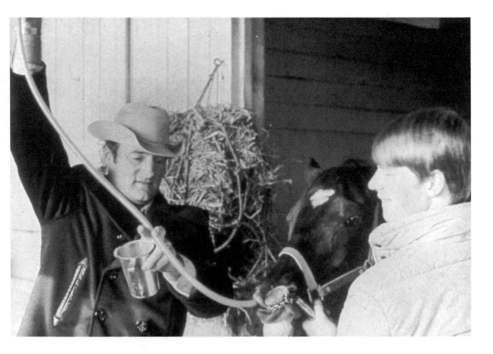

Fig. 6 Administration of liquid oral medication to a horse by means of an esophageal delivery device (stomach tube). (Courtesy of Merck & Co., Inc., Rahway, New Jersey.)

Drenching Syringes

Drenching (dosing) syringes are used to dispense liquid medication for oral or rectal administration to animals. These syringes have either preset volumes or a dosage dial that can be set to deliver the desired volume of the liquid product. The preset volume syringe can be either all metal (usually heavy chrome plating over brass) ranging in size from 2 to 32 oz, or it may consist of a metallic dose pipe attached to a 2-oz rubber bulb (Fig. 7, top and middle).

Drenching syringes are loaded by placing the dose pipe or the nozzle in the liquid and drawing the liquid up into the chamber. For a successful application, the product should have sufficient viscosity so that after it is pulled into the syringe, it does not drip during transfer to the animal's mouth. Viscosity adjustments can be made by using appropriate thickening agents, which promote thixotropy.

The medicine dropper is a single dose drenching device in its simplest form. This device is most suitable for small pets (i.e., cats and dogs as shown in Fig. 8) and neonates of larger species.

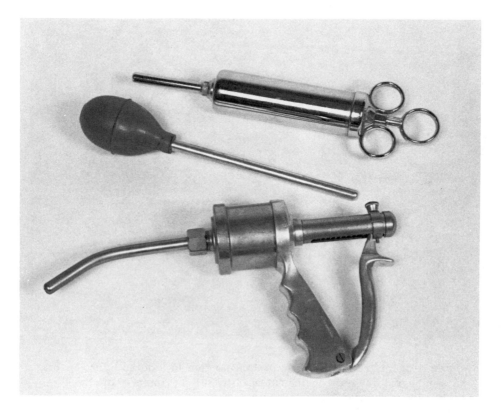

Fig. 7 Examples of drenching devices. Top: 4 oz. drenching (dose) syringe with metal plunger; plunger rod is calibrated in 1/2 oz. increments. This device is easily disassembled for cleaning and sterilization. Middle: 2 oz. bulb syringe consisting of rubber ball and chrome-plated dose pipe. Bottom: 2 oz. single-dose drenching gun with plunger calibrated in 1/2 oz. increments. Dose volume adjustment is by handle screwing into the barrel via special bushing. (Courtesy of Ideal Instruments, Chicago.)

Drenching Guns

Drenching guns can be single-dose or multidose depending on the application and the number of animals to be treated. A single-dose drenching gun is loaded the same way as the drenching syringe. A slightly viscous solution or suspension reduces dripping. A very viscous product is undesirable because it is difficult to draw into the chamber, and the operator can be rapidly exhausted trying to eject the dose. Addition of a wetting agent may help wet the inside walls of the chamber

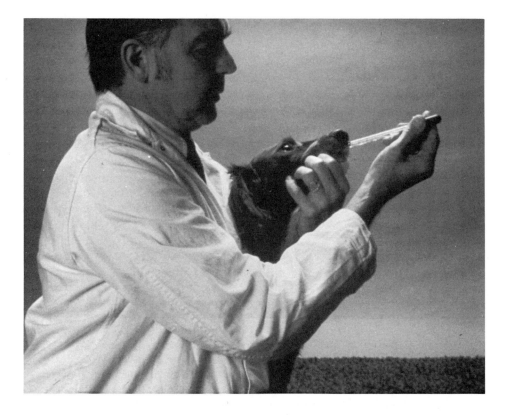

Fig. 8 Administration of liquid oral medication to a dog using the medicine dropper type of single-dose syringe. (Courtesy of Merck & Co.,
Inc., Rahway, New Jersey.)

and the nozzle, making it easier to operate the gun. A multidose drenching gun is fed from a bulk pack strapped on the operator's back
or attached to the belt. The product is expected to flow readily from
the reservoir to the gun and completely refill the measuring chamber
after each dose is ejected.

Single-Dose Gun

The single-dose gun is primarily designed for large-volume administration. It is filled by pushing the piston to the end of its stroke and
then drawing it back after dipping the nozzle into the liquid product.
The nozzle is then introduced into the mouth of the animal. When using
a shoulder-activated gun, the handle is held by one hand and the operator's shoulder is placed against the plunger end to push the piston

forward and discharge its contents. The other hand is free to manipulate the animal.

Single-dose guns are available in versions with maximum capacities of 30, 60, 120 and 150 ml. They are ideal for use with dairy herds or small flocks. In some single-dose drenchers, the dose can be set by adjusting the movement of the plunger by either the handle screwing into the barrel via a special bushing (Fig. 7, bottom) or by a sliding scale locked by a screw with a revolving pad.

Multi-Dose Gun

Large-volume, single-dose drench guns can be used to administer doses of product in step quantities. Several animals may be dosed before the gun is refilled by setting the gun to deliver small quantities with each trigger pull.

Automatic Gun

Automatic drench guns are designed for quick administration of liquids to a large number of animals. The chamber fills directly from a large-volume reservoir after ejection of the dose. Automatic guns have calibrated chambers and some means of volume adjustment. Some guns are designed to deliver fixed doses of liquid. Automatic drenchers are available in 30, 60, and 120 ml models; the last two drenchers are designed primarily for use with cattle, while the 30 ml unit is suitable for either cattle or sheep. The movement of the drench gun piston either in its intake or discharge stroke is limited by axially staggered stops projecting from the piston rod and engaging a dose-selecting disc mounted on the tool body. This adjuster has apertures to allow all the projections to pass unhindered except for a selected projection which limits the piston movement to give the required dose. Figures 9 and 10 show a drench gun-backpack assembly and the administration of medication to cattle using such a unit. Fig. 11 shows a Phillips 20-mL MKII automatic drencher.

Liquid drench formulations to be used with automatic drench guns must remain fluid at field use temperature conditions. The average hand grip strength for repeated dosing is 50 lbs/in^2. Formulations requiring higher strength can cause operator exhaustion. Extensive testing of the formulation and the dosing device is needed to evaluate the ease of use and the compatibility with the device components [2].

Current changes in the nature of veterinary chemicals and their method of administration have led to the design of specific devices and the use of appropriately selected materials for the component parts that come in contact with these chemicals. Developments have modified the drench guns for versatile applications. Figure 12 shows a precision, low volume syringe capable of switching from drenching to injecting. Specialized applicators with different nozzle spray patterns

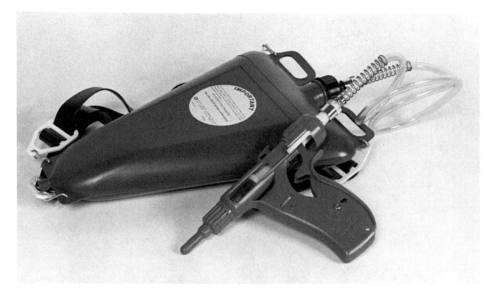

Fig. 9 Automatic drench gun-backpack assembly. This Sure-Shot applicator gun with dose volume adjustment is connected to a backpack via flexible draw-off tubing. (Courtesy of Instrument Supplies, Ltd, Hamilton, New Zealand, and Mesa, Arizona.)

and quick-change dosage adjustment mechanism have enabled drenchers to be used for topical application of products to animals (Fig. 13).

IV. SEMISOLID ORAL MEDICATIONS

Paste and gel products have gained popularity over some other dosage forms such as the bolus primarily because they are easier to handle and quicker to administer. Moreover, they lend themselves to pet owner treatment. Pastes and gels are adaptable dosage forms for all animals. It is important that this type of medication be tenacious or sticky so that it cannot be worked out of the animal's mouth. The formulation must also be fluid at all use temperatures so that an administration time of not more than 2 or 3 sec is possible. Ideally the paste or gel formulation should be as tasteless as possible, since new or strange tastes tend to be objectionable to most animals, making the administration process more difficult. The type of administration device used for pastes is a function of the number of animals to be treated at a single time and the ease of restraining the animals.

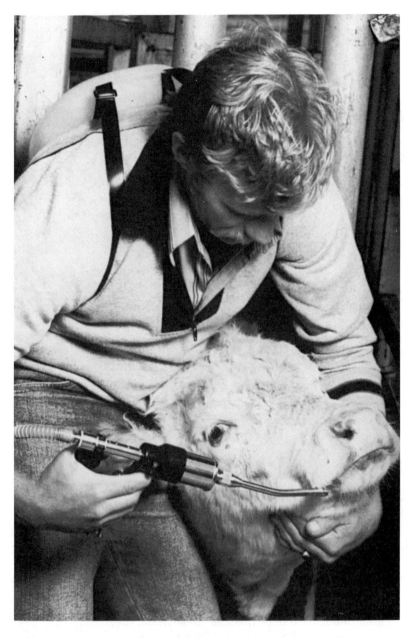

Fig. 10 Administration of liquid oral medication to cattle, demonstrating the use of the Phillips Automatic Drencher. (Courtesy of N. J. Phillips Pty Ltd, Dee Why, Australia.)

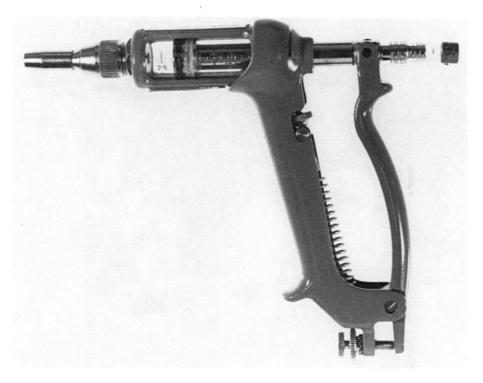

Fig. 11 The Phillips 20 ml MK-II Automatic Drencher, a dosing gun
made for administration of all solution and suspension drenches. Dose
volume can be checked on the calibrated transparent cylinder, where
adjustable doses of 0 to 20 ml are marked. (Courtesy of N. J. Phillips
Pty Ltd, Dee Why, Australia.)

A. Single-Dose Syringes

A convenient device configuration for administering paste formulations
to large animals such as horses is that of a syringe. This may be either
a single dose (i.e., one syringe per animal) for use by the pet owner
or a multiple-dose syringe for use by the professional. Single-dose
syringes are typically capable of treating horses weighing up to 1250
lb in 250 lb subdivisions. The syringe tip is placed through the interdigital space and the paste formulation expelled within 2 to 3 sec. Figures 14 and 15 show typical paste dosing syringes, while Fig. 16 shows
a horse receiving a dose of an anthelmintic from its owner, using a
single-dose syringe.

Anthelmintics are administered to piglets as paste formulations
because this administration technique does not induce significant trauma

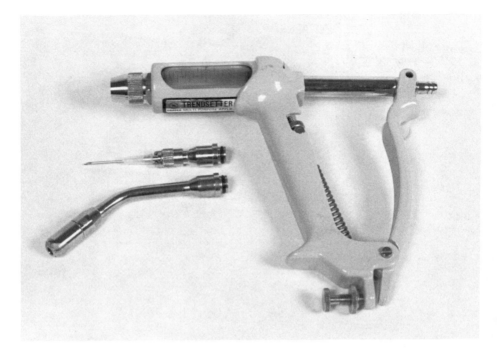

Fig. 12 The Trendsetter Multipurpose Applicator, an example of inter-changeable injection needles and drenching nozzle. (Courtesy of Coopers Animal Health, Inc., Kansas City, Missouri.)

to small animals. The delivery devices are designed for treatment of as many as 10 piglets per syringe. Figure 17 presents a typical 10 dose syringe. The sawtooth rail or notch is flexible and extends into the syringe barrel when a dose is expelled. The individual notches on the syringe barrel are spaced equidistant, so that the dose of paste displaced between notches provides a predetermined quantity of drug. The user pushes the plunger with enough force to bend the notch or sawtooth, which in turn enters the syringe barrel. The differential force encountered as the next plunger notch (tooth) pushes against the syringe barrel indicates the completion of delivery of the desired dose. The multidose syringe system depicted requires a paste formu-lation that is highly thixotropic, to preclude inadvertent expulsion or leakage of the formulation between administrations. This device presents the important attributes for a veterinary dosing: accuracy, convenience, and economy. Delivery devices with other dose-setting configurations (e.g., interlocking rings) are available for low dose rate treatment. These devices must be set for each dose.

B. Multiple-Dose Cartridges

Large animals, such as cattle which are easily restrained, can be conveniently dosed with a multidose cartridge system that is delivered
by use of paste guns not unlike ordinary paste caulking guns (see
Fig. 18). Figure 19 shows a multiple-dose paste cartridge for professional administration to horses. The paste gun has been modified so
that the pistol grip, when fully depressed, delivers sufficient drug
formulation to treat a full-grown animal. The number of notches advanced per plunger depression can be reduced for dosing animals of
lower body weights. The accuracy and precision of such a device is
excellent provided there are no air pockets present in the filled cartridge. A paste cartridge generally delivers approximately 20 full dose
treatments (for cattle approximately 20 g each). It is not unusual
for a cartridge to contain some air bubbles—from extemporaneous filling
or during a manufacturing operation. Product quality standards dic-
tating maximum deviation in individual dose weights of (mean ± 15%)
are readily achievable with this delivery device.

Administration of a paste formulation with the cartridge system
requires that the animal be restrained in a stanchion. The paste is
delivered on the posterior portion of the tongue, and unless the product has an objectionable taste, the animals swallows the dose with a
detectable enjoyment (Fig. 20). The paste cartridge nozzle can be
removed and interchanged with nozzles of different configurations if
desired. Additional paste cartridge gun units are available which are
modifications of the basic caulking gun as shown in Fig. 21.

V. INJECTABLE MEDICATIONS

Medications are administered to animals parenterally when an immediate
action is needed, when it is difficult to administer medication by the
oral route, or when the drug is ineffective by other routes. For most
animals, administration of a drug by intramuscular or subcutaneous
injection is a convenient means adaptable for the treatment of large
numbers of animals.

Injectable medications are acceptable if they:

1. Cause minimum irritation at the site of injection
2. Cause no permanent damage to the tissues
3. Are safe and efficacious

Injectable medications are usually isotonic aqueous solutions with
pH between 7 and 8. Other forms, such as suspensions or emulsions,
may be considered when the drug lacks sufficient aqueous solubility.
When suspensions or emulsions are used as injectables, the bioavailabil-

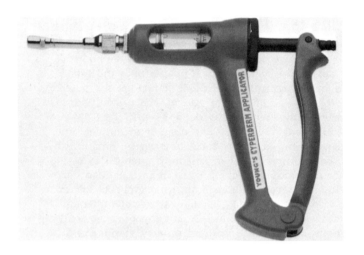

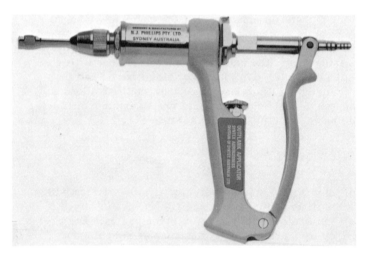

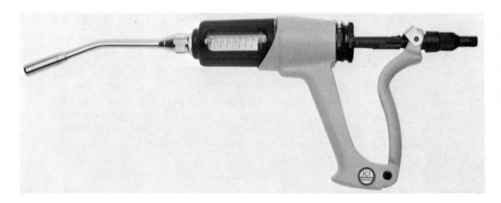

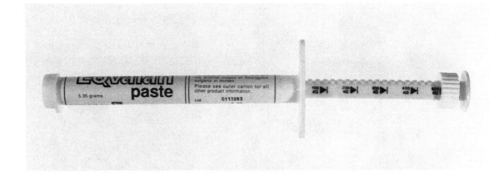

Fig. 14 Single-dose syringe for horse anthelmintic product. The constant bore barrel (including the tip) permits rapid delivery of paste product. Lock nut on plunger is for setting administration dose by animal weight. (Courtesy of Merck & Co., Inc., Rahway, New Jersey.)

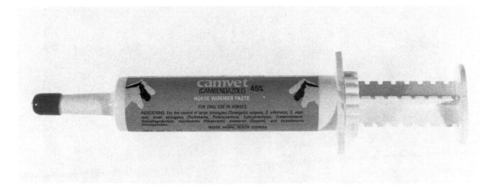

Fig. 15 Single-dose paste syringe, featuring removable protective tip cap and adjustable ring on plunger rod for dose adjustment. (Courtesy of Merck & Co., Inc., Rahway, New Jersey.)

Fig. 13 Automatic drench guns with specialized applicators: examples of different nozzles, which provide variable spray patterns with quick-change dosage adjustment mechanism. Special spray patterns offer a convenient means for application of topical products to animals. (Courtesy of N. J. Phillips Pty Ltd, Dee Why, Australia.)

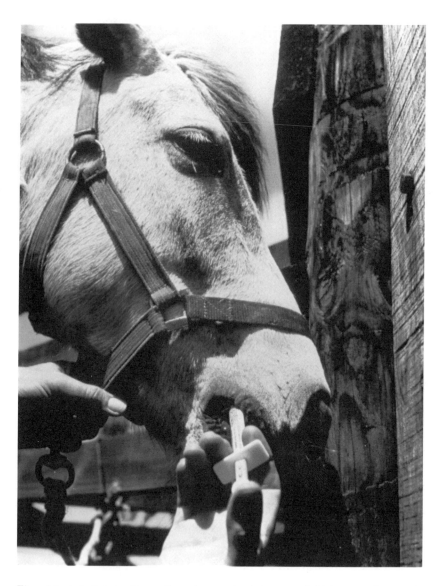

Fig. 16 Administration of paste product to an adult horse via a unit dose syringe. Note syringe placement into the interdigital space. (Courtesy of Merck & Co., Inc., Rahway, New Jersey.)

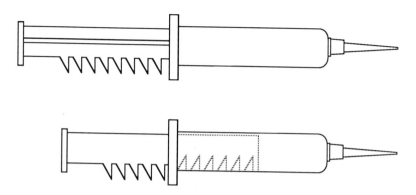

Fig. 17 Single-dose syringe for piglet anthelmintic product showing sawtooth rail on plunger and removable tip cap (top) and sawtooth rail inserted within the barrel (bottom). Each tooth is equivalent to one dose. This same syringe design (sawtooth plunger) may also be used with other species. For instance, horses, for administration of anti-inflammatory agents in pastes which mask objectionable tastes and other medication requiring discrete dosages. (Courtesy of Merck & Co., Inc., Rahway, New Jersey.)

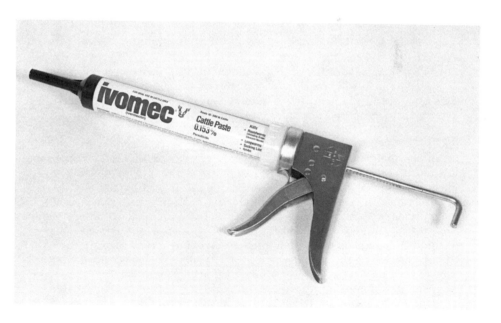

Fig. 18 Multiple-dose paste cartridge with dosing gun. Each full depression of the trigger expels sufficient paste product to treat 300 lb of animal body weight. (Courtesy of Merck & Co., Inc., Rahway, New Jersey.)

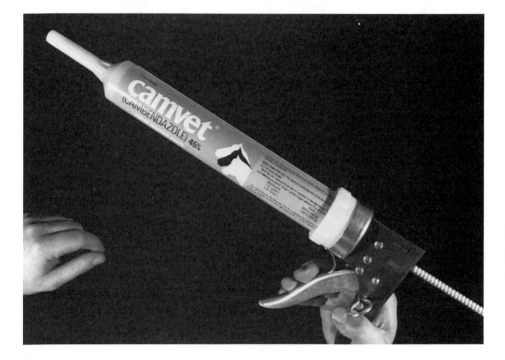

Fig. 19 Multiple-dose horse paste cartridge with paste cartridge in holder. Each full depression of the trigger expels the required dose. The ring-pin in the handle is a safety feature. (Courtesy of Merck & Co., Inc., Rahway, New Jersey.)

ity of the drug may be affected (delayed effect may be seen as opposed to the immediate action), and encapsulation at the site of injection is likely. Water solubility of the drug may be improved by the addition of cosolvents such as alcohol, propylene glycol, glycerol formal, and polyethylene glycol. In case of drugs that are unstable in water, water-miscible solvents may be used. However, this approach becomes complicated if the animal receiving such a solvent is a food animal; then, the disposition of the vehicle as well as the drug may need to be determined, and long-term toxicity studies must be conducted.

The selection of appropriate equipment for parenteral administration should be based on the following considerations.

1. Number of animals to be treated at one time
2. Volume of formulation to be administered

   (a) Dose volume specification (calibration) and flexibility

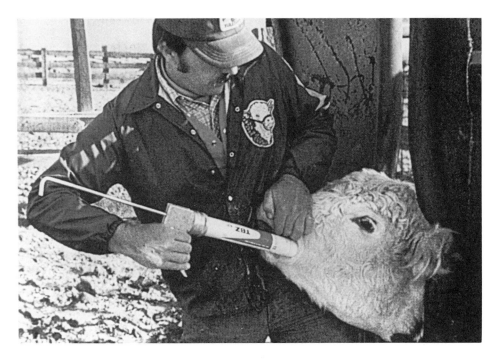

Fig. 20 Administration of anthelmintic paste product. Nozzle of paste gun is inserted into mouth to permit placement of paste at the base of the tongue. (Courtesy of Merck & Co., Inc., Rahway, New Jersey.)

      (b) Dose volume precision and accuracy
      (c) Dose volume setting: (i) Screw-type mechanism with a lock nut or (ii) Locking mechanism

3. Contact stability/physical compatibility of product with the components of the equipment and with the materials of construction
4. Viscosity of the formulation to be administered

      (a) Ease of volumetric chamber filling
      (b) Ease of expulsion of formulation

5. Ease of use and cleaning
6. Ease of adjusting tension on return spring
7. Ease of sterilization

Administration devices can be classified into four groups: unit dose syringes, multidose syringes, automatic syringes, and jet injectors.

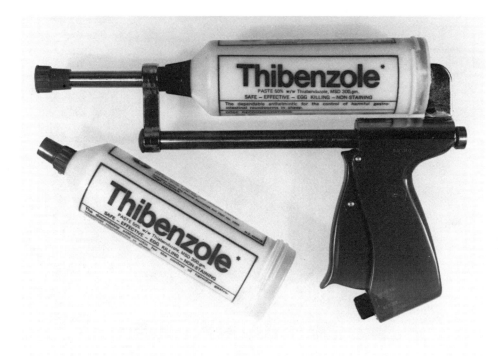

Fig. 21 Multiple-dose paste cartridge with dosing gun for sheep, showing interchangeable nozzle with tip cap. (Courtesy of Merck & Co.,
Inc., Rahway, New Jersey.)

A. Unit Dose Syringes

Unit dose syringes are used for injection of small number of animals
with a small volume of formulation. Unit dose syringes are available
as disposable or resterilizable nylon, polypropylene, or glass with
centered or eccentric, and slip or Luer-lock tips. Unit dose prefilled
and sterilized packs are also available.

Multicompartment syringes have been designed to mix drug powder
and liquid components before administration so that a drug that is unstable in solution or suspension form can be maintained until needed
in its most stable form. These syringes usually have two separate
compartments where the drug and the liquid are kept. Then the liquid
is mixed with the drug by piercing a separating diaphragm, pressure
rupture of the diaphragm, or pressure dislodgement of a separating
system [3-5].

B. Multidose Syringes

Multidose syringes are designed to treat small herds or isolated animals when an automatic syringe is not necessary. Most multidose syringes have the dose metered by slots or striations on the plunger. Some systems utilize a plunger with a track and a barrel with a track follower. Each stage of the track and groove corresponds to a move of the plunger that dispenses a set dose [6]. Multidose syringes enable the administration of several doses without the need for reloading the syringe or measuring the plunger movement against a graduated scale. Figure 22 shows a multidose syringe with a graduated, transparent cylinder that is virtually unbreakable; a simple rotary dial permits dose settings of 1, 2, 3, 4, or 5 ml.

C. Automatic Syringes

Automatic syringes are used for treating a large number of animals with large volumes of medication. In automatic syringes return and filling to a preset volume are accomplished automatically so that the process is quick and not very tiring. The bulk formulation is usually stored in plastic containers, and the formulation is fed to the automatic syringe either directly into the chamber or through the handle via plastic tubing.

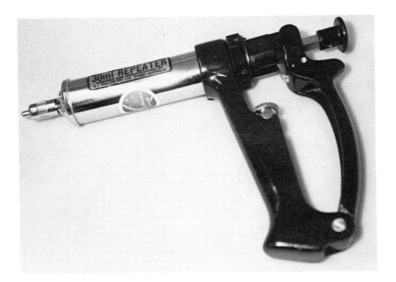

Fig. 22 The Phillips 30 ml Repeater, a multidose syringe designed for vaccination of small herds or isolated animals. (Courtesy of N. J. Phillips Pty Ltd, Dee Why, Australia.)

Fisons Limited's Automatic Multidose Injector uses the chamber-fill method; a bulk dose pack is attached directly to the barrel of the syringe [7]. N. J. Phillips (Australia) also uses the chamber-fill method in their 1 ml Automatic Poultry Injector MK-II (Fig. 23) and the Phillips 2 ml Automatic Vaccinator (Fig. 24). The 2 ml Automatic Vaccinator is available in three different versions: with 100 ml bottle adapter, with flexible pack adapter, and with connecting attachment to draw-off systems.

With the handle-fill design, the formulation is fed into the chamber through the handle via plastic tubing dipped into a bulk formulation container. Bulk containers can be carried around the neck or the waist, or as a harness backpack. This design is commonly used with automatic syringes. A handle-fill automatic injector being used to dose sheep is shown in Fig. 25.

Specialized automatic syringes have been developed to satisfy the needs of animal growers. High-rate vaccination injectors are available for use in stock farms raising many small animals or birds. Such injectors provide accurate dosage and precision in the point and angle of injection by electronic or pneumatic movement of the syringe. Agri-Bio Corporation (Ithaca, New York) markets the Biojector high-speed vaccinator, which increases chick vaccination rate by two to three times over hand or automatic injection techniques. Another specialized automatic injector has been designed by Agrimatic Corporation (Cerritos, California) for inoculation of fowl eggs with a heater [8]. The heater serves to sterilize the area of the shell when the hole is made, seals the hole by coagulating egg albumin, and sterilizes the needle between inoculations.

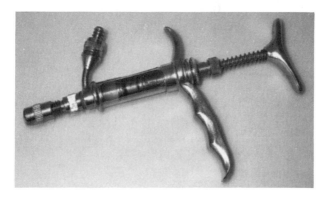

Fig. 23 The Phillips 1 ml Automatic Poultry Injector MK-II, an automatic syringe with a chamber-fill design specially made for mass treatment of poultry. (Courtesy of N. J. Phillips Pty Ltd, Dee Why, Australia.)

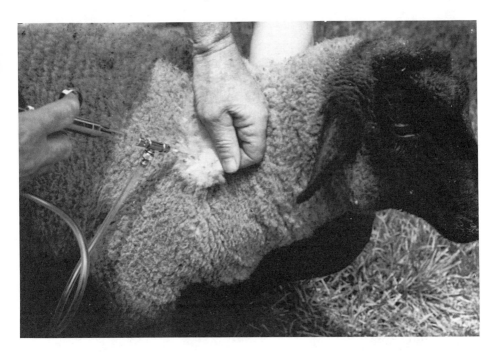

Fig. 24 The Phillips 2 ml Automatic Vaccinator, used in the inoculation of sheep. This automatic syringe with a chamber-fill design and connecting attachment to the draw-off system is used for the administration of sera and vaccines to sheep, cattle, swine, and poultry. (Courtesy of N. J. Phillips Pty Ltd, Dee Why, Australia.)

Breakage of needles may be a problem when vaccinating active livestock. A syringe with a flexible needle coupling that allows lateral needle deflection has been designed to alleviate this problem. Western Instrument Company (Denver) markets the Flexible Luer-Lock Needle Adaptor, which reduces the incidence of bent, broken, or embedded needles, yet is rigid enough to hold the needle and penetrate tough hides.

D. Jet Injectors

In a jet injector, a dose of liquid medication is expelled under extremely high pressure through an orifice disposed against or adjacent to the epidermis of the animal. The hypodermic jet injection apparatus commonly used on humans can also be used in veterinary medicine, but only with small animals. A modified jet injector (Vet-Jet) has been developed for use with larger animals. Vet-Jet uses a "crowned" jet

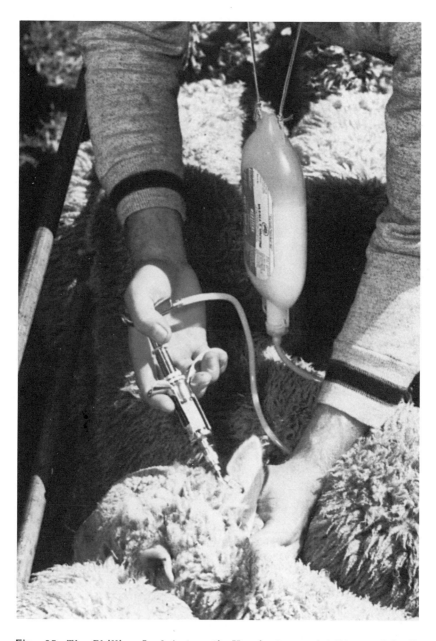

Fig. 25 The Phillips 5 ml Automatic Vaccinator model 74, used in the inoculation of sheep. This automatic syringe, exemplifying the handle-fill design, is used for all sera and vaccines for mass treatment of live-stock. Dose adjustment is variable through a range from 0.5 to 5.0 ml. (Courtesy of N. J. Phillips Pty Ltd, Dee Why, Australia.)

nozzle, which is optimal for use on fur of animals. A force intensifier
is added to double the injection force, and a larger (2.25 ml) accessory
vaccine pump section is used to supplement the 1 ml human vaccine
section. A backpack frame permits the foot-operated injector to be
back mounted and operated by hand while in this position. This provides freedom of motion to the operator working in an animal pen [9].

The advantage of the jet injector is that it provides a fast, sterile
technique for vaccinating large numbers of animals. Simplicity of operation provides speed equal to or surpassing conventional-type injectors.
Front-end and feed-needle assemblies can be cold sterilized or auto-
claved [9].

VI. IMPLANT MEDICATIONS

Implants are dosage forms in which multiple doses of drug are stored
at a site in body tissues to release active drug over a period of time.
Implant candidates must have high potency, so that the size of the
implant can be kept at a minimum to provide a practical means of medication. Implants are designed to maintain a constant blood level and
tissue concentration of an active ingredient above the minimum effective
concentration. Such a dosage form reduces the sawtooth oscillations
of drug levels that accompany periodic dosing. Implantable systems
represent a practical dosage form for use in animals. This approach
minimizes the number of times the animal must be handled and does
not suffer from the cosmetic factors, which tend to minimize the use
of this route of administration for human dosage forms.

Historically, the subcutaneous implantation of drug pellets was
the first approach to prolonged drug activity. Pellets are made by
compressing drug powders—with or without excipients—into small
cylindrical masses, which are then implanted into subcutaneous tissue
by means of a pellet injector (implanter). Subcutaneous tissue is rich
in fat but poor in nerve network and hemoperfusion; these properties
make it an ideal location for implants. It is readily accessed, drug
absorption is slow, and the introduction of implants (foreign materials)
causes low reactivity. One problem with pellet implants is the lack of
control of the drug release.

Techniques of controlled drug delivery have been utilized in preparing implants for animals. The Compudose implant (marketed by
Eli Lilly) releases estradiol for up to one year. It is composed of a
drug-free Silastic cylinder coated with a layer of Silastic containing
20% estradiol. Such a design warrants a relatively constant release
rate since the coating is thin and the loading is high.

Synovex C and S implants, marketed by Syntex, release progesterone and estradiol benzoate for growth promotion in calves and steers,

respectively. Synovex H implants release testosterone and estradiol benzoate for growth promotion and feed efficiency in heifers. The release rate of the drug is a function of the dissolution of the pellet in the ear, with growth promotion effect lasting approximately 90 to 120 days.

Ralgro implants (International Minerals and Chemical Corp.) release the nonsteroidal anabolic agent zeranol, which is widely used commercially for increasing the rate of weight gain and improving feed conversion in cattle and sheep. Zeranol has been approved for use in cattle as a 36 mg dose for subcutaneous ear implantation with a 65 day withdrawal period, and for use in feedlot lambs as a 12 mg implant with a 40 day withdrawal period [10].

Syncro-Mate-B (marketed by Ceva Laboratories) is a hydrogel implant fabricated from a hydrophilic polymer of polyethylene glycomethacrylate to contain 6 mg of Norgestomet for estrus synchronization. This small (2 × 21 mm) device can be easily inserted into the animal's ear by a specially designed implanter. The implant is used together with an injection containing Norgestomet and estradiol valerate in sesame oil; the combined treatment leads to much higher incidence of pregnancy in treated animals.

Osmotic drug delivery devices have also been evaluated as implants. Osmotic devices are fabricated by encapsulating a concentrated drug solution inside a collapsible compartment with a delivery orifice and impermeable flexible walls with a sealed layer of osmotic active salt on its external surface, which is contained within a semipermeable membrane. When an osmotic system is implanted, the semipermeable membrane controls the rate at which the osmotic agent imbibes extracellular fluid. The osmotic pressure exerted on the collapsible compartment forces the contents of the drug reservoir through the orifice. These types of systems are dealt with in Chapter 4, Osmotic Pumps.

An implant may be perceived by the body as a foreign agent and cause irritation at the site. The acute phase of the inflammatory reaction leads to the formation of exudate and fibrinous network at the affected site. The presence of an implant requires major adaptation by the host; the implant may remain as an incompletely covered foreign body with a barrier of connective tissue forming between it and the surface epithelium. This may block the release of the drug from the implant or change the release properties. Leaching out of any additives from implants may also lead to toxic reactions. The problem of device rejection from the implant site has been encountered; oxytetracycline has been incorporated into the Compudose implant to prevent infection at the site of implantation. This addition has significantly improved the overall retention of the implant and its performance.

Implants are available in various shapes and sizes, and the devices for this purpose differ in configuration and in mechanism of action. The most common implant sites are the ear and the neck.

A. Pellet Implant Devices

Pellet implanting devices are designed to administer a specific size of pellet. Pellets are stored singly or as groups in a cartridge. Depending on the implant device used, cartridges can be manually fed to the device individually, gang loaded, or multidose loaded. The choice of cartridge loading depends on the number of animals to be dosed, the availability of the particular cartridge, and the implant devices on the market. Figure 26 shows an automatic pellet implanter equipped with a plastic clip containing 10 implants. The device is being used for the Synovex implants. A new design in pellet implanters is seen with the SX10 gun for Synovex implants (see Fig. 27). This implant gun features a needle that deposits implant pellets in proper position and automatically retracts from the ear, eliminating the need to withdraw the needle manually. Figure 28 shows the multidose implant gun with cartridge load used with the Ralgro implant system. The specially designed implant gun used with Syncro-Mate-B implants is shown in Fig. 29.

Implantation to the ear using pellet implanters (see Fig. 30) entails the following steps.

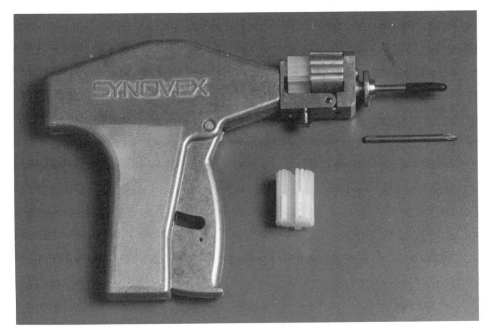

Fig. 26 The Synovex implanter, an automatic implanter with a plastic clip containing 10 implants. (Courtesy of Syntex Animal Health, Inc., West Des Moines, Iowa.)

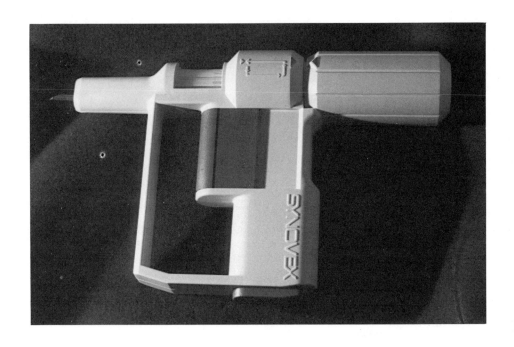

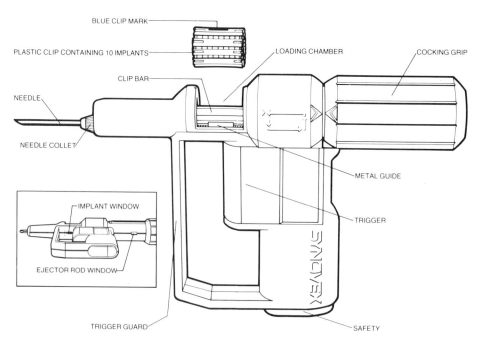

BLUE CLIP MARK

PLASTIC CLIP CONTAINING 10 IMPLANTS

CLIP BAR

LOADING CHAMBER

COCKING GRIP

NEEDLE

NEEDLE COLLET

METAL GUIDE

IMPLANT WINDOW

TRIGGER

EJECTOR ROD WINDOW

TRIGGER GUARD

SAFETY

Fig. 27 The SX10 gun for Synovex implants. (Courtesy of Syntex Animal Health, Inc., West Des Moines, Iowa.)

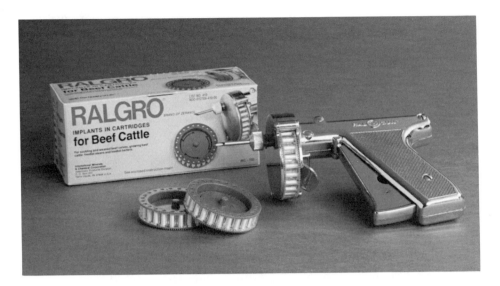

Fig. 28 The Ralogun implanter gun, an automatic pellet implanter with cylindrical implants in plastic cartridge disks. (Courtesy of International Minerals and Chemical Corp., Terre Haute, Indiana.)

1. *Restraint.* Confine the animal in a squeeze chute or head gate. Restrain the animal's head to restrict movement.

2. *Site preparation.* Select an implant site on the outer surface of the ear. The site should be approximately midway between the tip and the fleshy base. Clip the hair and scrub the site with a brush and disinfectant.

3. *Affix sterile needle.* Take needle from tray of disinfectant solution and affix to implanter.

4. *Load the implanter.* Remove the sheathed implant from its foil pack. Be sure to keep the implant dry at all times. Pull implanter plunger back, place implant in slot, and release plunger to rest on the implant. To activate for implantation, push implant out of the sheath a distance of 1/16 in.

5. *Insert implant* (a) With beveled side of needle away from the skin, pick up skin of the ear and penetrate skin surface. Do not penetrate cartilage. Expect the animal to flinch as skin is pricked and penetrated. (b) With needle parallel to the ear surface, push needle between skin and cartilage (subcutaneously) until all the needle is under the skin. (c) Holding the needle all the way in to the hub, push the plunger all the way in, ejecting the implant under the skin of the ear. Be careful not to let the needle be forced back as the plunger

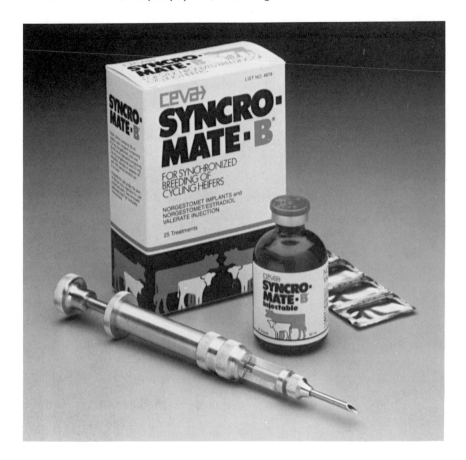

Fig. 29 The Syncro-Mate-B implanter, a single-dose-loading implant gun. Implants are packaged in foil, as shown; also shown is the injectable solution used in conjunction with the implant. (Courtesy of Ceva Laboratories, Inc., Overland Park, Kansas.)

is pushed forward. . . hold the needle all the way in until the implant has been ejected from the syringe.

6. *Withdraw needle.* Withdraw the needle and make sure the implant is in place, a half-inch from the needle hole. Pull plunger back to remove empty sheath. Remove needle and place in disinfectant solution.

To remove an implant from the ear, restrain the animal as for implantation. Then locate the implant entry point in the ear by feel or

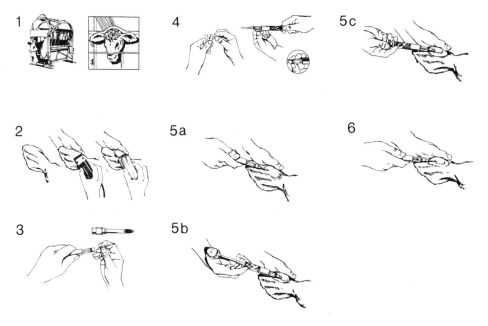

Fig. 30 Implantation of implants to the ear using pellet implanter. See text for details of steps 1 to 6. (Courtesy of Ceva Laboratories, Inc., Overland Park, Kansas.)

by sight, disinfect the area, and proceed with the following steps (Fig. 31).

1. With the tip of a pair of forceps, suitably disinfected, open the partially healed entry point. Insert the forceps, and follow along the "old" needle path to open the path until you reach the implant.
2. Most implants can be pushed out with the thumbnail; or, grasp the implant with the forceps and remove it [11].

B. Ball Implant Devices

Ball implants are constructed to be 1/8 in. in diameter and are shaken down into the chamber to load. The depth of the plunger push determines the number of implants delivered. Figure 32 shows a ball implant device [12]. Newer implant devices are constructed in the shape of guns for ease of use; every pull of the trigger delivers one ball-type implant. Depending on the weight of the animal, one to several ball implants may be used.

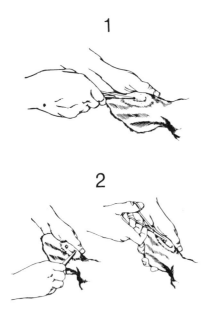

Fig. 31 Removal of implants from the ear; see text for detail. (Courtesy of Ceva Laboratories, Inc., Overland Park, Kansas.)

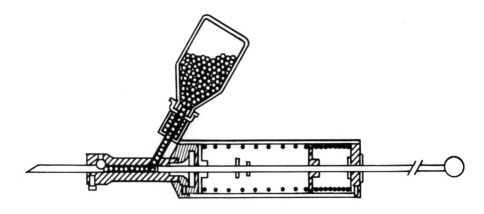

Fig. 32 Ball implant device. (From Ref. 10.)

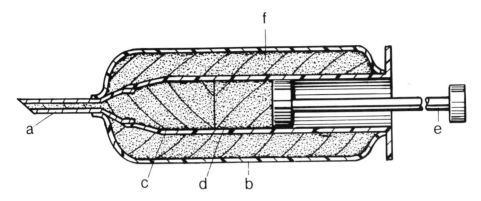

Fig. 33 Molten implant applicator: a syringe with heating means for liquefying the solid implant composition. Key: a = injecting needle, b = fluid-tight jacket, c = medication situated in a solid condition, d = second medication (if needed), e = plunger, and f = thermal mass, which changes from solid to liquid form while remaining at a constant temperature to maintain the medication (c and d) in molten form. (From Ref. 13.)

C. Molten Implant Devices

Molten implant devices are used to inject the animal with liquid, which subsequently solidifies at body temperature. The implant usually contains waxes or hydrogenated oils in which the active ingredient can be dispersed. The implant apparatus (modified syringe: see Fig. 33) contains the implant composition in the solid state [13]. A heating element on the syringe transforms the thermoplastic composition into a molten fluid prior to injection. Once the implant has been deposited within the body (subcutaneously or intramuscularly), the implant will return to the solid state or remain in the plastic state, depending on the thermal characteristics of the composition.

VII. CONCLUSIONS

The development of specialized dosage forms to treat a variety of animals results in the need for specialized administration devices. For the administration of conventional dosage forms such as compressed tablets (boluses), solutions, suspensions, and vaccines, the industry has developed multipurpose administration devices—simple balling guns, nasogastric tubes, and single- and multiple-dose dosing guns suitable for drenching or inoculation. For paste dosage forms the success of the treatment is related to both the formulation and the specially de-

signed single- or multiple-dose syringe, the syringe design being species specific. The advent of controlled release implantable devices
and rumen retention devices has hastened the need for the development of product-specific administration devices. Innovation in the
administration device area will continue to satisfy the needs of the
veterinary drug formulator and drug user to provide the tools that
will permit precise administration of the desired drug to the animal in
need of treatment.

The administration devices discussed above do not represent an
exhaustive list. A review of the patent literature reveals that a steady
flow of novel delivery and administration tools is being invented to
support the growing needs of the industry.

ACKNOWLEDGMENTS

The authors would like to thank Drs. G. W. Benz, Y. M. Joshi, R.
L. Seward and E. Vadas for their editorial recommendations and technical comments during the development of the text. A special note of
appreciation to the Visual Communications department and to Ms. Nancy
Bell, MSD-Agvet Marketing Communications, Merck & Co., Inc. for
their assistance in preparation and collection of photographic materials.

REFERENCES

1. D. Mann, U.S. Patent 4, 637, 816 (1987).
2. J. R. Zingerman, D. G. Pope, P. K. Wilkinson, and L. Perfetto,
    Int. J. Pharm., 36:141 (1987).
3. E. A. Zackheim, U.S. Patent 3, 494, 359 (1970).
4. E. A. Tischlinger, U.S. Patent 4, 059, 109 (1977).
5. G. Lataix, U.S. Patent 4, 067, 440 (1978).
6. A. M. Sanchez, U.S. Patent 4, 050, 459 (1977).
7. D. G. Pope, in *Formulation of Veterinary Dosage Forms* (J.
    Blodinger, ed.), Dekker, New York, 1983.
8. G. E. Miller, U.S. Patent 4, 040, 388 (1977).
9. Instructions for the Operation and Maintenance of the Hypodermic
    Jet Injection Apparatus, Ped-O-Jet, manufactured by Ped-O-Jet
    International, Carlstadt, NJ.
10. R. S. Baldwin, R. D. Williams, and M. K. Terry, *Regulatory
    Toxicology and Pharmacology*, 3:9 (1983).
11. Ceva Laboratories, Overland Park, KS. Product literature
    Syncro-Mate-B. (1987).
12. R. Uclaf, French Patent 2, 287, 894 (1976).
13. L. Bucalo, U.S. Patent 4, 030, 499 (1977).

Index

A

Absorption, 19
Acrylic adhesives, 412-414
Active transport test, 47
Active transport, 46
Adhesive matrix, 404
Alloxanization, 438
Alzet osmotic pumps, 139-140, 142-144
Ambulatory continuous infusion, 227
Ambulatory infusion pump, 181, 204, 205
Ambulatory insulin pump, 204
Ambulatory pump, 180, 184, 207
Area under the concentration-time curve, 23
Area under the first-moment curve, 25
Arterial infusions, 215

Avascular membrane, 422

B

Ball implant devices, 597-598
Balling gun, 564, 567
Balloon reservoir function, 215
Balloon reservoir, 215
Bands and tail tags, 542, 543
Banned device, 105
Bioactive agents, 138
Bioavailability, absolute, 23
Biocompatibility, 12
Biocompatible materials, 286
Biocompatible plastic, 289
Biodegradable-implants, 308
Biopharmaceutical aspects, 51
Biopharmaceutical characteristics, 33
Bolus, 560